A. Cano Sanchez · J. Calaf i Alsina · J.-L. Dueñas-Díez

Selective Estrogen Receptor Modulators

A New Brand of Multitarget Drugs

Antonio Cano Sanchez
Joaquim Calaf i Alsina
José-Luis Dueñas-Díez
(Editors)

Selective Estrogen Receptor Modulators

A New Brand of Multitarget Drugs

With 74 Figures, Including 40 in Color

Springer

Antonio Cano Sanchez
Department of Pediatrics
Obstetrics and Gynecology
School of Medicine
University of Valencia
Valencia, Spain

Joaquim Calaf i Alsina
Servei d'Obstetricia i Ginecologia
Hospital de la Santa Creu i Sant Pau
C/ Sant Antoni M. Claret 167
08025 Barcelona
e-mail: jcalaf@santpau.es

José-Luis Dueñas-Díez
School of Medicine
University of Sevilla
Department of Obstetrics and Gynaecology
Hospital Universitario Virgen Macarena
Sevilla, Spain

ISBN-10 3-642-44552-7 Springer Berlin Heidelberg New York
ISBN-13 978-3-642-44552-1 Springer Berlin Heidelberg New York

Springer is a part of Springer Science+Business Media
springeronline.com

Softcover re-print of the Hardcover 1st edition 2006

Editor: Dr. Ute Heilmann, Heidelberg
Desk Editor: Wilma McHugh, Heidelberg
Cover design: Frido Steinen-Broo, eStudio Calamar, Spain
Typesetting and production: LE-TEX Jelonek, Schmidt & Vöckler GbR, Leipzig, Germany
Printed on acid-free paper 21/3100/YL – 5 4 3 2 1 0

Preface

The increasing awareness on the varied consequences of hypogonadism in distinct organs and systems has supported the notion of estrogens as systemic agents. This observation is congruent with the variety of tissues affected by estrogens when used in hormone therapy formulations on hypogonadic women. Apart from the genital tract and the breast, recognized as traditional targets for estrogens, the skeleton, the vascular tree, or the central nervous system, are good examples of territories that have demonstrated sensitivity to estrogens. This evidence has created great interest, as shown by the great amount of literature that has been produced on the benefits and risks associated with the use of estrogens.

In parallel to the clinical interest, basic research has improved our knowledge on the complexities involved in estrogen action at the molecular level. Together with effects mediated through specific receptors, a concept that has been the mainstay of the interpretation of estrogen action for years, there is enough evidence to hold the notion of receptor-independent effects. The substantial advances in modern technology applied to research have helped in enlightening the particulars of this versatile action of estrogens. This more detailed knowledge on the sophisticated mechanism of action of estrogens has nourished the emergence of multiple hypotheses speculating with the possibility of manipulating estrogen action. The notion that a widely extended regulatory system of cell function, as it is the estrogen receptor machinery, might be modulated at wish has arisen as an attractive, although still elusive postulate.

Increasing support for this concept has evolved from the developments of classical pharmacology in the field of agonists/antagonists for receptors, together with the extensive basic and clinical knowledge acquired with the use of tamoxifen, originally considered as an estrogen receptor antagonist. It has been the great experience with tamoxifen, plus the accompanying basic research, which have led to the actual notion that tamoxifen is, as perhaps any compound capable of binding to the estrogen receptor, nothing but a selective estrogen receptor modulator (SERM). Today, the biological steps set in motion by the activation of the estrogen receptor are sufficiently intricate to convert into a difficult exercise the definition of compounds that respond to the concept of pure agonism or antagonism. Instead, it seems that there is a wide, increasing variety of ligands capable of binding to distinct species of receptors and determining effects whose profile will depend on the compound as well as on the target tissue.

The corollary of these premises is that modern medicine faces a great challenge but at the same time a wonderful opportunity. The hypothesis of governing a physiological, an often powerful, regulatory system of cellular functions is starting to become a tangible reality. Accordingly, the new concept of multitarget drugs has been created. From the veteran tamoxifen, which proved efficacious as an antagonist in breast but created concern due to its agonistic effects in the uterus, the list of SERMs has not interrupted its continuous growth. Raloxifene has defined a landmark in this sequence as a consequence of the abundant basic and clinical studies forming a solid body of doctrine that warrants his actual indication in osteoporosis as well as its possible role as chemopreventive against breast cancer. Many other SERMs, distributed in different families, are already under research in experimental and clinical studies.

This book represents the effort of a group of scientists and clinicians to offer the reader an updated view of the main advances occurred in the field in the recent years. Every author has been selected because of his/her experience with modulators of estrogen receptors, either in basic or clinical grounds. This explains the structure of the book, which reviews the main basic concepts in the first part, to immediately concentrate in the recent news on the many uses of SERMs in clinical practice. We are very grateful with all of them for his excellent contribution. To conclude, we also would like to express our gratitude to Springer-Verlag for the excellent technical support as well as to those who, from different perspectives, are at the base of our work, our patients and our families.

Antonio Cano
Joaquin Calaf
José-Luis Dueñas-Díez

Contents

Part I Basic Area

List of Contributors

M.I. Acién
Service of Obstetrics
and Gynecology
San Juan University Hospital
and Dept/Division of Gynecology
School of Medicine
"Miguel Hernández" University
Campus of San Juan
Alicante, Spain

P. Acién
Service of Obstetrics
and Gynecology
San Juan University Hospital
and Dept/Division of Gynecology
School of Medicine
"Miguel Hernández" University
Campus of San Juan
Alicante, Spain

Rafael Alonso
Laboratorio
de Neurobiología celular
Departamento de Fisiología
Universidad de La Laguna
38206 Tenerife, Spain
and
Instituto
de Tecnologías Biomédicas
Universidad de La Laguna
38206 Tenerife, Spain

C. Bellido
Department of Cell Biology
Physiology and Immunology
University of Córdoba
Córdoba, Spain

María Carmen Barbancho
Department of Obstetrics
and Gynecology
Santa Cristina University Hospital
Madrid, Spain

Joaquim Calaf i Alsina
Servei d'Obstetricia i Ginecologia
Hospital de la Santa Creu i Sant Pau
C/ Sant Antoni M. Claret 167
08025 Barcelona

Antonio Cano Sanchez
Department of Pediatrics,
Obstetrics and Gynecology
School of Medicine
University of Valencia
Valencia, Spain

Mario Díaz
Laboratorio de Fisiología Animal
Departamento de Biología Animal
Universidad de La Laguna
38206 Tenerife, Spain
and
Instituto
de Tecnologías Biomédicas
Universidad de La Laguna
38206 Tenerife, Spain

B. Nicolás Díaz Chico
Canary Islands Cancer
Research Institute
Department of Biochemistry
and Physiology
Universidad de Las Palmas
de Gran Canaria

Juan C. Díaz Chico
Canary Islands Cancer
Research Institute
Department of Biochemistry
and Physiology
Universidad de Las Palmas
de Gran Canaria

Adolfo Díez-Pérez
Department of Internal Medicine
and Infectious Diseases
Hospital del Mar
Autonomous University
of Barcelona
Unidad de Investigación
en Fisiopatología Ósea
y Articular (IMIM)
Barcelona, Spain

José Luis Dueñas-Díez
School of Medicine
University of Sevilla
Head
Department of Obstetrics
and Gynaecology
Hospital Universitario Virgen
Macarena
Sevilla, Spain

Eduardo Escrich Escriche
Multidisciplinary Group
for the Study of Breast Cancer
Department of Cellular Biology,
Physiology and Immunology
School of Medicine
Universidad Autónoma
de Barcelona

Benito García Marrero
Instituto de Productos Naturales
y Agrobiología
CSIC
38206 Tenerife, Spain
Instituto
de Tecnologías Biomédicas
Universidad de La Laguna
38206 Tenerife, Spain

Miguel Angel García-Pérez
Research Unit
Hospital Clínico Universitario
de Valencia
and Department of Genetics
Faculty of Biology
Valencia, Spain

Tomás Gomez
Laboratorio de Fisiología Animal
Departamento de Biología Animal
Universidad de La Laguna
38206 Tenerife, Spain
Instituto
de Tecnologías Biomédicas
Universidad de La Laguna
38206 Tenerife, Spain

M. González
Departments of Physiology
and Animal Biology
& Institute
of Biomedical Technologies
University of La Laguna
La Laguna, Spain

P. Guelmes
Departments of Physiology
and Animal Biology
& Institute
of Biomedical Technologies
University of La Laguna
La Laguna, Spain

Carlos Hermenegildo
Research Unit
Hospital Clínico
Universitario of Valencia.
Unidad Central de Investigación
School of Medicine and Dentistry
University of Valencia
Avda. Blasco Ibañez, 17
46010 Valencia, Spain

G. Hernández
Departments of Physiology
and Animal Biology
& Institute
of Biomedical Technologies
University of La Laguna
La Laguna, Spain

Fernando Marín
Eli Lilly and Company
Lilly Research Center
Windlesham, Surrey, UK

Raquel Marín
Laboratorio
de Neurobiología celular
Departamento de Fisiología
Universidad de La Laguna
38206 Tenerife, Spain
Instituto
de Tecnologías Biomédicas
Universidad de La Laguna
38206 Tenerife, Spain

Jorge Marrero-Alonso
Laboratorio de Fisiología Animal
Departamento de Biología Animal
Universidad de La Laguna
38206 Tenerife, Spain
Instituto
de Tecnologías Biomédicas
Universidad de La Laguna
38206 Tenerife, Spain

Domingo Navarro Bosch
Canary Islands Cancer
Research Institute
Department of Biochemistry
and Physiology
Universidad de Las Palmas
de Gran Canaria

Santiago Palacios
Institute Palacios
of Woman's Health
Calle Antonio Acuña, 9
28009 Madrid, Spain

Stefano Palomba
Department of Obstetrics &
Gynecology
University "Magna Greacia"
of Catanzaro
Italy

F. Quereda
Service of Obstetrics
and Gynecology
San Juan University Hospital
and Dept/Division of Gynecology
School of Medicine
"Miguel Hernández" University
Campus of San Juan
Alicante, Spain

J.E. Sánchez-Criado
Department of Cell Biology,
Physiology and Immunology
University of Córdoba
Córdoba, Spain

Fulvio Zullo
Department of Obstetrics &
Gynecology
University "Magna Greacia"
of Catanzaro
Italy

Part I

Basic Area

Chapter 1

Molecular Mechanisms of Estrogen Action in Target Tissues

B. Nicolás Díaz Chico · Domingo Navarro Bosch ·
Juan C. Díaz Chico · Eduardo Escrich Escriche

1.1 Introduction

The majority of signals that govern cell operations have their origin in the plasma membrane. They proceed from membrane receptors that respond to substances of diverse origins. An important part of these signals arrives at the cells via blood circulation, as it is the case of endocrine signals transmitted by hormones. Another essential group of signals originates in the neighborhood of the cells, or even in the cell itself. This is the case of paracrine and autocrine signals transmitted by an extensive assemblage of growth and differentiation factors.

The interaction of external signals with membrane receptors generates second messengers. These messengers either modify the cell concentration of ions or metabolites or alter the functional state of a chain of several molecules that act as intermediaries. These intermediaries may modify the intensity of determined biochemical reactions or, in other cases, are integrated into the machinery of gene transcription and alter the expression of specific genes. The consequences of these activities can lead to the induction of cell division.

An important group of endocrine signals does not require membrane receptors, second messengers, or intermediaries in signaling chains. They proceed from substances that seem to penetrate into the interior of cells without difficulty, where they join with intracellular receptors, and through which they act on the cell genome. These substances are small liposoluble molecules, of which several are of a hormonal nature: the steroid hormones – androgens, estrogens, progestagens, glucocorticoids, and mineral corticoids – the thyroid hormones, and vitamin D3. There are also nonhormonal substances, such as retinoic acid, prostaglandin J2, or fatty acids, which utilize intracellular receptors and exert powerful genomic effects. All these substances share common mechanisms of action through soluble intracellular proteins that are members of the nuclear hormone receptor family (Evans 1988; Vaseduvan et al. 2002).

Once nuclear hormone receptors are bound to their hormone, they are capable of being integrated directly into the machinery that regulates the transcription of specific genes. This action is more direct, and apparently more primitive, than that originating in membrane receptors. By controlling gene expression, the hormones regulate more the abundance of determinate, specific proteins rather than their biochemical activity. Those hormone–receptor complexes are also efficient regulators of cell proliferation.

Nuclear hormone receptors accumulate several functions in a single molecule. They are capable of recognizing and binding small molecules like steroids with high affinity and specificity. These hormone–receptor complexes are capable of recognizing and joining with specific sequences of DNA present only in genes that are the object of hormonal regulation. They are capable, in short, of interacting with other proteins – coactivators or corepressors – that participate in the regulation of the machinery of gene transcription and of initiating or modifying the expression of specific genes. The meeting of all these functions, and others not mentioned, in a single molecule make these receptors an extremely elaborate product from the point of view of evolution.

This chapter reviews the main characteristics of two of the better known members of the nuclear hormone receptor family: estrogen receptors α and β (ERα and ERβ). First, the different functional regions harbored by the molecule of the receptor are described. These properties will be used to describe the cellular, molecular, and other consequences that derive from the interactions of receptors with their own hormone, other proteins, or DNA.

The interaction of estrogen receptors with signaling systems of the cell membrane that respond to growth factors and mediate nongenomic, fast actions of estrogens will be reviewed as well. These mechanisms have a growing importance in the comprehension of phenomena like the induction of endothelial NOS (nitric oxide synthase) by estrogens (Rubanyi et al. 2002).

1.2 General Aspects

The hypothesis that hormones act through cell receptors is as old as the concept of the hormone. Nevertheless, and as usually occurs in science, hormone receptors were only discovered when the required technology became available.

1.2.1 The Discovery of Hormone Receptors for Steroid Hormones

Hormone receptors for steroids were discovered in the early 1960s, when the technology to radioactively mark steroids became available. By obtaining tritium-labeled estradiol, Jensen could show the existence of an intracellular protein component that bound specifically to this hormone and that was called the estradiol receptor (ER).

Shortly thereafter, O'Malley obtained an autoradiography image in which an accumulation of estradiol was observed within the nuclei of cells from chicken oviduct (O'Malley et al. 1974). It had been known that estradiol significantly altered the synthesis of RNA within a few minutes. With these scant initial data, the theory that steroids act through intracellular receptors, by means of which they carry out the regulation of specific genes, was established (Toft et al. 1966). The use of radioactively marked compounds permitted the discovery of receptors for the other steroid hormones, vitamin D3, and the thyroid hormones (Bouillon et al. 1995; Navarro et al. 2002; Evans 1989; Evans 1988). For many years, the only available technology to determine concentrations of receptors and to study their properties was based on the use of radioactive hormones.

It was not until 1995 that news emerged of the existence of a second type of ER, the ERβ, described almost simultaneously in two European laboratories (Nilsson et al. 2001; Kuiper et al. 1996). Since then , the original ER has been called ERα. Both receptors are independent biological entities, encoded by different genes that respond to the same denomination. Both genes have different patterns of tissue expression, with exclusive expression in some cell types and joint expression in others (Palmieri et al. 2002; Kuiper et al. 1996; Krege et al. 1998). ERα dominates in the reproductive tract, while in other tissues, especially the nervous, digestive, and ovary tissues, ERβ dominates (Nilsson et al. 2001; Krege et al. 1998; Couse et al. 1999a; Couse et al. 1999b).

1.2.2
Nuclear Hormone Receptors?

The intracellular distribution of steroid hormone receptors has long been the object of controversy. The first theoretical formulation on the intracellular location of the ERs was elaborated by Jensen in 1968 and is known as the "two-step theory." Its execution was based entirely on biochemical observations obtained by means of tritium-marked estradiol. The ERs, in cells not exposed to hormones, are found abundantly in the soluble cell fraction, or cytosol (Fig. 1.1). Treatment with hormones confines the receptors to the particulated or nuclear fraction and causes their disappearance from the cytosol. The two-step theory established that the receptor is found in the cytoplasm naturally and upon the arrival of a hormone it is transformed into a complex hormone–receptor (first step) capable of translocating itself to the nucleus and of modifying gene expression (second step).

In the 1980s, Jensen and others obtained monoclonal antibodies against several of the nuclear hormone receptors (Díaz-Chico et al. 1988; Jordan et al. 1990). These antibodies permitted the introduction of immunohistochemical techniques in the study of receptors. Consequently, King and Greene verified

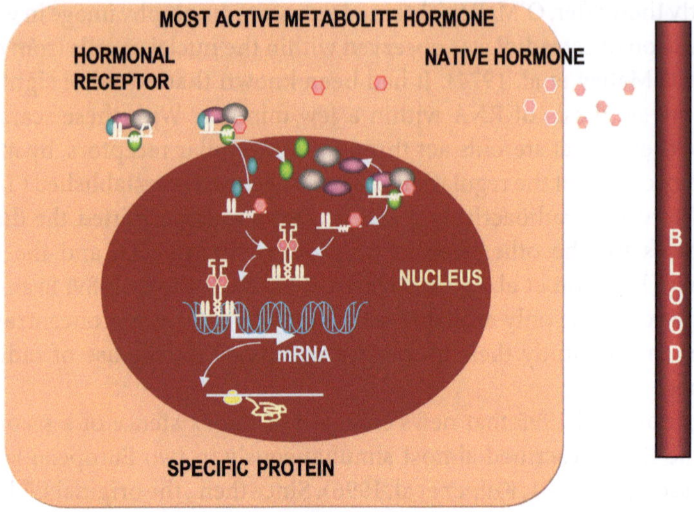

Fig. 1.1. General mechanism of action of steroid hormones. Steroid hormones cross through the plasmatic membrane without apparent difficulty favored by gradient. Some, which can be considered prohormones, are metabolized and transformed into more active products. This is the case with testosterone, which becomes dihydrotestosterone (DHT) in the target tissues of androgens, through the 5-alfa-reductase enzyme. The hormone binds to the receptor, a soluble protein of the cellular cytosol that, in the absence of hormone, is found associated with other proteins (hsp90 and others) that maintain the receptor in an inactive state. The hormone–receptor bond causes the other proteins to separate and a homodimer to be formed. The homodimer is the activated form of the receptor since it is capable of recognizing the genes that depend on that steroid hormone as well as of activating its expression, which leads to the synthesis of specific proteins

that there were receptors in the nuclei of cells sensitive to estrogens, regardless of whether or not the cells had been exposed to hormones (King et al. 1984).

Simultaneously, Gorski's group (Welshons et al. 1984), utilizing a type of cell fractionation that permits separating the cytoplasm from the nucleus, was also able to detect the presence of nuclear ER, even if the cell had not been exposed to hormones. These findings led to a different theoretical formulation, according to which the native receptors would be found in the cell nucleus, to which the hormone would accede directly.

At present, the two-step theory is still accepted, but it leaves out the question of receptor location within the cell so as to be able to cover all members of a family. The receptor, in the absence of hormone, is found associated with other proteins (hsp90, p59, and perhaps others) and very weakly bound to cell structures (nuclear or cytoplasmatic). The arrival of hormones transforms the receptor, freeing it from other proteins, giving it a greater affinity for nuclear structures, and causing it to achieve an active state as a transcription factor (Beato et al. 1996; Beato 1989). The difference is that the receptors not bound to estradiol are soluble, and they can be extracted also from the nucleus during homogenization: they are "cytosolic", not "cytoplasmatic".

1.3
Structure of Estrogen Receptors

Knowledge of the molecular structure of ERs was initiated from the cloning of the complementary DNA for the messenger RNA (mRNA) that encodes ERα. This was possible thanks to the explosive evolution of the recombinant DNA technology during the 1970s and to the production of monoclonal antibodies against ERα. In 1986 the sequence of amino acids of ERα was published by the Chambon group (Green et al. 1986a; Green et al. 1986b).

ERβ was cloned by chance, since it was found through the use of probes aimed at hybridizing with the most conserved part of the nuclear receptors – the DNA binding domain (DBD) – trying to find related sequences. This procedure has expanded the family of nuclear receptors to more than 100 members. Thus, the discovery of ERβ in rat prostate by the Gustafsson group was a surprise (Kuiper et al. 1996; Nilsson et al. 2001).

1.3.1
Primary Structure of Estrogen Receptors

The receptor molecule, that is to say the protein that interacts directly with the hormone, is formed of a single polypeptide chain in not only ERα and ERβ but also in the remainder of the known nuclear receptors (Evans 1989; Evans 1988; Krege et al. 1998; McDonnell et al. 2002; McEwen et al. 1999; Nilsson et al. 2001).

The idea that nuclear receptors belong to the same molecular family arose upon discovery of the considerable homology in the amino acid sequences among the receptors (Evans 1989). These homologous sequences affect six regions of the respective molecules, labeled with the letters A to F. The functions assigned to each homologous region were deduced from the comparison with the known functions of amino acid sequences in other proteins. The final confirmation was obtained from the analysis of the alterations in the function of the receptors that were produced after their structures were altered by means of controlled mutations.

Human ERα has 565 amino acids, greater therefore than the dominant isoform of ERβ, which has 530 amino acids (Kuiper et al. 1996), the isoforms are products of the same gene and are generated by alternate processing of mRNA. Nevertheless, the structure in the domains of both types of ER reflect the general pattern described, except that ERβ lacks the carboxyterminal F region (Kumar et al. 1987; Nilsson et al. 2001). Both ERα and ERβ, as well as their isoforms, can have different functions, inasmuch as they can activate different genes and even carry out antagonistic functions (Fuqua et al. 1992; Fuqua 2001; Pettersson et al. 2000). This is a field of extraordinary activity, where research has tried to find the different degrees of implication of every hormone and isoform in carcinogenesis and in tumor response to hormone treatment (Palmieri et al. 2002).

1.3.2 Activity Domains in the Molecules of Estrogen Receptors

ERs are transcription factors that are activated by means of a high affinity reaction (Kd between 0.01 and 1 nM) with a ligand (hormone or antihormone). The reaction transforms the receptor from a native state that is genetically inactive to an activated state capable of identifying the genes susceptible of responding specifically to each receptor. The functional organization of the ER is carried out through particular structures of the receptor molecule. These are formed by means of a series of folds of the molecule that permit reaching the (tertiary) spatial structure adequate for carrying out each function. Each one of the structures of the molecule that can carry out one of the particular functions is called a molecular domain. Molecular domains are not always formed by consecutive sequences of amino acids. They can be formed by several short sequences of amino acids, separated from each other by amino acids that are not part of a given domain.

ERs have domains responsible for nuclear location, hormone binding, dimerization, DNA binding, and transcription activation (Figs. 1.2 and 1.3) (Beato et al. 1996; Beato 1989; Fawell et al. 1990; Hall et al. 1999; Kumar et al. 1987).

1.3.3 Genetic Encoding of Estrogen Receptors

As in any another protein, the synthesis of an ER begins with the transcription of the gene that encodes it in RNA as a primary transcript (Chin 1995; Ponglikitmongkol et al. 1988). This forms a very long strand that is then processed to give mature mRNA. The maturation process includes the elimination of the exons and the modification of the ends of the RNA strand. The genes of the ER include 8 exons, some of them very large (> 26 kilobases). The mature mRNA has an open reading frame that encodes for the sequence of amino acids of the receptor, flanked on both ends by long sequences of nucleotides that are not translated.

The elimination of exons during RNA maturing requires two cuts and a coupling for each exon. Occasionally errors are produced, providing a source of

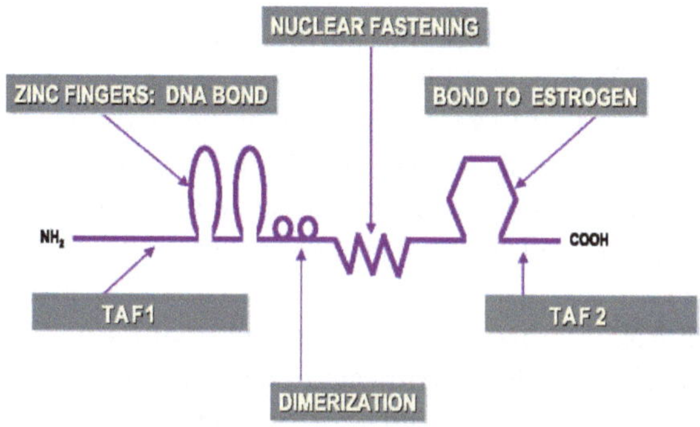

Fig. 1.2. Structure and domains of the estrogen receptor. ERs have a structure that couple several functions in a single protein. The aminoterminal region of the receptor contains a binding domain to DNA, with two zinc fingers that confer upon the receptor the capacity to recognize short sequences of DNA, called estrogen response elements (ERE), in the promoter region of the estrogen-dependent genes. That region also contains a transcription activator region or transactivator, TAF1, which binds with nuclear transcription factors to complete the gene transcription machinery. The carboxyterminal region of the receptor contains a large binding domain to the hormone that occupies more than half the molecule and through which the receptor interacts with estrogens and antiestrogens. That same zone contains another transactivator region, TAF2, which only becomes activated in the presence of estrogen, a zone of dimerization, and another for binding to hsp90. Between the hormone and the DNA binding domains there is the hinge region, which contains a short sequence of basic amino acids that confer nucleophylia to the receptor and one of the zones that participates in the dimerization of the receptor

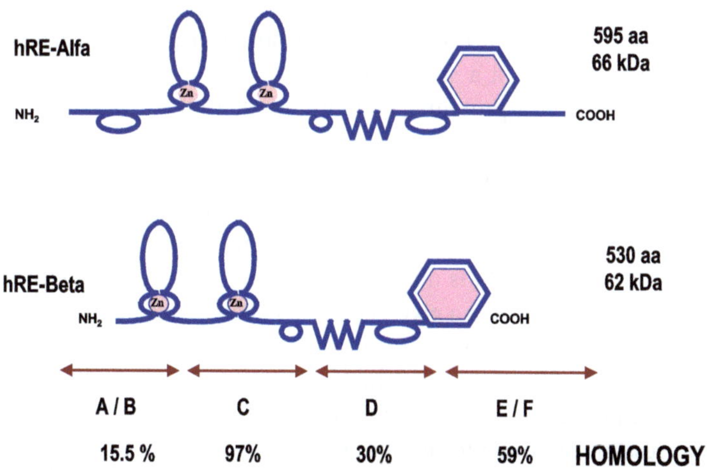

Fig. 1.3. Comparison of alpha and beta estrogen receptors. The alpha and beta ERs are products of different genes, but they maintain a similar structure. The figure shows that both receptors share different degrees of homology in their amino acid sequences, the highest one being that corresponding to the DNA binding domain. The beta receptor lacks the carboxyterminal zone, called zone F, which is absent in other members of the nuclear receptor family and is considered a peculiarity of the alpha ER

receptor variants. The receptors thus formed can be truncated, that is, they lack the amino acids encoded by some of the exons. Additionally, receptor molecules can appear that have in duplicate amino acids encoded by some of the exons. These products of alternate mRNA maturation, called isoforms, exist for both types of ER and are produced in normal tissue, but their functional significance is not known (Fuqua et al. 1992; Fuqua 2001; McGuire et al. 1991; Scott et al. 1991).

Alternative mRNA maturation is frequent in tumor tissue expressing ER. In some cases it would give rise to truncated receptors that would maintain the capacity to bind hormones but would have lost their capacity as a transcription factor. Additionally, truncated receptors would be produced that would lack the capacity to bind hormones but would conserve intact their capacity to interact with DNA. In this case, the truncated receptors can become tumorigenic by stimulating the proliferation of cells uncontrolled by hormones. These receptor variants have been the object of exhaustive study at the level of mRNA in tumors of the breast, mainly estrogen-dependent tumors (Clemons et al. 2001; García et al. 1988; Palmieri et al. 2002), but tests for the existence of receptor protein with these characteristics have not corroborated the expectation created by their theoretical interest.

1.3.4 Native Receptor

In cell cultures deprived of hormones or in target organs of ovariectomized animals, ERs are found in a state known as "native", characterized by their association with several proteins (Redeuilh et al. 1987). The best known are hsp90 and p59.

hsp90 is a chaperone protein that accompanies the ER from receptor synthesis and is indispensable in the acquisition by the receptor of the appropriate three-dimensional conformation. This protein, induced by heat or by cell stress (Redeuilh et al. 1987), is ubiquitous and much more abundant than the group of nuclear receptors of a given cell. hsp90 continues bound to the receptor until the receptor itself binds to the hormone. At this point, the receptor loses affinity for hsp90 and undoes the bond between both molecules.

p59 is an immunophyline, characterized by its specific binding with the immunosuppressant rapamicine (Ratajczak et al. 1993). It is unknown whether this property is related to the biology of the receptors. The native structure in vivo has been studied by means of substances that enter the cell and, once inside, establish covalent bonds between protein structures that were previously associated by noncovalent interactions (Segnitz et al. 1995). Studies carried out by the Ghering group have verified that the structure of glucocorticoid, estrogen, and progestin receptors is identical: a receptor molecule, two of hsp90 and one of p59. Other proteins, such as hsp70, have been identified in the native complexes of receptors in vitro (Smith et al. 1993). Nevertheless, the presence of these proteins has not been verified in vivo.

The formation of the structure of the native receptor depends essentially on the hsp90–receptor interaction. This is produced among specific sequences of both proteins in three dimensions; one of them is found in the DBD and the other in the ligand binding domain (LBD, domain E). When lacking a 24-amino-acid chain between the end of domain C, that of binding to DNA, and the beginning of domain D, the ER does not join with hsp90 and, therefore, does not form the hetero-oligomeric structure of the native receptor and remains a monomer. The binding of the ER with hsp90 is produced soon after the synthesis of the receptor and precedes the incorporation of the other proteins.

1.3.5 Estrogen Transforms the Native Receptor

The binding of hormone transforms the receptor in vivo, freeing it from the accompanying proteins. The transformation involves the conversion of the receptor into a more nucleophylic form, which can be extracted from the nuclei only with solutions of high salinity (0.4 M KCl). The transformation of the receptor can be verified through centrifugation of cytosol in a sucrose gradient of density. The native receptor complex has a coefficient of sedimentation of 8S, which changes to 4S when the hormone transforms the receptor (Fig. 1.5). This change of coefficient of sedimentation reflects the rupture of the hetero-oligomer of the native receptor (8S), which frees the receptor monomer (4S) from its bond with hsp90 and p59 (Redeuilh et al. 1987; Navarro et al. 1998).

From what has been discovered, it can be deduced that part of the functions of ERs remains hidden in the native state. Interaction with hormone causes this structure to come apart. This process of activation or transformation permits the receptor to exhibit all the potential of interaction with DNA and makes the receptor exhibit the properties that were hidden by the proteins that accompanied it in the 8S form (McGuire et al. 1991).

1.3.6 Domain of Nuclear Location

All nuclear receptors have sequences known as domains of nuclear location (Picard et al. 1987). These sequences, rich in arginine and lysine, confer upon the many proteins that contain them the capacity to bind to nonhistone nuclear proteins. Receptors have up to four of these sequences, whose cooperation is necessary for nuclear location. When these sequences are exposed, the receptor tends to be located in the nucleus. When covered by other proteins, receptors are distributed throughout the cell.

In the case of the ER, when a region of 20 amino acids between 250 and 270 is missing, the receptor is located strictly in the cytoplasm. Domains of similar size and function have also been located in the receptors of glucocorticoids and of progesterone. The zone of nuclear location overlaps with one of the sequences for interacting with hsp90, which at the same time is next to the DBD. The coincidence of the three functions in a space so restricted implies that they are totally or partly incompatible sterically (Evans 1989; Gruber et al. 2002).

1.4 Hormone–Receptor Interaction

The recognition of each receptor by its respective hormone is a highly specific process occurring at the LBD. The small hormonal molecule enters a hydrophobic cavity of the receptor molecule, forming a high affinity bond.

1.4.1 Ligand Binding Domain

The binding domain for the hormone, or LBD, is situated in the carboxyl half of the receptor, the final portion of which is critical. For example, the deletion of 12 amino acids in the carboxyl end of the androgen receptor suppresses its capacity to bind hormone (O'Malley et al. 1974). The LBD has an amino acid composition that confers upon it a net hydrophobic character, suitable for interacting with organic molecules of low molecular weight, such as steroids.

In spite of the extensive homology in the key amino acids of the LBD (Fig. 1.3), each of the two ER isoforms has different affinities for natural and synthetic ligands (Table 1.1). This suggests that the responses are very different in tissues dominated by one or another receptor (Kuiper et al. 1996).

It is noteworthy that such a long portion of ERα is required (more than 220 aa.) to interact with a structure as small as a steroid. Nevertheless, the whole structure seems necessary since this domain includes a transcription activation function through which the receptor binds with the cofactors (coactivators and corepressors). It is considered that amino acids kept among different members of the nuclear receptor family form a hydrophobic cavity that lodges the hormone. Amino acids not preserved among different members of the family but preserved by the same receptor in different species can be important for discriminating among structurally similar hormones and provide specificity for the binding of each receptor with its hormone (Mester et al. 1995).

Table 1.1. Relative binding affinity of ligands to estrogen receptors α and β

Ligand	RE-α	RE-β
17-β Estradiol	100	100
17-α Estradiol	58	11
Estriol	14	21
Estrone	60	37
4-OH-Estradiol	13	7
2-OH-Estrone	2	0.2
Tamoxifen	4	3
Raloxifen	69	16
Genistein	4	87
Cumestrol	20	140
Daizdein	0.1	0.5
4-Octylphenol	0.02	0.09
Nonylphenol	0.05	0.09

Data from Kuiper et al. Endocrinology 138:863 (1997)

At the time the hormone is introduced into the LBD (Fig. 1.4), a conformational change is produced in the three-dimensional structure of the receptor, a change that is key to the subsequent steps in hormonal action. This change is produced by a few contacts (between 6 or 7 and 15) of the receptor's amino acids with related groups from the hormone's structure. Some basic amino acid residues, particularly from arginine, which are preserved virtually intact among receptors, are critical in the execution of this function (Quingley et al. 1995).

The LBD harbors a zone of interaction with hsp90. When the hormone binds with the corresponding domain in the receptor, the protein changes its conformation, losing its affinity for hsp90. As a result, the receptor loses its affinity for hsp90.

As previously noted, the LBD of the receptor presents a series of functions that are not very well delimited such as those of dimerization with another receptor, nuclear translocation, and activation of the ligand-dependent gene transcription. As was just mentioned, the interaction of a ligand with its receptor has as its immediate consequence the conformational change of the molecule, a change that also determines the molecule's functionality. The importance of this point is that the stated conformational change is predetermined by the chemical nature of the ligand and the form in which it interacts with the receptor.

This can be verified easily if one analyzes the changes that take place in this zone when both the ERα and ERβ bind to agonist or antagonist ligands. By means of crystallography studies, it has been verified that the binding of agonists such as estradiol or diethylethylbestrol (DES), or even partial antag-

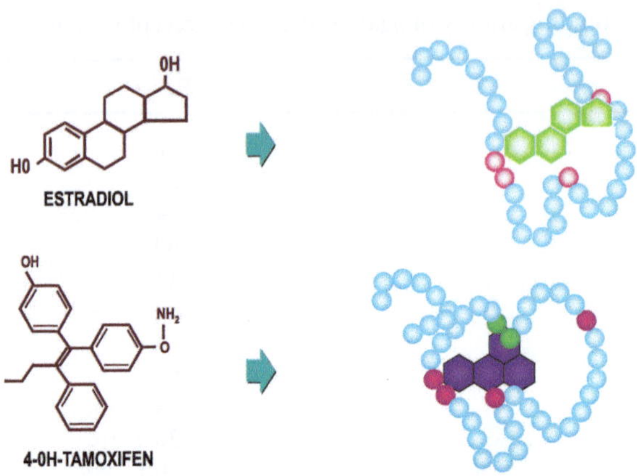

Fig. 1.4. Hormone-binding domain. Estrogen receptors concentrate in the extensive hormone-binding domain (> 300 amino acids) several functions with a common characteristic: they only manifest themselves when the receptor has been bound to the hormone and a change in its three-dimensional structure has been produced. The hormone-binding domain forms a bag-shaped structure, hydrophobic in nature, that lodges the hormone. The interaction occurs between specific atoms of the hormone and residues of specific amino acids of the receptor that at times are very distant in the primary sequence but that are next to each other in the three-dimensional structure of the receptor. Estrogens interact with a few concrete amino acids of this domain, while antiestrogens and SERM (selective estrogen receptor modulators) are in contact with some of the same amino acids as well as with some others. The result is a structural folding different for the receptor as a function of the ligand with which it interacts

onists like raloxifene or 4-OH tamoxifen, induces different three-dimensional conformations in both isoforms, affecting the spatial disposition of the LBD zone and, therefore, the functionality of the molecule. This could explain why a drug such as tamoxifen behaves like a partial agonist in the case of ERα and, in contrast, like a complete antagonist when interacting with ERβ, or why the phytoestrogen agonist genistein has 30 times more affinity for ERβ than for ERα, when the homology between both isoforms in terms of their tertiary structure is very high (Barkhem et al. 1998).

1.4.2 Structure of Receptor and Hormonal Antagonism

As was previously established, the spatial structure of the receptor domains is altered by interaction with the hormone, with DNA, with other proteins, and by the state of the receptor phosphorylation. Different states of folding suppose that the receptor exhibits different surfaces that permit it to gain or to lose affinity for DNA sequences or for proteins, as they are components of the native receptor or of the transcriptional machinery. The different properties that

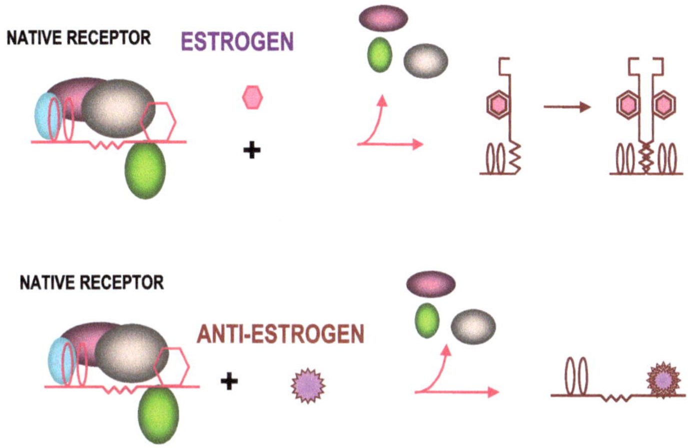

Fig. 1.5. Activation of the native receptor by the hormone. The hormone–receptor interaction determines a very strong bond that attracts distant amino acid residues, which alters the three-dimensional structure of the receptor. As a consequence, the receptor loses its affinity for the proteins that were originally close but that no longer find their zones of contact with the receptor. Simultaneously, the receptor reorganizes other hormone-dependent zones: it acquires dimerization capacity and exhibits a capacity to bind to DNA and to transcription factors. The interaction with antiestrogens also produces a conformational change, which can give rise or not to the formation of dimers, in any case with a different conformation

characterize the receptor are fully manifested only when the adequate spatial distribution of the molecule is reached (Brzozowski et al. 1997; Castellano-Díaz et al. 1989; Edwards et al. 1995; Edwards et al. 2002; Jordan et al. 1990).

The interactions of the receptor with structural analogs of the natural hormone give rise to conformation changes that can be similar, slightly different, or totally different from those produced by interaction with its natural ligand. A structural analog that produces a folding of the receptor that is very different from the normal one will give rise to nonproductive configurations from a transcriptional point of view. This would occur in the case of hormonal antagonists or antihormones that would blockade the receptors into a state of incapacity to induce gene expression. As a consequence, they would not manifest the physiological effects of the hormone (Gruber et al. 2002; MacGregor et al. 1998; McDonnell et al. 1994; Nilsson et al. 2001; Shiau et al. 1998; Wakeling 1993).

On the contrary, if the structural analog structure produces a folding sufficiently similar to the normal one, it can give rise to interactions with diverse degrees of transcription capacity. This is the case of analogs that function like partial agonists. In this case, the context of the gene promoter plays an important role, so that the complexes formed are capable of inducing the transcription of some genes but not of others. The cell context is also important since different cell lineages contain distinct transcription factors. This way, the same product behaves like an agonist in some cells and in others like an antagonist. Everything depends on whether or not the configurations attained are capable of interacting with the present transcription factors. Tamoxifen is the paradigm par excellence of the partial estrogen agonist. It functions like an antiestrogen in human breast cancer and as estrogen in the liver (MacGregor et al. 1998; Shiau et al. 1998; Tzukerman et al. 1994).

It is precisely in the so-called transcription activation zone-1 (TAF1) where we find significant differences between both kinds of ER. If in ERα this function represents a fundamental role in the specific activation of various genes in experiments carried out with cell lines, it has been verified that, in the same conditions, the TAF1 of ERβ practically does not intervene in such processes (Cowley et al. 1999). Similarly, the interaction of both receptors with specific ligands presents certain similarities and differences. Thus, synthetic antiestrogens such as tamoxifen, raloxifene, and ICI 164.384 present partial estrogen activity when they are bound to ERα, since they manage to induce the gene transcription mediated by this receptor. Meanwhile, they are pure antagonists for ERβ (McDonnell et al. 1995). The contrast may be explained by differences found in the TAF1 zone for both receptors. It is known that two different zones exist inside the TAF1 in the alpha isoform, both of which are necessary for the agonism with estradiol and for the partial agonism with tamoxifen, while in the beta form this dual function of the AF1 zone has not been detected (McInerney et al. 1998). Therefore, it is fitting to conclude that, based on these observations, the exact function of the TAF1 zone in ERβ, as opposed to that in the alpha isoform, still remains without clarification.

1.4.3 Receptor Folding in Separate Domains

A truncated ER lacking domains A, B, and C still grasps estradiol with high affinity. This indicates that these regions do not participate in the binding to hormone. It also indicates that domains D, E, and F fold themselves autonomously, reaching the necessary configuration to bind with the hormone. It is presumed that region D, which connects the LBD with the DBD, functions like a hinge pin, keeping apart two areas functionally separated in the protein. Region C tends to form a partly autonomous, very compact structure with regard to domains A and B. It is possible to idealize the receptor as an assembly of three separate structures of folding, where the LBD would be able to rotate with ample freedom with regard to the other two structures (Evans et al. 1988).

The simultaneous presence of several functions in the same zone of the molecule is something that should not surprise. The LBD is sufficiently extensive so that different amino acids participate in distinct functions. When these functions reside in neighboring sequences that overlap, functions demonstrate themselves successively: the receptor binds the hormone, then it loses affinity for hsp90, soon after that it gains affinity for another receptor and dimerizes, and finally it earns affinity for other cofactors of transcription. Each step is necessary so that the following can be taken in the process of activation.

1.4.4 Dimerization Domains

The formation of dimeric structures - homodimeric in the case of the ER, heterodimeric in the case of the thyroid hormone with a retinol receptor - is very common among the proteins that regulate gene transcription. The dimers embed themselves in the greater furrow of the DNA double helix and in this way facilitate the interaction between specific amino acids and nucleotides. It has been shown that the receptor dimers, and those of other regulating proteins, produce angulation of the double helix. This process facilitates the fixation of other components of the transcription machinery and the initiation of the transcription (Lee et al. 1989). The formation of dimers plays a central role in the recognition of genes regulated by the hormones.

Dimerization is a process necessary for the receptor to carry out its interaction with DNA and to initiate the response to the hormone. Dimerization occurs when the receptor monomer has freed itself of hsp90 and the other accompanying proteins forming the structure of the native receptor. Moreover, binding to the hormone provides the receptor with the necessary three-dimensional structure to produce the interaction between the two receptor monomers (Kuiper et al. 1996; O'Malley 1990).

At least three regions of the receptor participate in the process of dimer formation. One of them is unspecific and is made up of the sequences of hydrophobic amino acids of the LBD. These form hydrophobic contact surfaces that facilitate, in a general way, the interactions among proteins. The other two are specific sequences of amino acids. One of them is situated immediately after the DBD. It is comprised of a group of some 20 amino acids, and its capacity to intervene in the dimer is independent of binding to the hormone. The other dimerization region is found inside the LBD. It is poorly located, and it is possible that noncontiguous sequences of amino acids participate in it. It is exhibited only when the receptor has been already bound to a hormone.

The formation of ER dimers can be favored once the first monomer has bound to the DNA, since this presents positive cooperation in binding the next monomer. In any case, DNA binding creates a greater compaction of the dimer that results in a subsequent spatial restructuring of the receptor molecules.

1.5 Receptor–Genome Interaction

Cell differentiation during the embryonic period has as consequences that the majority of genes remain definitively silenced and that only a reduced number can be expressed in each cell (Beato et al. 1996; Beato 1989). The last group of genes constitutes the patrimony of each differentiated cell lineage and includes two subgroups: the genes that are expressed constitutively and those that are inducible and/or repressible. The latter are the object of regulation by factors internal or external to the cell, for example the hormones. It is the task of the nuclear hormone receptors to recognize which genes are susceptible to respond to a specific hormone.

1.5.1 Specific DNA Sequences for the Hormone Response

The identification of the few genes regulated by hormones, among the multitude of the genes that are expressed in each cell, is a first-order problem. What makes the identification possible is the existence of some short specific sequences of DNA, situated in the promoter region of each gene, that are recognized by the dimer of the hormone receptor. These sequences are called hormone response elements (HRE) (Seiler-Tuyns et al. 1986; Tzukerman et al. 1994).

The genes that respond to a specific hormone contain identical HRE (Fig. 1.6). Normally, it is a matter of short nucleotide sequences: pentamers or hexamers. In the case of the ER, the sequences are found repeated in inverse order in the same strand of DNA (palindromic, or symmetrically legible sequences: 5′GGACA–*nnn*–ACAGG 3′; *n* is any nucleotide). In the case of the thyroid hormones and retinoic acid, the HRE at times are presented like two repeated sequences in the same order (direct repetition: GGACA–GGACA).

Generally, between the two halves of the palindrome (or of the direct repetition) there are from one to five nucleotide spacers whose sequence varies from one gene to another. The sequence in which these nucleotides are found is irrelevant, as they do not directly participate in the dimer–DNA interaction. It is very important, however, that the number of nucleotide spacers be fixed to allow for correct binding to its corresponding receptor dimer.

Note that there is a great similitude among all the known HRE for nuclear receptors. Two subgroups have been established in which the sequences are practically identical: the subgroup of the glucocorticoid receptor, which utilizes the pentamer sequence GGACA and also includes the progesterone, mineralocorticoid, and androgen receptors (Seiler-Tuyns et al. 1986) and the subgroup of the ER, which utilizes the pentamer GGTCA and also includes the

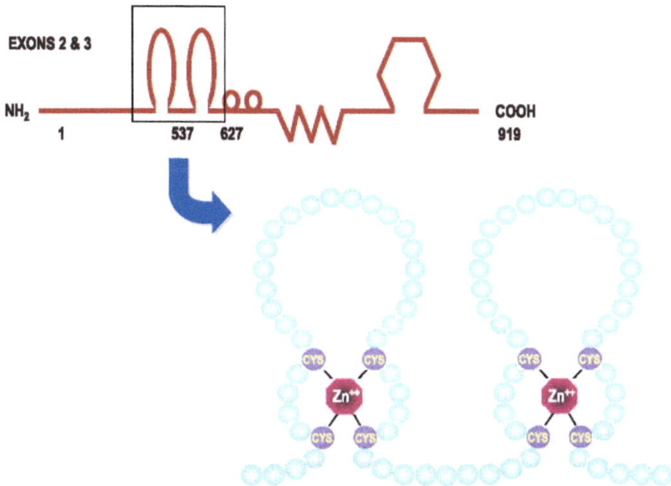

Fig. 1.6. Binding domain to DNA. ERs contain two structures called zinc fingers, typical of proteins that interact with DNA. One zinc atom forms four links of coordination with four cysteine residues of the protein structure, which occupy nearby positions, thus leaving a loop of some 15 to 22 aminoacids. The zinc fingers of the receptor are capable of interacting with specific sequences of DNA, the hormone response elements, with which they establish hydrogen bridges and form stable structures

receptors for vitamin D3, thyroid hormones, and retinoic acid (Bouillon et al. 1995; Tora et al. 1988). The first two utilize the palindromic system, and the last two can utilize the palindrome or the direct repetition, depending on the receptor subclass (α, β, or γ).

The structure in palindrome or in direct repetition and the size of the spacing sequence between the two pentamers are the critical variables in establishing the specificity of response to each one of the receptors that share the same pentamer. For example, the elements of estrogen and thyroid response can share the same palindrome and be differentiated only by the number of nucleotide spacers: three for the first one, none for the second.

HRE are not always a perfect palindrome, nor are pentamers repeated perfectly. It is frequently sufficient that one of the pentamers be the one that corresponds to an HRE. In the second pentamer, there can be a different nucleotide without altering the interaction with the receptor in a noticeable way.

1.5.2 DNA-Binding Domain

The interaction of the receptor with the HRE is produced once the dimer of the receptor has been formed. Given that the majority of HRE are palindromic, the interaction requires that the dimer be formed symmetrically facing both receptor monomers.

The DBD resides in a zone rich in cysteine in domain C of the receptor. This region is characterized by an interaction among four cysteines next to an atom of zinc (Fig. 1.6). The zinc atom stabilizes the structure by means of four coordination links to form what are called zinc fingers. The nuclear receptors form two zinc fingers per molecule. The zinc fingers contain a quite constant number of amino acids (18 to 22), and the space between the fingers is filled by a group of amino acids that varies from one type of receptor to another (Evans et al. 1988; Klug et al. 1987).

The zinc fingers are common structures among the transcription factors. Nevertheless, the coordination with zinc is more frequently produced between two histidine residues and two neighboring cysteines than when it is among four cysteine residues, as occurs in the nuclear hormone receptors. The zinc fingers provide an optimum architecture for the mutual recognition between specific sequences of amino acids and nucleotides. In the case of the nuclear receptors, the interaction occurs between particular amino acids of the DBD and guanine residues of the DNA sequence (Fig. 1.7).

In the recognition of each pentamer of the HRE participate two groups of amino acids, one from each zinc finger, perfectly preserved along evolution. The first, or proximal, group is situated in the nodule of the zinc finger and participates with three amino acids. The distal group participates with three other amino acids and seems to be essential to the recognition of the segment

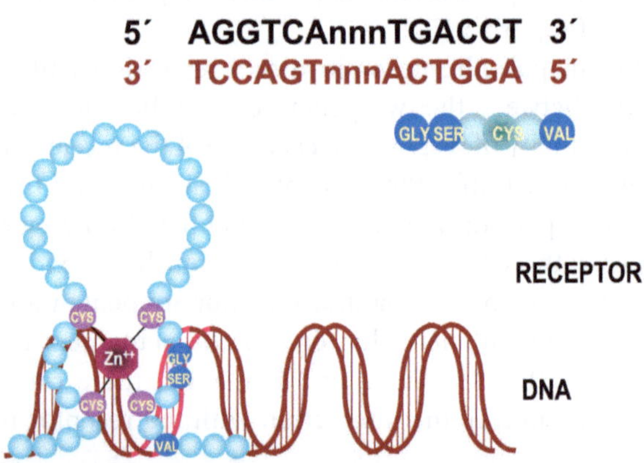

Fig. 1.7. Interaction of receptor with hormone response element. The hormone response elements are located in the promoter region of genes regulated by hormones with nuclear receptors. They are constituted of sequences from 13 to 15 nucleotides. The elements of estrogen response are formed by two semi-elements, which are sequences of 5 nucleotides, and a spacer of 3 unspecific nucleotides (*n*). The interaction is produced so that the section of the zinc fingers of the receptor lodges in the main furrow of the DNA double helix

spacer between the two pentamers of the palindrome (Freedman et al. 1988; Filardo 2002).

The interaction between the receptor dimer and DNA is produced in an orderly manner. First, the dimer is placed in the main furrow of the double helix, and the first monomer interacts with the first pentamer of the HRE in the main furrow of the double helix. Later the second molecule of the receptor dimer binds to the second pentamer. The distance between both pentamers is minimum: from zero to five nucleotides, depending on the type of receptor. This implies that the dimer assures a sufficiently compact and symmetrical structure among both receptor molecules, so that a similar intimacy can be produced in the association with the palindrome.

1.5.3 Recognition of Hormone Response Element

The native receptors of steroid hormones, in the absence of hormone, have little affinity for nuclear structures. Contact with the hormone augments this affinity to an extraordinary degree. This fact does not necessarily show that the hormone has caused the receptors to enter into contact with specific DNA sequences in the genes that respond to the hormone in question (Beato et al. 1996; Beato 1989). It has been calculated that in a normal target cell there are only a few genes that can respond to a hormone. Each target cell contains from 1000 to 10,000 receptors, which become activated in increasing number, in function with the concentration that the hormone reaches in the cell. It is not possible, therefore, for all the activated receptors to find specific genes with which to interact.

The excess of the activated receptor, at least in the case of the progesterone, binds with acid proteins that function like acceptors. Two possible functions are attributed to these proteins that have not been confirmed: that of being an active receptor reservoir and that of being responsible for directing the excess of the receptor toward degradation (Filardo 2002; Gruber et al. 2002).

The dimer of the hormone–receptor complex should scrutinize an infinity of sequences before finding its HRE. The role of the hormone in the recognition of the HRE seems to be that of dramatically increasing the velocity of DNA sequence recognition, that is to say, it binds and disconnects more quickly to sequences of nonspecific DNA. When it finds the sequence of its HRE, a bond of affinity is formed that is similar to that of hormone–receptor interaction (Kd in the nM range).

The state of the chromatin has influence as well on the velocity with which is produced the recognition between the receptor dimer and the HRE sequences. The inactive heterochromatin has methylated histones, so that a different compactment from that of the nucleosomes is produced that is characteristic of genetic inactivation. The active chromatin presents different degrees of acetylation, and those regions are more relaxed and permit the dimer to move more freely to scrutinize until it finds the HRE. These are found in accessible places of the nucleosome so it is not necessary for the dimer to travel the entire length of the DNA strand.

The normal form of interaction between receptor and DNA requires the hormone to have broken the native structure of the receptor and the dimer to have been formed. That is to say, the receptor–DNA interaction comes after the hormone–receptor interaction. Nevertheless, situations have been described in vitro in which the receptor is able to be previously associated to the HRE. This situation occurs in vivo for the thyroid hormone receptors, in which case it seems that the hormone-free dimer acts as an expression repressor of genes dependent on these hormones (Evans et al. 1988). The arrival of the hormone activates the dimer in situ and inverts its role as regulator.

1.5.4
Role of Receptor–Hormone Response Element Complex

The sequences of the HRE are situated in the promoter region of the gene. In a zone close by (less than 100 nucleotides away) and always between the HRE and the point of initiation of the transcription, there is a sequence rich in thymidine and adenosine (TATA, or its equivalent) on which the RNA polymerase II attaches itself (Beato et al. 1996; Beato 1989; Chin 1995; Gruber et al. 2002; Nilsson et al. 2001).

Once the interaction receptor dimer–HRE of the DNA occurs, a very fast progression of events is produced (Fig. 1.8). The receptor dimer causes a curvature in the structure of the double helix in the neighborhood of the region next to the starting point of the gene transcription. This curvature implies a structural change that permits the RNA polymerase II to accede to the TATA-rich sequence of DNA. The RNA polymerase II recruits some transcription factors and forms the transcription preinitiator complex on the sequence of TATA (or its equivalent one) (Klug et al. 1987; Nilsson et al. 2001).

The receptor dimer, associated with the HRE, will attract other transcription factors, with which the protein–protein interaction is produced. Finally, they will come together with the RNA polymerase II and the remaining transcription factors that formed the preinitiator complex to complete the machinery of gene transcription. The role of the receptor dimer is, therefore, that of assuring the correct anchorage of the transcription factors in the promoter region of the gene so that the functional assembly of the machinery of gene transcription is produced.

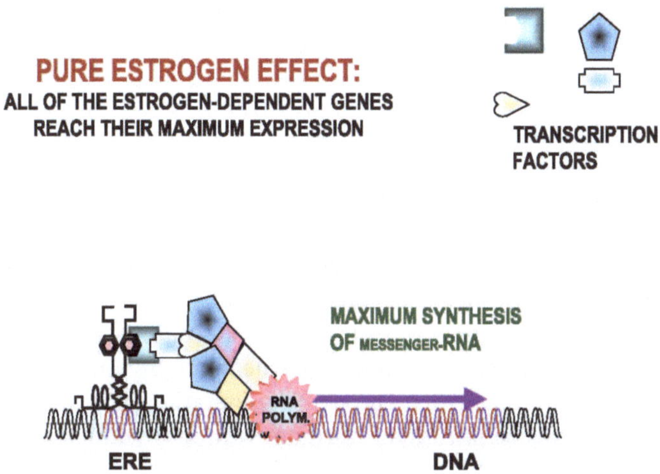

Fig. 1.8. Activation of gene expression. The interaction of the receptor dimer with the estrogen response element, located in the promoter region of the genes that are estrogen activatable, enables the recruitment of cofactors (coactivators) of transcription. The dimer of the receptor establishes a connection through coactivators with the basic transcription machinery that is associated with the promoter region of the gene in the TATA region (or similar region, depending on the gene). The consequence is that the transcription machinery becomes activated by one or two orders of magnitude and multiple copies of the mRNA of the gene begin to appear. In the case of a pure estrogen, like estradiol or DES, the activation will affect all of the estrogen-dependent genes and in all the estrogen target cells, although in varying intensity depending on the gene since not all are equally sensitive to estrogen

The structure of the chromatin and their state of acetylation are important at the moment of initiating the gene transcription. Indeed, some of the transcription factors recruited by the receptor dimer have histone-acetyltransferase activity that permits the gene transcription after diminishing the condensation of the chromatin (Gruber et al. 2002; Nilsson et al. 2001; Vigushin et al. 2002).

Well-documented cases exist where the estrogens inhibit the expression of some genes. These are usually transcribed by means of the constitutive activity of powerful promoters. The inhibition is a result of the steric interposition of the receptor dimer in the development region of the gene, which thereby recruits corepressors that interrupt the prior instigator effect in the absence of receptor (McKenna et al. 1999; Mester et al. 1995; Smith et al. 1997; Tora et al. 1989).

1.6 Hormonal Regulation of Gene Transcription

The final phase of action of the hormones that utilize nuclear hormone receptors lies in the modification of the gene transcription. In spite of the enormous effort expended, it is a process that remains only partly understood. This is due to its extraordinary complexity and to the multiple varieties that show up as gene or tissue specific.

1.6.1 Domains of Transcription Activation (Transactivators)

The participation of the nuclear receptors in the machinery of gene transcription takes place by means of specific domains of the molecule known as transactivators (abbreviation for transcription activators). These are made up of sequences of amino acids that interact by means of protein–protein contacts with other transcription factors. The artificial alteration of these sequences has as a consequence the inability of the hormone to induce gene expression (Beato et al. 1996; Klug et al. 1987; Lones et al. 1995).

At least seven proteins, besides the RNA–polymerase II, participate in the transcription machinery. The initiation of the transcription occurs when the transcriptional complex in the promoter region of the gene has been stabilized. The receptor dimer forms a complex of high affinity with the sequence of the HRE. This binding provides a firm base for the anchorage and stabilization of the transcriptional complex. The dimeric structure of the receptor acquires affinity to attract different coactivators that bring together the proteins of the transcriptional complex (Fig. 1.9).

As mentioned in a previous section of this chapter, there are two fully identified transactivator domains in the family of nuclear hormone receptors. One of them resides in the region preceding the DBD and is independent of the binding to the hormone. It is called TAF1 (trans-activation factor 1) and is transcriptionally active in the absence of the LBD (Tora et al. 1989). TAF1 is regulated by means of phosphorylation and can form part of signal transmission systems from the cell membrane. These can recruit the ER to activate some genes that have elements of estrogen response in the absence of estrogens (Filardo 2002; Lee et al. 2002; Osborne et al. 2001; Segars et al. 2002).

The other transactivator domain, TAF2, is found immersed in the LBD and acts only when the hormone–receptor complex is formed. A sequence of 15 well-conserved amino acids from the different members of the family of nuclear receptors, and situated very close to the carboxyl end of the receptors, participates in it (Gruber et al. 2002; Nilsson et al. 2001).

The transactivation domains only make their accessibility evident in the dimer bound to the HRE. It is very probable that, in this way, the spatial structure (tertiary) optimizes itself so that the contact surfaces between the receptor and the other cofactors of transcription are formed.

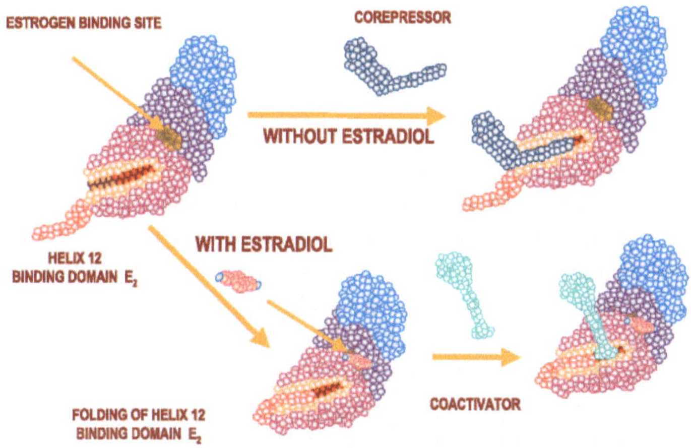

Fig. 1.9. Coactivators, corepressors, and the binding domain to the hormone. It has been possible to express the hormone binding domain in bacteria and to obtain great quantities in a pure state. This has made it possible to analyze its crystalline structure bound to ligands and to determine how this influences the recruitment of coactivators and corepressors. Several parts of the domain experience changes that justify its activity, but the most important one is helix 12. In the absence of estrogen, helix 12 leaves a hydrophobic cavity uncovered where corepressors containing zipper sequences of leucines lodge. In the presence of estrogens, helix 12 blocks that cavity and the corepressor does not fit. At the same place (or in the neighborhood) a new site is created that interacts with the complementary domains of the coactivators, thus initiating the bridge that connects with the transcription machinery, which is finally activated

1.6.2 Intermediary Transcription Cofactors

Among the proteins that form part of the transcription machinery are found some cell factors that are produced in limited quantities. They are called cofactors of transcription (NCoA, for nuclear-receptor coactivator; NCoI, for nuclear-receptor coinhibitor), formerly known as transcription intermediary factors (TIF) (McDonnell et al. 2002; McKenna et al. 1999). They constitute one of the classes of proteins that form part of the transcription machinery. These proteins are utilized by diverse types of intensifiers, that is to say, by sequences of DNA that anchor transcription factors, of which HRE are a particular case (Gruber et al. 2002; Mester et al. 1995). They do not interact directly with the DNA, but they do with the receptors and with the other elements of the transcription apparatus (Fig. 1.9).

The participation of the different cofactors that form part of the transcription machinery is not homogeneous. Some, like p160, can interact with both transcription activator domains of the receptor, TAF1 and TAF2, even though they utilize different p160 domains. Others, like CBP/p300, do not enter into contact with the receptor, but do with other coactivators, such as p160. It seems clear that each protein–protein contact causes conformational changes in them, so that new affinities for other coactivator proteins arise (Fig. 1.10). The final result of those contacts is the assembly of a transcription machinery that functions at full steam (McKenna et al. 1999).

In the moments prior to initiation of the transcription, a true rivalry is established by the transcription coactivators. The affinity with which the receptors are capable of interacting with the coactivators is decisive at the moment of including these in the transcription machinery and inducing the gene expression. If at the same time other machineries are themselves configuring transcriptions that capture these intermediary factors more efficiently than do the receptors, then the hormone-regulated transcription of the gene does not occur. In this case, the expression of such genes will have to wait for more favorable conditions for the transcription to appear.

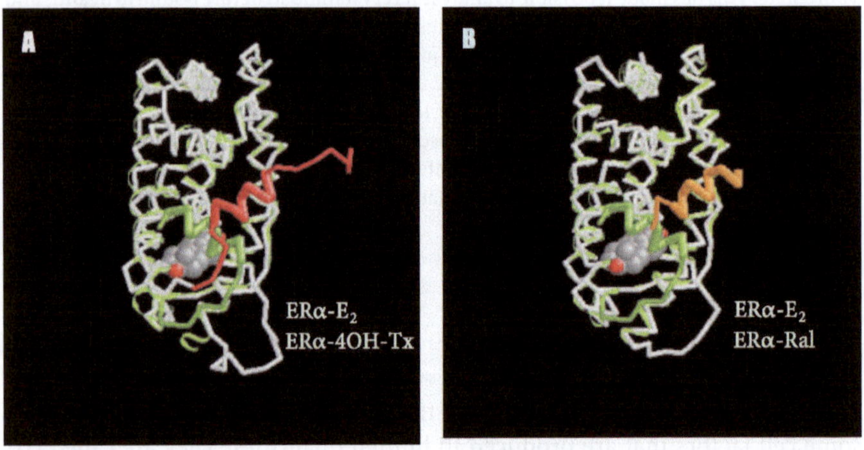

Fig. 1.10. Crystallography of receptor bound to estradiol or SERMS. **A** Crystallographic structures of binding domain to hormone of estrogen receptor alpha bound to estradiol (E2) and to 4-OH-tamoxifen. *Gray*: Parts of domain that do not experience changes bound to ligand. *Green*: Changes induced by estradiol. *Red*: Changes induced by 4-OH-tamoxifen. Notice that helix 12 of the domain bound to 4-OH-tamoxifen occupies a position salient and perpendicular to that occupied by the same helix in the case of binding to estradiol. **B** Changes induced by estradiol (*green*) and by raloxifene (*yellow*) in the crystalline structure of the binding domain to the hormone. Raloxifene causes a change in the position of helix 12 that is different from that of estradiol, although it is not as dramatic as in the case of 4-OH-tamoxifen. In each cell type, interactions by coactivators or corepressors with the new structures of the domain formed will be produced, a process that will depend on which of those coregulators are present

1.6.3 Interaction of Receptor with Transcription Cofactors

In the absence of hormone, the three-dimensional configuration of the receptor favors binding to corepressors present in the cell nucleus. The interaction is produced at the level of zipper-type sequences of leucines (–L–X–X–L–), present in the corepressors, with the LBD of the receptor. This has a structure that is complementary to the leucine zipper, which remains accessible while the receptor itself does not bind to the hormone (Gruber et al. 2002; Nilsson et al. 2001).

The spatial conformation that the ligand–receptor acquires, particularly the spatial disposition that helix 12 of the LBD attains when it binds to estradiol, is key for the subsequent recruitment of the transcription cofactors (Fig. 1.9). Indeed, the arrival of estradiol restructures the entire domain, making helix 12 rotate and close the hole where the leucine zipper sequence of the corepressor had been lodged before (Fig. 1.10). Consequently, both molecules, corepressor and receptor, lose their affinity and their bond is undone. Another structure capable of interacting with gene transcription coactivators is formed at the same place on the receptor (MacGregor et al. 1998; McDonnell et al. 2002).

Hormone agonists share various contacts with the amino acids of the LBD, although these are of variable intensity. The result of these interactions is a ranking of hormonal power the different agonists display (Cosman et al. 1999; Kelly et al. 1999; Jordan 2001; McDonnell 1999; Shang et al. 2002). The antagonists interact with a part of the same amino acids as the agonists, but these interactions include other contacts (Chan 2002; Jordan 2002; Riggs et al. 2003). From this interaction of the antagonists a structure of the receptor is created that varies as a function of the ligand, and this is reflected in the resulting crystallographic aspect of the LBD when occupied by different agonist or antagonist compounds (Fig. 1.10).

When bound with pure antagonists, the configuration of the LBD is such that helix 12 does not rotate to undo the binding site of the corepressor (Jordan 2002; Riggs et al. 2003) (Fig. 1.11). On the contrary, the binding of an agonist to the receptor causes the production of a structure that is more similar to that formed upon binding to estradiol. Nevertheless, each agonist creates a different tertiary structure that, consequently, presents slight variations as to the spatial conformation in which the coactivators need to lodge.

1.6.4 Coactivators in Cellular and Gene Promoter Context

Depending on the type of coactivator(s) present in each particular cell type, a productive or unproductive receptor–agonist–coactivator bond can be cre-

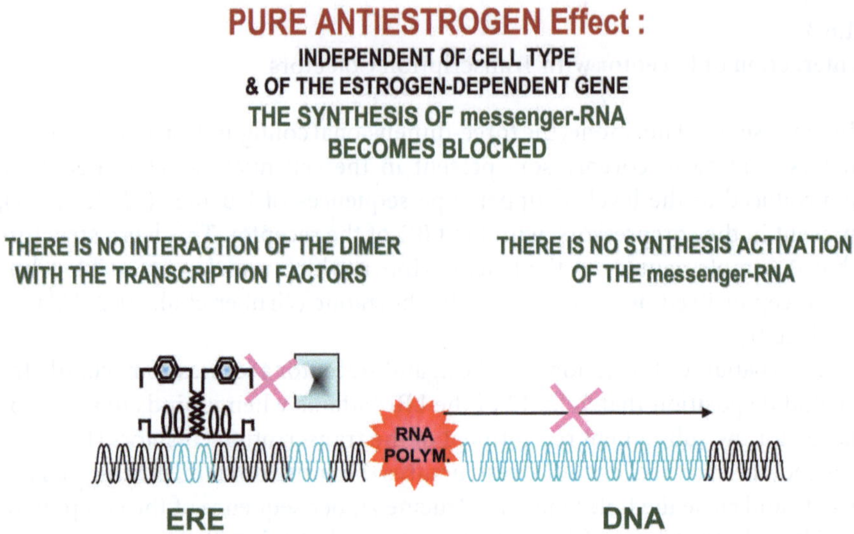

Fig. 1.11. Pure antiestrogen effect. The conformational change produced in the zone of binding to the hormone by a pure antiestrogen can be of a nature that incapacitates the receptor for dimerizing, making it fragile to the attack of intracellular proteases (Faslodex). It is also possible that the pure antiestrogen confers upon the receptor a conformation that incapacitates it from interacting with coactivators so that it cannot form the bridge with the transcription machinery. Finally, it is possible that the conformation acquired by the receptor recruits corepressors instead of coactivators, thus inhibiting the synthesis of mRNA. For a compound to be considered a pure antiestrogen, it must interfere with the estrogen-dependent gene expression in all cell types

ated. If the bond is productive, the compound behaves like an estrogen in that cell type; on the contrary, if the bond is unproductive, the compound can block the activity of a concurrent estrogen compound in the cell, and therefore the compound behaves like an antiestrogen (Jordan 2001; Riggs et al. 2003).

An additional variable to consider is how the subsequent interaction of the coactivators with other proteins of the transcription machinery is affected. This interaction occurs in the context of the promoter of each particular gene.

The bond of the receptor dimer with the nucleotide sequence of the HRE in the promoter region of the gene is what directs the assembly of the proteins (up to 19) that yields the transcription machinery. The operation of the machinery depends on the continual, sequential reestablishment of protein–protein contacts. Each new interaction depends on whether the previous proteins had assembled themselves correctly in such a way that the protein under consideration does not bind unless the prior interactions have created the appropriate surface of contact.

Agonist and antagonists not only modify the three-dimensional structure of the receptor, they also modify the three-dimensional structure of the coactivator and help to create the contact surface with the following protein. It is easy to imagine that small variations in the conformation of the site of interaction between the receptor bound to the agonist and the coactivator can create spatial orientations that can be incorrect in the context of the promoter of each particular gene (Jordan 2001; Riggs et al. 2003).

1.6.5 Concept of SERM from Point of View of Coactivator

For any substance with potential estrogen activity it is necessary to consider whether the configuration that the receptor acquires upon binding is capable of interacting correctly with the coactivators present in the cell. It is also necessary to consider whether from an imperfect interaction between receptor and coactivator the capacity to activate can be deduced from the expression of some, several, or all the genes that have HRE.

The concept of SERM (Selective Estrogen Receptor Modulator) refers to compounds capable of binding to the ER and to have an extensive range of cell responses that go from the net estrogen to antiestrogen activity (McDonnell 1999; Riggs et al. 2003; Shang et al. 2002). From what has previously been presented, it can be deduced that depending on the cell context, there will be coactivators that are either capable or incapable of binding to each receptor–SERM complex or of doing it in such a way that these can activate some genes with determinate promoter conformation, but not others (Fig. 1.12).

What will occur with a SERM in a particular tissue is unpredictable. Its behavior depends on at least two factors:

- The availability of coactivators in that cell line that recognize the receptor–SERM complex that, at the same time, is subject to a regulation of its expression, to competition, as they may be in the process of being recruited by other receptors, etc.
- The context of the gene promoter being considered that has some specific conditions for accepting activation by particular conformations of the transcription machinery.

1.6.6 Structure of Chromatin and Hormone Response

The curvature effect of the double helix of DNA, caused by the binding of dimers of active receptors to the HRE sequences, has been obtained by means of experiments of transfection of lineal DNA structures to cells that previously did not express the gene under study. The reality of the cells in vivo must be

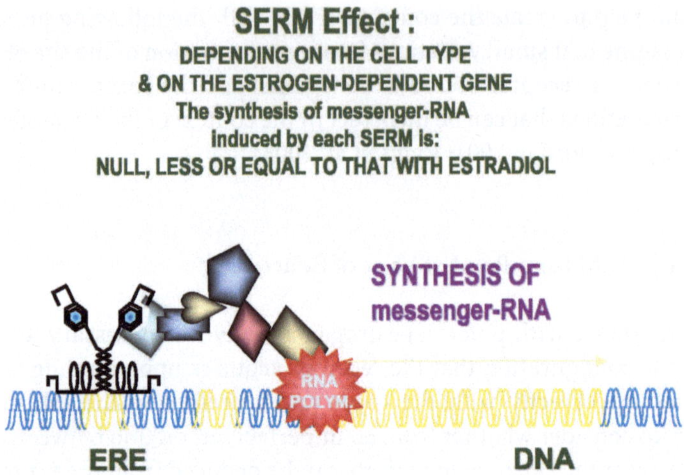

Fig. 1.12. SERM or not SERM, that is the question. The spatial conformation that a compound with SERM activity confers to the estrogen receptor gives it the capacity to interact with determinate coactivators or corepressors, but not with others. Depending on the cell lineage, and therefore on the collection of coactivators and corepressors present in that cell, this will activate the expression of some estrogen-dependent genes and the repression of others. One gene induced by estrogens in several cell types containing different coactivators is activated by SERMs in some cell types but not in others. In this case, the promoter context of each gene plays a determining role in whether that gene is or is not activatable by a determinate SERM

much more complex (Nilsson et al. 2001; Vigushin et al. 2002). In the regulation of gene expression in vivo, the structure of the chromatin participates decisively. This represents the effect of cell differentiation on the accessibility of only determinate genes to induction by hormones.

The Beato group has studied in depth the influence of the nucleosome structure in response to glucocorticoids (Beato 1989). Nucleosomes are formed by segments of 120 nucleotides of the double helix of DNA that make two twists around an octamer of histone. There are 200 nucleotides between two consecutive nucleosomes, so that a gene normally has tens of nucleosomes.

The structure of the promoter region of some of the genes studied overlaps a nucleosome in such a way that the RNA polymerase II cannot get to its binding site. The interaction between the receptor dimers and the HRE causes the nucleosomes to have their structures altered, either by being displaced or by having their structure come partly undone. This change in the configuration permits the fixation of the RNA polymerase II, with which the transcription can be initiated.

The histones, which provide the nucleosomes with their structural base, are susceptible to acetylation. Receptors bound to antagonists, or even hormone-free ones, are available to bind with corepressors that recruit histone-deacetylase, a process that provokes the contraction of the nucleosomes and impedes gene transcription. In contrast, the agonist-receptor dimer attracts coactivators, some of which directly have acetyltransferase activity, or even recruit other coactivators that have that enzymatic activity. The result is the acetylation of the histones and the consequent relaxation of the nucleosome structure, which permits the transcription of the gene regulated by the hormone.

1.6.7
Specificity of Gene Transcription Induced by Hormones

The specific transcription of the genes depending on each hormone runs up against the evident similarities among HRE for each hormone. For example, HRE are identical for androgens and progesterone (Navarro et al. 2002). This seems to introduce a certain degree of confusion at the moment of assuring a correct hormone-specific gene transcription. In other words, since the resemblance among HRE does not offer guarantees of specificity in the response, other elements have to exist that guarantee it.

The fact that a receptor dimer identifies a HRE does not assure, by itself, the transcription of the gene. This is a necessary, but insufficient, condition. Once the dimer–HRE interaction has been produced, the machinery of transcription needs to be assembled, requiring the binding of other intermediary cofactors. Some of these are tissue specific, and others recognize only a particular receptor dimer, thus obviating others that could recognize the same HRE.

1.6.8
Multiple Regulation of Gene Expression

Various elements of response to regulating transcription factors concur in a real promoter region of a gene. This reflects the complexity of situations influencing transcription in response to different signals. One of these, necessary but not totally sufficient for the induction of maximum transcription, is the receptor dimer. Others may be the protein that mediates the transcriptional response to cyclic AMP or the AP1 that recognizes fos-jun dimers (Gruber et al. 2002; Nilsson et al. 2001). Each one of these DNA sequences recognizes its own coactivators, and all can be simultaneously present in the promoter region of the gene, offering a variety of possible interactions.

The situation is still more complex. Thus the presence of elements of response from signaling pathways that regulate the expression of the gene in different directions may be detected in the promoter region. These elements recruit coactivators and corepressors, repression being one form of hormonal regulation of gene expression. It is obvious that the transcription machinery of such genes will couple or uncouple as a function of the relative influence of the cofactors that intervene in each moment.

The formation of a transcriptionally active complex requires the interaction of all transcription cofactors with their respective specific DNA sequences. Once they have bound to their specific sequences, it is on these that the remaining elements of the complex that do not interact directly with the DNA are assembled (Chin 1995; Filardo 2002). The elements of the complex that do not come into direct contact with DNA have their own specificity of interaction with the remaining proteins of the complex. Therefore, they include important restrictions so that a fully active transcriptional complex can be assembled with difficulty on a receptor dimer that has incorrectly recognized a HRE. Indeed, an incorrect interaction can imply a noticeable degree of transcription inhibition.

Many aspects relating to the specificity and intensity of gene transcription in response to hormones remain open. Nevertheless, a prudent conclusion permits establishing that two definite elements are intervening: the interaction of the receptor dimer with the palindrome and several protein–protein interactions that are produced between the dimer and the remaining components of the transcription machinery (Beato 1989).

1.6.9 Nuclear Hormone Receptors and Endocrine Disruptors

The chemical structure of the substances capable of interacting with a determinate nuclear receptor is tremendously varied. For now no pattern exists that permits one to assure that a particular substance is going to interact with the receptor to produce an agonist or antagonist effect. In recent years the concept of "endocrine disruptors" has been introduced to describe the substances that are capable of modifying the endocrine equilibrium. Some of them act by binding with nuclear hormone receptors, while others interfere with the processes of regulation of hormone secretion (Lathers 2002; Melnick et al. 2002; Nakata 2002; Powles 2002; Brown et al. 2002; Sonnenschein et al. 1998).

Endocrine disruptors apparently affect all nuclear receptors. Thus, a notable increment in impotence, alterations of the libido and of oligospermia in workers exposed to pesticides has been described. These alterations are due to the action of some compounds with estrogen-mimetic action and to their interaction with the androgen receptor. Additionally, alterations of thyroid function have been detected in rats exposed to dioxin and other toxic agents, though it is not sure if this effect is produced by direct interaction with the thyroid hormone receptor.

Among the endocrine disruptors that interact with the nuclear hormone receptors are the chemical substances that have an estrogen character. Thus, it has been discovered that substances as dissimilar as polychlorated biphenyls used as pesticides, numerous vegetable compounds (phytoestrogens), and components of plastic, paint, and detergent have weak estrogen activity. Given the abundance of these compounds in the diet or in western lifestyles, the substances are partly blamed for the growing incidence of breast cancer (Anderson 2002; Badger et al. 2002; Clemons et al. 2001; Colditz 1998; Jacobs et al. 2002; Safe 1998).

1.7 Regulation of Intensity of Hormone Response

The molecular details of the mechanism of hormonal action do not always clarify the numerous unknowns of the way in which the intensity of the hormone response is regulated from cell to cell and from minute to minute. There are numerous factors implicated in this process directed at achieving the greatest functional equilibrium of the organism. From the entry of the hormones into the cell to the conclusion of hormonal action, an ensemble of factors arises that intervenes in the process in a decisive way.

1.7.1 Membrane Receptors for Steroid Hormones

The entrance of steroid hormones into the cells has always been assumed to be a passive phenomenon, based on its solubility in the phospholipids of the cell membrane. Nevertheless, the existence of specific fixation of steroid hormones to cell membranes has opened the possibility of their entrance into the cells mediated by proteins of the membrane (Levin 2002). Nevertheless, it has not been possible to verify that they participate in some way in the transportation of steroids to the interior of the cell (Beato et al. 1996; Beato 1989). For them, other possible extragenomic actions have been postulated such as enzymes that participate in the metabolism of hormones or even membrane receptors (Beato et al. 1996; Chirino et al. 1991; Fernández et al. 1994; Gruber et al. 2002; Revelli et al. 1998).

There is growing evidence that the membrane receptors for estrogens are very important in tissues as the vascular endothelium (Chambliss et al. 2002; Hodgin et al. 2002; Mendelsohn 2002; White 2002). In the endothelial cells ERs appear to be located in specific zones of the membranes called caveolas, but not in the greater part of the membrane. Such receptors mediate rapid responses to estrogens, such as the activation of NOS (nitric oxide synthase) in the vascular endothelium (Chambliss et al. 2002).

There are also numerous enzymes anchored in membranes of the microsomal cell fraction that participate in the metabolism of steroid hormones. Thus, those of the p450 family, which carry out molecular oxidation, or the sulfatases and sulfotransferases, more or less specific to several hormones (Pasqualini et al. 1995). The affinity of steroid hormones for proteins of the membrane (Kd between 10 and 100 nM) is frequently greater than that which some of these enzymes present for their substrates (Luzardo et al. 2000). Therefore, it is unlikely that a part of the proteins of the membrane that bind steroids is in reality enzymes metabolizing these hormones.

In the case of vitamin D3, there is a membrane receptor that, after being bound to this compound, and by the mediation of a G-protein, activates the opening of channels for the entrance of calcium into the cell (Bouillon et al. 1995). There are also membrane receptors for progesterone that mediate, among other processes, the reaction of acrosomes in spermatozoa. Finally, evidence of extragenomic participation of estrogens in exocytosis does exist (Machado et al. 2002).

1.7.2
Regulation of Concentration of Receptors per Cell

Abundance of receptors is one of the most important factors in the regulation of the intensity of hormone response. This depends on the degree of expression of their respective genes and on the speed with which the receptors are eliminated.

During embryonic development, profound changes are produced in the expression of the genes for receptors and in the corporal distribution of the cells capable of expressing them. The thyroid hormone receptors are among the more ubiquitous of this family of receptors and are present in all cells. Nevertheless, both their abundance and the type of receptor that is expressed vary with age and from one tissue to another. The other receptors vary extensively among the different tissues. This unequal cell distribution conditions the response to the hormone, which has given rise to the concept of the target cell.

The gene that encodes for a receptor can be subjected to regulation by signals of diverse origin, as occurs with any other gene. The regulation of gene expression of the nuclear hormone receptors does not follow a single pattern. The hormone itself acts to negatively regulate the gene transcription of the receptor, particularly when the hormone is in excess. This diminishes the protein excess in the interior of the cell. There are, however, some exceptions since physiological doses of estrogens or androgens induce the synthesis of their own receptors.

There are numerous examples of how hormones regulate other receptors. Of recognized physiological importance, the synthesis of progesterone receptors is induced by estrogens in the endometrium, a process that regulates the transition of the proliferative phase to the secretory phase in the menstrual cycle. Additionally, androgen receptors are induced by FSH in Leydig cells in a process that is decisive in the regulation of testicular steroidogenesis (Mester et al. 1995).

An example of the complexity involved in the regulation of nuclear hormone receptors is shown in the case of the ER in the liver. Its synthesis is induced by estradiol, growth hormone, thyroid hormones, and glucocorticoids.

1.7.3 Receptor Destiny After Activation

The regulation of transcription by hormones requires a controlled limitation in order to guarantee that the protein is produced in adequate amounts. This process, nevertheless, is very poorly understood for members of the family of nuclear receptors.

The receptors are continuously subjected to a process of synthesis and destruction, which achieves a steady state. The concentration of receptors in the cell only reflects the situation of the steady state at that moment. As a consequence of hormone action, the number of receptors per cell drastically diminishes in the hours that follow. This observation has led to the postulation that the receptors undergo a process of destruction, or "processing", induced by the hormone. Despite all efforts, receptor processing has not been deciphered. The destruction of receptors implies the existence of a proteolysis process. Nevertheless, signs of proteolysis, in the form of small peptides of degradation originating in the receptor, have not been detected in the cell. Therefore, if there is a process of receptor proteolysis, it has to be very fast and complete (Beato 1989; Edwards et al. 2002; Kassis et al. 1983).

The possibility of receptor reutilization, once its function has been performed, has been advanced for a long time, but it has been verified only in the case of glucocorticoid receptors (Munck et al. 1995). Very little is known of the details of that process.

1.8 **Cross-Talk Signaling**

Numerous intracellular signaling pathways initiated in the membrane receptors include processes of phosphorylation (Aaronica et al. 1993; Munck et al.

1995). Eventually, nuclear receptors can act as substrata of phosphorylation–dephosphorylationin response to signals originating in other pathways. The state of phosphorylation of the nuclear receptors integrates them within the system of cell membrane signaling.

In this way, the gene transcription activity induced by the nuclear receptors modifies the abundance and activity of the proteins that participate in the pathways of membrane signaling. There also is evidence that the steroid hormone receptors activated by their ligands can interact with elements of the membrane signaling system by activating the pathway in the absence of a corresponding extracellular signal. In this way, a real crisscross of signals from membrane and nuclear receptors is produced, originating in membrane and in nuclear receptors, that maintains the cellular activity integrated into the individual whole.

Cross-talk signaling is an area of very recent investigation that is acquiring greater importance each day. As an example, cyclic AMP, under very specific conditions, enlarges the transcription capacity of ERs (Aaronica et al. 1993). Indeed, the members of the hormone receptor family are the object of phosphorylation. It has been described that this occurs in serine residues for all of them, although it has been described in serine and in tyrosine for ERs (Gruber et al. 2002; Powles 2002).

Regulation of the proteic activity by means of phosphorylation and dephosphorylation is well known. In the case of nuclear receptors, it has been described that the state of phosphorylation affects not only their affinity for the hormone, but also their transcription activity. The process of phosphorylation seems to occur after the receptor binds with the hormone and frees the hsp90, which is a phosphoprotein (Mester et al. 1995).

The enzymes that carry out the processes of receptor phosphorylation are kinases belonging to the signaling pathways of membrane receptors. The pathway of the MAP kinases, activated by different growth factors (EGF, Heregulin, IGF-1, TGF-ALPHA), phosphorylate specifically the ER in the serines S118 and S167 (Gruber et al. 2002; Nilsson et al. 2001; Powles 2002). These serines form part of the TAF1 region of the receptor and are activated by this procedure independently of the binding of the receptor to estrogen. Once phosphorylated, the receptor is capable of dimerizing and activating the expression of some genes in the absence of estrogen.

The cycline-dependent kinases (complex cyclines A/E and CDK2) are able to phosphorylate the ER in serine, particularly in the S104 and S106 belonging to TAF1, and with consequences similar to those of the pathway of the MAP kinases (Osborne et al. 2001; Powles 2002).

Some signal pathways that activate the adenylate cyclase phosphorylate tyrosine residues (Y535) of the TAF2 domain, which, as previously mentioned, is dependent on hormone binding. In this case, modulation of the transcription induction activity is produced in the presence of the hormone (Lee et al. 2002; Osborne et al. 2001).

Inversely, the ER bound to estradiol may be capable of binding with src proteins that form part of the signals transmission complex from the EFG. The consequence is that activation of the EGFR-dependent pathway is produced in the absence of EGF, with the consequent cascade of reactions due to such active agents. It is very probable that this type of reaction mediates the induction of cell proliferation in the endometrium, where estrogen and EGF play dominant, mutually dependent roles that are hardly separable (Lee et al. 2002; Osborne et al. 2001; Powles 2002). Moreover, cross-talk between proteins of the src family and the ER has been described. This signaling includes the phosphorylation of the receptor, in a process initiated by the interaction of src-1 with progesterone (Lee et al. 2002; Miglaccio et al. 1998; Powles 2002).

Experimental evidence exists that some mutated receptors that cannot bind the hormone are constitutionally active from a transcriptional point of view. In these cases, the phosphorylation of the receptor can play an important role in the transcription of some genes in the absence of the hormone.

These findings complete the panorama relative to the mechanisms of hormonal action mediated by nuclear receptors. Thus, gene activation mediated by nuclear receptors can respond to three clearly differentiated modalities: (1) receptor bound to hormone and not phosphorylated, (2) receptor bound to hormone and phosphorylated, and (3) receptor not bound to hormone and phosphorylated (Filardo 2002; Lee et al. 2002; Powles 2002).

Although it is difficult to establish firm conclusions in this area, a prudent formulation of the concept of cross-talk should stress that phosphorylation is a prominent process in the regulation of the activity of the different members of the family of nuclear receptors. This knowledge opens new perspectives in the global comprehension of the processes of cell regulation and illustrates the points of contact among the pathways of intracellular signaling of steroid hormones on the one hand and of the growth factors and peptide hormones on the other. Both pathways were, until recently, considered separate and relatively independent.

1.9
Silencing of Genes for Nuclear Hormone Receptors

The technology for the production of animals completely lacking the gene of one of the receptors (knockout mice) has erupted with extraordinary force in the generation of knowledge on multiple facets of hormonal action (Korach 1994). The coincidental discovery of human subjects with a deficit of some of these genes has brought, moreover, the possibility of verifying up

Table 1.2. Principal effects of knocking out genes for estrogen receptors α and β in the mouse

RE-α-KO	RE-β-KO
Not lethal	Not lethal
Both sexes infertile	Male fertile; female subfertile
Normal RE-β expression	
Normal prenatal development of reproductive tract, insensitive to estrogens and anti-estrogens	Normal uterus
Normal prenatal and postnatal ovarian development, with multiple nonovulatory hemorrhagic follicles as an adult, 30–40% incidence of ovarian cancer in 18 months	Ovary apparently normal in its development, but does not present normal frequency of spontaneous ovulations.
Normal prenatal development, but insensitive to the development promoted by estrogens during puberty. Sensitive to progesterone and prolactin.	Breast indistinguishable from normal type in virgin mice. Normal differentiation during pregnancy and lactation.
Normal pre- and postnatal male reproductive tract development. Progressive atrophy with age of rete testis and seminal tubules. Diminution of fertilizing capacity of sperm.	Normal development of masculine tract. No evidence of problems related to sperm or to fertility.
Females: Neuroendocrine system apparently normal, except for an excess of transcription of gonadotropin genes. Elevated levels of estradiol, and testosterone and LH, but normal for FSH and progesterone. Rapid hypocampal response to estradiol maintained.	Normal level of circulating estradiol.
Males: Neuroendocrine system apparently normal, except for an excess of transcription of the gonadotropin genes. Elevated levels of estradiol, and testosterone and LH, but normal for FSH and progesterone.	Normal level of circulating estradiol.
Females: Mating behavior response lacking under influence of estradiol. Greater aggressiveness and infanticide.	No apparent defects in sexual behavior.
Males: Normal mounting, but without penetration or ejaculation.	No apparent defects in sexual behavior.

Data from Couse JF, Korack SK, Endocr Rev 20:358 (1999)

to what point the conclusions obtained in mice are applicable to the human species.

Particularly exciting are the advances in techniques of molecular biology applied to human endocrinology. The case of a man homozygous for a type of ER truncated at the beginning of the molecule is a good example. The receptor lacked all the functionally relevant domains (Smith et al. 1994). The characteristics of this subject, and the subject's data as compared with those of "knockout" mice, have revealed the determinant role of estrogens on aspects such as inhibiting growth (the individual continued growing at the age of 27), spermatogenesis (he had oligospermia), or hypothalamic feedback (he secreted an excess of LH despite a normal level of androgens).

The majority of descriptions on the effects of ER gene suppression are anatomical (Table 1.2), although the functional studies in mice are already erupting with force (Couse et al. 1999a; Couse et al. 1999b; Krege et al. 1998). An important surprise from these experiments includes fewer incidents than expected when one receptor is absent, for example, the viability of gametes lacking ERα or the scarcity of defects produced by the absence of a thyroid hormone receptor (Kastner et al. 1995; Korach et al. 1996; Mangelsdorf et al. 1995).

Globally, those experiments with knockout mice suggest that the implication of more than one member of the nuclear receptor family may have prominent effects in organogenesis, even if their expression is for a brief period during embryonic life. The mice with double or triple knock-outs, lacking two or three receptors, will surely contribute to finally clarifying the roles of each hormone and each receptor.

1.10 Summary

Steroid hormones regulate a very extensive assembly of functions in numerous corporal tissues. Estrogens, the steroid hormones to which the majority of this chapter is dedicated, regulate from basic functions related to reproduction, the development of the skeleton, the maintenance of arterial tension, or diverse nervous functions. The molecular studies on the mechanism of action of estrogens have set the foundations that will permit us to understand how they carry out such diverse functions in such dissimilar tissues as well as how some substances that act through the estrogen signaling pathway can exercise opposite functions in different tissues. In this respect, there are five facts of particular importance that constitute the central nucleus of this revision:

1. There are two types of intracellular ER (ERα and ERβ) that are the product of different genes, have different patterns of tissue expression, have different pharmacological properties, activate different groups of genes, and can even carry out opposite actions when they are simultaneously present in the same cell.
2. The vast majority of the actions for which the estrogens in tissues are known are mediated by one of their intracellular receptors and imply the modification of the expression of extensive groups of genes that vary from one

tissue to another. The estrogen–receptor complexes recognize the genes regulated by estrogens through short sequences of nucleotides (estrogen response elements) in their promoter region that specifically anchor the receptor. Once the receptor is bound to DNA, cofactors of transcription (coactivators or corepressors) capable of influencing the efficiency of the gene transcription machinery are recruited.
3. Target cells have different collections of coactivators and corepressors that
   a) are not functionally equivalent,
   b) are not recruited with the same efficiency by the hormone–receptor complex,
   c) do not influence the transcription machinery of each cell with the same efficacy, and
   d) do not behave identically in each gene promoter regulated by estrogens.
4. There is growing evidence on the existence of ERs anchored to specific regions of the plasmatic membrane of target cells. These receptors mediate fast actions of estrogens that are executed by their own signaling mechanisms and that are different from the actions used at the genome level by the intracellular receptors.
5. Evidence is also accumulating on the existence of a system of interconnected signals among ERs and signaling systems originating in membrane receptors for growth factors. The use of ER free of ligand as one of the steps in the signaling pathways of membrane receptors for growth factors has also been observed.

In this way, although ERs participate in all cases and in all cells capable of responding to estrogens, the nature and intensity of the response is conditioned by the receptor interaction with three different types of molecules: estrogen (steroid or not), DNA (through the HRE sequences), and the protein–protein interactions, including cofactors of transcription as well as elements of the signaling pathway from membrane receptors.

In the West, where demographic trends suggest that women will live on average 30 years after menopause, the need to replace the ovarian source of estrogens has become evident. The Gordian knot (Diamanti-Kandarakis et al. 2003) rests in finding drugs (SERMs) that replace the functions of estrogens without producing estrogen-dependent tumors and other adverse consequences.

Only in-depth knowledge of the mechanisms of the action of estrogens and of other ligands for their receptors will permit a deeper understanding of the foundations on which the specificity of action on tissue for each SERM are based. This is perhaps among those challenging frontiers of knowledge that carry with it the potential to impact society in a profound way.

References

1. Aaronica SM, Katznellenbogen BS (1993) Stimulation of estrogen receptor-mediated transcription by estrogen, cyclic-AMP and IGF-1. Mol Endocrinol 7:743
2. Akner G, Wikström AC, Gustafsson JA (1995) Subcellular distribution of the glucocorticoid receptor and evidence for its association with microtubules J Steroid Biochem Mol Biol 52:1
3. Ali S, Metzger D, Bornert JM, Chambon P (1993) Modulation of transcriptional activation by ligand-dependent phosphorylation of the human oestrogen receptor A/B region. EMBO J 12:1153
4. Anderson E (2002) The role of oestrogen and progesterone receptors in human mammary development and tumorigenesis. Breast Cancer Res 4:197
5. Badger TM, Ronis MJ, Hakkak R, Rowlands JC, Korourian S (2002) The health consequences of early soy consumption. J Nutr 132:559S
6. Beato M, Sánchez-Pacheco A (1996) Interaction of steroid hormone receptors with the transcription initiation complex. Endocr Rev 1:587
7. Beato M (1989) Gene regulation by steroid hormones. Cell 56:335
8. Bouillon R, Okamura HO, Norman AW (1995) Structure-function relationship in the vitamin D endocrine system. Endocr Rev 16:200
9. Brann DW, Hendry LH, Mahesh V (1995) Emerging diversities in the mechanism of action of steroid hormones. J Steroid Biochem Mol Biol 52:2
10. Brzozowski AM, Pike AC, Dauter Z (1997) Molecular basis of agonism and antagonism in the oestrogen receptor. Nature 389:753
11. Brzozowski AM, Pike ACW, Dauter Z, Hubbard RE, Bonn T, Engstrom O, Ohman L, Greene GL, Gustaffson JA, Carlquist M (1997) Molecular basis of agonism and antagonism in the estrogen receptor. Nature 389:753
12. Castellano Díaz E, Gonzalez Quijano MI, Limiñana JM, Díaz Chico BN (1989) Tamoxifen decreases the estradiol induced progesterone receptors by interfering with nuclear estrogen receptor accumulation. J Steroid Biochem 33:133
13. Chambliss KL, Shaul PW (2002) Estrogen modulation of endothelial nitric oxide synthase. Endocr Rev 23:665
14. Chan S (2002) A review of selective estrogen receptor modulators in the treatment of breast and endometrial cancer. Semin Oncol 29:129
15. Chin WL (1995) Hormonal regulation of gene expression. In: DeGroot L (ed) Endocrinology. Saunders, Philadelphia, p 6
16. Chirino R, Fernández L, López A, Navarro D, Rivero JF, Díaz-Chico JC, Díaz-Chico BN (1991) Thyroid hormones and glucocorticoids act synergistically in the regulation of the low affinity glucocorticoid binding sites in the male rat liver. Endocrinology 129:3118
17. Clemons M, Goss P (2001) Estrogen and the risk of breast cancer. N Engl J Med 344:276
18. Colditz GA (1998) Relationship between estrogen levels, use of replacement theraphy and breast cancer. J Natl Cancer Inst 90:814
19. Cosman F, Lindsay R (1999) Selective estrogen receptor modulators: clinical spectrum. Endocr Rev 20:418
20. Couse JF, Hewitt SC, Bunch DO, Sar M, Walker VR, Davies BJ, Korack K (1999a) Postnatal sex reversal of the ovaries in mice lacking estrogen receptors alpha and beta. Science 286:2328
21. Couse JF, Korack KS (1999b) Estrogen receptor null mice: what have we learned and where will they lead us? Endocr Rev 20:358

22. Diamanti-Kandarakis E, Sykiotis GP, Papavassiliou AG (2003) Selective modulation of postmenopausal women: cutting the Gordian knot of hormone replacement therapy with breast carcinoma. Cancer 97:12
23. Díaz-Chico BN, Ogasawara Y, Chamness GC, Salman M, McGuire WL (1988) A 46 kDa antigen associated with estrogen receptors in human breast cancer. J Steroid Biochem 30:315
24. Edwards DP, Altaman M, DeMarzo A, Zhang Y, Weigel N, Beck CA (1995) Progesterone receptor and the mechanism of action of progesterone antagonists. J Steroid Biochem Mol Biol 53:449
25. Edwards DP, Wardell SE, Boonyaratanakornkit V (2002) Progesterone receptor interacting coregulatory proteins and cross talk with cell signaling pathways. J Steroid Biochem Mol Biol 83:173
26. Evans RM, Hollenberg S (1988) Zinc fingers: gilt by association. Cell 52:1
27. Evans RM (1989) Molecular characterization of the glucocorticoid receptor. Rec Prog Horm Res 45:1
28. Evans RM (1988) The steroid and thyroid receptor family. Science 240:889
29. Fawell SE, Lees JA, White R, Parker MG (1990) Characterization and colocalization of steroid binding and dimerization activities in the mouse estrogen receptor. Cell 60:953
30. Fernández L, Chirino R, Boada LD, Navarro D, Cabrera N, Del Río I, Díaz-Chico BN (1994) Stanozolol and danazol, unlike natural androgens, interact with the low affinity glucocorticoid binding sites from male rat liver microsomes. Endocrinology 134:1401
31. Filardo EJ (2002) Epidermal growth factor receptor (EGFR) transactivation by estrogen via the G-protein-coupled receptor, GPR30: a novel signaling pathway with potential significance for breast cancer. J Steroid Biochem Mol Biol 80:231
32. Freedman LP, Luisi BF, Korszum ZR, Basavappa R, Sigler PB, Yamamoto KR (1988) The function and structure of the metal coordination sites within the glucorticoid receptor DNA binding domain. Nature 334:543
33. Fuqua SA, Fitzgerald SD, Allred DC, Elledge RM, Nawaz Z, McDonnell DP, O'Malley BW, Greene G, McGuire WL (1992) Inhibition of estrogen receptor action by a naturally occurring variant in human breast tumors. Cancer Res 52:483
34. Fuqua SA (2001) The role of estrogen receptors in breast cancer metastasis. J Mammary Gland Biol Neoplasia 6:407
35. García T, Lehler S, Bloomer WD, Schachter B (1988) A variant estrogen receptor messenger ribonucleic acid is associated with reduced levels of estrogen binding in human mammary tumors. Mol Endocrinol 2:785
36. Green S, Kumar V, Theulaz I, Wahli W, Chambon P (1988) The N-terminal DNA-binding "zinc finger" of the oestrogen and glucocorticoid receptors determines target gene specificity. EMBO J 7:3037
37. Green S, Walter P, Kumar V, Krust A, Bornert JM, Argos P, Chambon P (1986a) Human oestrogen receptor cDNA: sequence, expression and homology to v-erb-A. Nature 320:134
38. Greene GL, Gilna P, Waterfield M, Baker A, Hort Y, Shine J (1986b) Sequence and expression of human estrogen receptor complementary DNA. Science 231:1150
39. Gruber CJ, Tschugguel W, Schneeberger C, Huber JC (2002) Production and actions of estrogens. N Engl J Med 346:340
40. Guiochon M, Loosfelt H, Lescop P, Sar S, Atger M, Perrot A, Milgrom E (1989) Mechanisms of nuclear localization of the progesterone receptor: evidence for interaction between monomers. Cell 57:1147

41. Hall JM, McDonnell DP (1999) The estrogen receptor beta-isoform of the human estrogen receptor modulates ER-alpha transcriptional activity and is a key regulator of the cellular response to estrogens and antiestrogens. Endocrinology 140:5566
42. Hodgin JB, Maeda N (2002) Minireview: estrogen and mouse models of atherosclerosis. Endocrinology 143:4495
43. Jacobs MN, Lewis DF (2002) Steroid hormone receptors and dietary ligands: a selected review. Proc Nutr Soc 61:105
44. Jensen EV (1991) Overview of the nuclear receptor family. In: Parker M (ed) Nuclear hormone receptor. Academic, London, p 1
45. Jordan VC, Murphy CS (1990) Endocrine pharmacology of antiestrogens as antitumor agents. Endocr Rev 11:578
46. Jordan VC (2001) Selective estrogen receptor modulation: a personal perspective. Cancer Res 61:5683
47. Jordan VC (2002) The secrets of selective estrogen receptor modulation: cell-specific coregulation. Cancer Cell 1:215
48. Kassis JA, Gorski J (1983) On the mechanism of estrogen receptor replenishment: recycling, resynthesis and/or processing. Mol Cell Biochem 52:27
49. Kastner P, Mark M, Chambon P (1995) Nonsteroid nuclear receptors: what are genetic studies telling us about their role in real life? Cell 83:859
50. Kelly MJ, Wagner EJ (1999) Estrogen modulation of G-protein-coupled receptors. Trends Endocrinol Metab 10:369
51. King WJ, Greene GL (1984) Monoclonal antibodies localize oestrogen receptor in the nuclei of target cells. Nature 307:745
52. Klug A, Rhodes D (1987) "Zinc finger": a novel protein motif for nucleic acid recognition. Trends Biochem Sci 12:464
53. Korach KS (1994) Insights from the study of animals lacking functional estrogen receptor. Science 266:1524
54. Korach SK, Couse JF, Curtis SW, Wahsburn TF, Linzdey J, Kimbro KS, Eddy EM, Miglacchio S, Snedeker SM, Lubhan DB, Schomberg DW, Smith EP (1996) Estrogen receptor gene disruption: molecular characterization and experimental and clinical phenotypes. Rec Prog Horm Res 51:159
55. Krege JH, Hodgin JB, Couse JF, Enmark E, Warner M, Mahler JF, Sar M, Korack K, Gustafsson JA (1998) Generation and reproductive phenotypes of mice lacking estrogen receptor beta. Proc Natl Acad Sci USA 95:15677
56. Kuiper GG, Carlsson B, Grandien K, Enmark E, Haggblad J, Nilsson S, Gustafsson JA (1996) Comparison of the ligand binding specificity ans transcript tissue distribution of estrogen receptor alpha and beta. Endocrinology 138:863
57. Kuiper GG, Enmark E, Haggblad J, Pelto-Huikko M, Nilsson S, Gustafsson JA (1996) Cloning of a novel estrogen receptor in rat prostate and ovary. Proc Natl Acad Sci USA 93:5925
58. Kumar V, Chambon P (1988) The estrogen receptor binds tightly to its responsive elements as a ligand-induced homodimer. Cell 55:145
59. Kumar V, Green S, Stack G, Berry M, Jin JR, Chambon P (1987) Functional domains of the human estrogen receptor. Cell 51:941
60. Lathers CM (2002) Endocrine disruptors: a new scientific role for clinical pharmacologists? Impact on human health, wildlife, and the environment. J Clin Pharmacol 2:7
61. Lee AV, Cui X, Oesterreich S (2002) Cross-talk among estrogen receptor, epidermal growth factor, and insulin-like growth factor signaling in breast cancer. Clin Cancer Res 7(12 Suppl):4429s

62. Lee MS, Gippert, GP, Soman KV, Case DA, Wright PE (1989) Three-dimensional solution structure of a single zinc finger DNA-binding domain. Science 245:635
63. Levin ER (2002) Cellular functions of plasma membrane estrogen receptors. Steroids 67:471
64. Lones D, Mark M, Mendehlson C, Dollé P, Decimo D, Chambon P (1995) Developmental roles of the retinoic acid receptors. J Steroid Biochem Mol Biol 53:475
65. Luzardo OP, Machín RP, Díaz-Chico BN, Fernández L (2000) Photoaffinity labeling identification of a specific binding protein for the anabolic steroids stanozolol and danazol: an oligomeric protein regulated by age, pituitary hormones, and ethinyl estradiol. Endocrinology 141:3377
66. MacGregor JI, Jordan VC (1998) Basic guide to the mechanisms of antiestrogen action. Pharmacol Rev 50:151
67. Machado JD, Alonso C, Morales A, Borges R (2002) A novel nongenomic action of estrogens: the regulation of exocytotic kinetics. Ann NY Acad Sci 971:284
68. Mangelsdorf DJ, Thrummel C, Beato M, Herrlich P, Schütz G, Umesono K, Blumberg B, Kastner P, Mark M, Chambon P, Evans RM (1995) The nuclear receptor superfamily: the second decade. Cell 83:835
69. McDonnell DP, Clemm DL, Imhof MO (1994) RU486 exerts antiestrogenic activities through a novel progesterone receptor A form-mediated mechanism. J Biol Chem 269:11945
70. McDonnell DP, Norris JD (2002) Connections and regulation of the human estrogen receptor. Science 296:1642
71. McDonnell DP (1999) The molecular pharmacology of SERMs. Trends Endocrinol Metab 10:301
72. McEwen BS, Alves SE (1999) Estrogen actions in the central nervous system. Endocr Rev 20:279
73. McGuire WL, Chamness GC, Fuqua SAW (1991) Estrogen receptor variants and clinical breast cancer. Mol Endocrinol 5:1571
74. McKenna NJ, Lanz RB, O'Malley BW (1999) Nuclear receptor coregulators: cellular and molecular biology. Endocr Rev 20:321
75. Melnick R, Lucier G, Wolfe M, Hall R, Stancel G, Prins G, Gallo M, Reuhl K, Ho SM, Brown T, Moore J, Leakey J, Haseman J, Kohn M (2002) Summary of the National Toxicology Program's report of the endocrine disruptors low-dose peer review. Environ Health Perspect 110:427
76. Mendelsohn ME (2002) Genomic and nongenomic effects of estrogen in the vasculature. Am J Cardiol 90:3F
77. Mester J, Baulieu EE (1995) Nuclear receptor superfamily. In: DeGroot L (ed) Endocrinology. Saunders, Philadelphia, p 93
78. Miglaccio A, Piccolo D, Castoria G, DiDomenico M, Bilancio A, Lombardi M, Gong W, Beato M, Auricchio F (1998) Activation of the Src/p21(ras)/Erk pathway by progesterone receptor via cross-talk with estrogen receptor. EMBO J 17:2008
79. Munck A, Tóth ANF (1995) Glucocorticoid action. In: DeGroot L (ed) Endocrinology. Saunders, Philadelphia, p 1642
80. Nakata K (2002) Theoretical approach to endocrine disruptors. Front Biosci 7:c68
81. Navarro D, León L, Chirino R, Fernández L, Pestano J, Díaz-Chico BN (1998) The two native estrogen receptor forms of 8S and 4S present in cytosol from human uterine tissues display opposite reactivity with tamoxifen aziridine and the estrogen response element. J Steroid Biochem Mol Biol 64:49

82. Navarro D, Luzardo OP, Fernández L, Chesa N, Díaz-Chico BN (2002) Transition to androgen independence in prostate cancer. J Steroid Biochem Mol Biol 171:1
83. Nilsson S, Mäkelä S, Treuter E, Tujangue M, Thomsen J, Anderson G, Enmark E, Pettersson K, Warner M, Gustafsson JA (2001) Mechanisms of estrogen action. Physiol Rev 81:1535
84. O'Malley B, Means AR (1974) Female steroid hormones and target cell nuclei. Science 183:610
85. O'Malley BW (1990) The steroid receptor superfamily: more excitement predicted for the future. Mol Endocrinol 4:363
86. Osborne CK, Schiff R, Fuqua SA, Shou J (2001) Estrogen receptor: current understanding of its activation and modulation. Clin Cancer Res 7(12 Suppl): 4338s
87. Palmieri C, Cheng GJ, Saji S, Zelada-Hedman M, Warri A, Weihua Z, Van Noorden S, Wahlstrom T, Coombes RC, Warner M, Gustafsson JA (2002) Estrogen receptor beta in breast cancer. Endocr Relat Cancer 9:1
88. Pasqualini JR, Chetrite G, Nguyen BL, Maoloche C, Delalonde M, Talbi M, Feinstein MC, Blacker C, Botella J and Paris J (1995) Estrone sulfate-sulfatase and 17β-hidroxisteroid dehydrogenase activities: a hypothesis for their role in the evolution of human breast cancer from hormone-dependence to hormone-independence. J Steroid Biochem Mol Biol 53:407
89. Pettersson K, Delaunay F, Gustafsson J-Å (2000) Estrogen receptor beta acts as a dominant regulator of estrogen signaling. Oncogene 19:4970
90. Picard D, Yamamoto KR (1987) Two signals mediate hormone dependent nuclear localization of the glucocorticoid receptor. EMBO J 6:3333
91. Ponglikitmongkol M, Green S, Chambon P (1988) Genomic organization of the human oestrogen receptor gene. EMBO J 7:3385
92. Powles TJ (2002) Anti-oestrogenic prevention of breast cancer – the make or break point. Nat Rev Cancer 2:787
93. Quingley CA, DeBellis A, Marschke KB, El-Awady MK, Wilson EM, French FS (1995) Androgen receptor defects: historical, clinical and molecular perspectives. Endocr Rev 16:271
94. Ratajczak T, Carrello A, Mark PJ, Warner BJ, Simpson B, Moritz RL, House AK (1993) The cyclophilin component of the unactivated estrogen receptor contains a tetratricopeptide repeat domain and shares identity with p59 (FKBP59). J Biol Chem 268:13187
95. Redeuilh G, Moncharmont B, Secco C, Baulieu EE (1987) Subunit composition of the molybdate stabilized 8-9S nontransformed estradiol receptor purified from calf uterus. J Biol Chem 262:6969
96. Revelli A, Massobrio M, Tesarik J (1998) Nongenomic actions of steroid hormones in reproductive tissues. Endocr Rev 19:3
97. Riggs BL, Hartmann LC (2003) Selective estrogen-receptor modulators – mechanisms of action and application to clinical practice. N Engl J Med 348:618
98. Rubanyi GM, Kauser K, Johns A (2002) Role of estrogen receptors in the vascular system. Vascul Pharmacol 38:81
99. Safe S (1998) Interactions between hormones and chemicals in breast cancer. Annu Rev Pharmacol Toxicol 38:121
100. Scott GK, Kushner P, Vigne JL, Benz CC (1991) Truncated forms of DNA-binding estrogen receptors in human breast cancer. J Clin Invest 88:700
101. Segars JH, Driggers PH (2002) Estrogen action and cytoplasmic signaling cascades. Part I: Membrane-associated signaling complexes. Trends Endocrinol Metab 13:349

102. Segnitz B, Ghering U (1995) Native structure of the estrogen receptor of MCF-7 cells "in vivo". Proc Natl Acad Sci USA 92:2179
103. Seiler-Tuyns A, Walker P, Martinez E, Merillat AM, Givel F, Wahli W (1986) Identification of estrogen-responsive DNA sequences by transient expression experiments in a human breast cancer cell line. Nucleic Acids Res 14:8755
104. Shang Y, Brown M (2002) Molecular determinants for the tissue specificity of SERMs. Science 295:2465
105. Shiau AK, Barstad D, Loria PM, Cheng L, Kushner PJ, Agard DA, Greene GL (1998) The structural basis of estrogen receptor/coactivator recognition and the antagonism of this interaction by tamoxifen. Cell 95:927
106. Brown SMT, Moore J, Leakey J, Haseman J, Kohn M (2002) Summary of the National Toxicology Program's report of the endocrine disruptors low-dose peer review. Environ Health Perspect 110:427
107. Smith CL, Nawaz Z, O'Malley BW (1997) Coactivator and corepressor regulation of the agonist/antagonist activity of the mixed antiestrogen, 4-hydroxytamoxifen. Mol Endocrinol 11:657
108. Smith EP, Boyd J, Frank GP, Lubhan DB, Korack KS (1994) Estrogen resistance caused by a mutation in the estrogen-receptor gene in a man. N Engl J Med 331:1056
109. Smith FS, Toft DO (1993) Steroid receptors and their associated proteins. Mol Endocrinol 7:4
110. Sonnenschein C, Soto AM (1998) An updated review of environmental estrogen and androgen mimics and antagonists. J Steroid Biochem Mol Biol 65:143
111. Toft DO, Gorski J (1966) A receptor molecule for estrogens: isolation from rat uterus and preliminary characterization. Proc Natl Acad Sci USA 5:1574
112. Tora L, Gaub MP, Mader S, Dierich A, Bellard M, Chambon P (1988) Cell-specific activity of a GGTCA half-palindromic oestrogen responsive element in the chicken ovoalbumin gene promoter. EMBO J 7:3771
113. Tora L, White J, Brou C, Tasset D, Webster N, Scheer E, Chambon P (1989) The human estrogen receptor has two independent nonacidis transcriptional activation functions. Cell 59:477
114. Tzukerman MT, Esty A, Santiso-Mere D, Danielian P, Parker MG, Stein RB, Pike JW, McDonnell DP (1994) Human estrogen receptor transactivational capacity is determined by both cellular and promoter context and mediated by two functionally distinct intramolecular regions. Mol Endocrinol 8:21
115. Vasudevan N, Ogawa S, Pfaff D (2002) Estrogen and thyroid hormone receptor interactions: physiological flexibility by molecular specificity. Physiol Rev 82:923
116. Vigushin DM, Coombes RC (2002) Histone deacetylase inhibitors in cancer treatment. Anticancer Drugs 13:1
117. Wakeling AE (1993) The future of new pure antiestrogens in clinical breast cancer. Breast Cancer Res Treat 25:1
118. Welshons WV, Lieberman ME, Gorski J (1984) Nuclear localization of unoccupied oestrogen receptors. Nature 307:747
119. White RE (2002) Estrogen and vascular function. Vascul Pharmacol 38:73
120. Cowley SM, Parker MG (1999) A comparison of transcriptional activation by ER alpha and ER beta. J Steroid Biochem Mol Biol 69:165
121. McDonnell DP, Clemm DL, Hermann T, Goldman ME, Pike JW (1995) Analysis of estrogen receptor function in vitro reveals three distinct classes of antiestrogens. Mol Endocrinol 9:659

122. McInerney EM, Weis KE, Sun J, Mosselman S, Katzenellenbogen BS (1998) Transcription activation by the human estrogen receptor subtype beta (ERb) studied with ERa and ERb receptor chimeras. Endocrinology 139:4513
123. Barkhem T, Carlsson B, Nilsson Y, Enmark E, Gustafsson J-Å, Nilsson S (1998) Differential response of estrogen receptor alpha and estrogen receptor beta to partial estrogen agonists/antagonists. Mol Pharmacol 54:105

CHAPTER 2

Clinical Pharmacology of Selective Estrogen Receptor Modulators (SERMs)

FERNANDO MARÍN · Mª CARMEN BARBANCHO

2.1 Introduction

Selective estrogen receptor modulators (SERMs) are a group of drugs with heterogeneous structural chemical characteristics that are characterized as high-affinity ligands (in the subnanomolar concentration range) to estrogenic receptors (ERs) but have the peculiarity of triggering estrogen-agonist or estrogen-antagonist actions, depending on the tissue in which they act. From a pharmacological perspective, SERMs should be differentiated from pure antiestrogens, such as fulvestrant (Chap. 6), which are molecules chemically related to estradiol and exclusively exhibit estrogenic antagonist activity. SERMs also should be differentiated from the so-called "gonadomimetic" drugs, such as tibolone, that act by means of nonselective binding to different types of sex steroid receptors.

The pharmacological development of these compounds has been closely connected, on one hand, to the vast experience that has been accumulated over decades in estrogen therapy (ET) and estrogen and progestin therapy (EPT) during menopause and, on the other hand, to the effects on nonbreast tissues of drugs traditionally classified as "antiestrogens", tamoxifen being the principal example. ET and EPT have proven to be effective in the prevention and treatment of the signs and symptoms of early estrogen deficiency associated with perimenopause and accelerated bone mass loss occurring after ovarian function ceases. Numerous observational studies have demonstrated that postmenopausal women receiving long-term treatment with ET/EPT show a reduced risk of osteoporotic fractures, cardiovascular diseases, and even Alzheimer's disease (Manson et al. 2001). However, the benefits suggested in the observational studies have not been confirmed in randomized, double-blind, placebo-controlled clinical trials, the design of which eliminates the significant selection bias presented in naturalistic studies. Recent clinical trials clearly have shown the lack of benefit from EPT or ET alone in primary and secondary prevention of ischaemic heart disease and cerebrovascular disease (Hulley et al. 1998; Writing Group for the Women's Health Initiative Investigators 2002; Women's Health Initiative Steering Committee 2004) and cast serious doubts on its safety in the deterioration of higher cognitive functions (Shumaker et al. 2004). Furthermore, treatment compliance tends to be very low because of the poor acceptance by many women regarding the return of menstrual bleeding or spotting and the fear of an increased risk of breast or uterine cancer. On the other hand, WHI trials suggest a positive effect of ET and EPT in reducing the risk for hip fracture and colorectal cancer, although the overall risk–benefit balance is not consistent with the requirements for a viable intervention for primary prevention of chronic diseases (Writing Group for the Women's Health Initiative Investigators 2002; Women's Health Initiative Steering Committee 2004).

Therefore, the primary objective for the pharmacological development of SERMs is to increase the benefit/risk ratio in comparison with ET and EPT in the prevention and treatment of several highly prevalent, chronic diseases in the postmenopausal period that are related to this physiological estrogen deficient state. As is often the case in medicine, the discovery of the pharmacological profile that gave grounds for hope in the development of this new drug class was the result of an unexpected paradox. Tamoxifen, a drug that was introduced over 35 years ago for hormone-dependent breast cancer treatment, has been considered an antiestrogen for decades because of its blocking action on the binding of endogenous estrogens to the estrogen receptor (ER) of neoplastic breast cells. However, several studies suggested that tamoxifen might have a protective action in bone tissue (estrogen agonist). For example, a study of postmenopausal women who previously had breast cancer but were clinically cancer free showed that tamoxifen increased lumbar spine bone mineral density compared to placebo (Love et al. 1992); that is, this study further suggested that tamoxifen was not purely antiestrogenic.

This drug class has an enormous potential in the primary and secondary prevention of several types of estrogen-dependent tumors, postmenopausal osteoporosis, and cardiovascular and neurodegenerative diseases.

In this chapter, a general review of SERMs will be given, highlighting some of the latest advances in the development of new SERMs and problems encountered during the clinical development of some of them. Details on the efficacy, safety, and clinical use of SERMs in which more clinical experience has been accumulated will be discussed in greater depth in other chapters.

2.2 Classification

There is an extensive list of compounds that can be considered SERMs for which there are available results in either *in vitro* cellular models or *in vivo* animal and human experiments. Approximately 70 molecules with a SERM-like pharmacological profile were described in a recent review (Meegan et al. 2003). Table 2.1 provides a summary of the main SERM groups, classified according to chemical structure. Certain phytoestrogens, such as genistein and daidzein, also appear to have a SERM-type pharmacological profile. Currently there are two main chemical classes of SERMs approved for clinical use: triphenylethylene derivatives, such as tamoxifen and toremifene, used to treat and prevent breast cancer, and clomiphene for ovulation induction; and the benzothiophene derivative raloxifene, indicated for the treatment and prevention of osteoporosis.

Table 2.1. Classification of SERMs

Chemical class	SERM	
Triphenylethylenes	Tamoxifen*	AstraZeneca
	Clomifene*	
	Toremifene*	Orion
	Droloxifene#	Pfizer
	Miproxifene (TAT-59)#	Taiho Pharm
	Idoxifene#	SmithKline Beecham
	Ospemifene (FC-1271a)†	Hormos Medical Corp
	Fispemifene	Hormos Medical Corp
	GW5638	Duke University
	MDL 103,323	Hoechst-Marion-Roussel
Benzothiophenes	Raloxifene (keoxifene)*,†	Eli Lilly & Co
	Arzoxifene†	Eli Lilly & Co
	LY-117018	Eli Lilly & Co
Naphthylenes	Lasofoxifene (CP-336, 156)†	Pfizer
	Nafoxidine	
	Trioxifene#	
Indoles	Bazedoxifene (WAY-140424)†	Wyeth
	Pipendoxifene (ERA-923)†	Wyeth/Ligand
Benzopyrans	EM-800 (SCH57050)†	Schering Plough
	Acolbifene (EM-652)†	Schering Plough
	SP-500263	Celgene Corp
	Ormeloxifene* (centchroman)	Indian Drug Research Inst.
	Levormeloxifene#	Novo-Nordisk
	NNC 45-0781 and derivatives	Novo-Nordisk

* Commercialized for different indications: breast cancer treatment, contraception, ovulation induction, prevention and treatment of postmenopausal osteoporosis.

† Phase III clinical research.

\# Clinical development cancelled.

2.3 Pharmacological Characteristics of SERMs

2.3.1 Triphenylethylenes

The primary objective of the initial clinical development of SERMs was the treatment of estrogen-dependent breast cancer, and it is in this disease in which the clinical benefit of these drugs has accumulated the largest amount of proof. Tamoxifen, a triphenylethylene derivative, has been used for over 35 years. The accumulated clinical experience in over 10 million women/year is proof of its beneficial effect in the treatment of disseminating breast cancer, in adjuvancy, and primary prevention of women at high risk of developing the disease (Fisher et al. 1998; Jordan et al. 1999; Wickherman 2002). It is important to emphasize that treatment with a first-generation SERM such as tamoxifen is efficient in all breast cancer subgroups except for ER-negative tumors in premenopausal women, which is not surprising considering its mechanism of action. The clinical problem of ER-positive breast cancer was the main driver for developing several new SERMs of the triphenylethylene family as toremifene (chlorotamoxifen), droloxifene (3-hydroxy-tamoxifen), idoxifene (4-iodo-pirrolidine-tamoxifen), ospemifene, fispemifene, miproxifene (TAT-59), and GW5638 (Fig. 2.1). Clomiphene, which may be considered the first SERM for clinical use, is also a triphenylethylene derivative, but it has been used since 1967 exclusively for ovulation induction, and no investigation for its clinical use in postmenopausal women has been carried out. Of all these drugs, only toremifene has been commercialized for the treatment of disseminated breast cancer, and from a clinical point of view it has not shown any advantage over tamoxifen in the benefit/risk ratio (Buzdar et al. 1998). In fact, although both drugs lead to similar significant reductions in serum lipids, their effects on bone mineral density in postmenopausal women are different.

In a head-to-head trial, tamoxifen showed a more potent effect in the preservation of bone mass than toremifene, with the latter causing a small but significant reduction in bone mineral density (Marttunen et al. 1999). On the other hand, as toremifene is not susceptible to α-oxidation by the P_{450} enzymatic system, it has not been shown to lead to hepatocarcinogenesis in rodent preclinical models, unlike tamoxifen. Unfortunately, both compounds present an estrogen-agonist action in the endometrium. This has been well demonstrated both in animal models (O'Regan et al. 1998) and in clinical experience, where the risk of developing premalignant and malignant endometrial lesions increases significantly by two to seven times with both drugs (Shapiro et al. 2001). In fact, long-term uterine safety is one of the key aspects that have to be closely monitored during clinical trials in humans. Thus, the clinical development of idoxifene, miproxifene, and droloxifene (compounds of the triphenylethylene

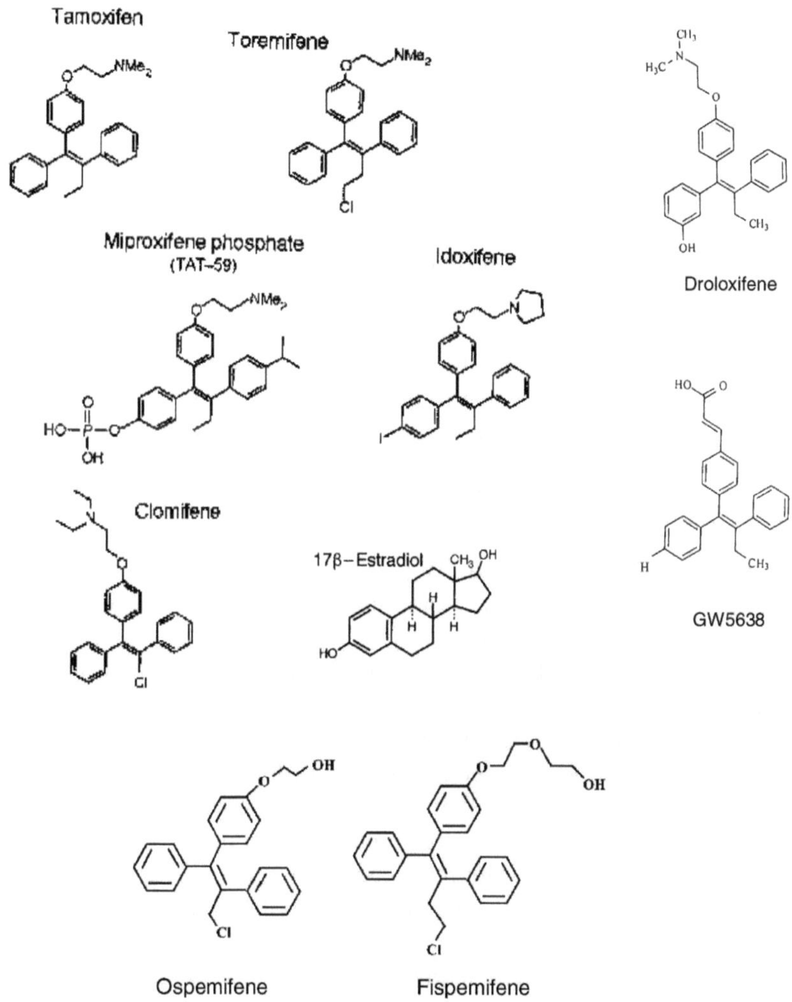

Fig. 2.1. Chemical structure of several SERMs in triphenylethylene group. The estradiol molecule is also included as a comparative reference

family that were in Phase II–III clinical trials for the treatment of breast cancer and postmenopausal osteoporosis) has been recently cancelled due to uterine safety issues. The unexpected adverse events found in the clinical studies in humans suggest that preclinical toxicological studies, mainly in rodents, may not necessarily predict the endometrial response to certain types of SERMs in women. Thus, although idoxifene had shown a potent activity in breast cancer cell lines that were resistant to tamoxifen, and in preclinical models had not shown estrogen-agonist activity in the endometrium (Nuttall et al. 1998; Gutman et al. 2002), it was associated with a dose-dependent increase in endometrial thickness, evaluated by transvaginal ultrasound after only 12 weeks of treatment in postmenopausal women. Furthermore, idoxifene was associated with an increased incidence of uterine prolapse (Hendrix et al. 2001), and this unexpected effect was unsuitable to evaluate in traditional preclinical models. Uterine prolapse has been a relatively frequent finding with other SERMs, as will be discused later.

Droloxifene (3-hydroxy-tamoxifen) behaves as an estrogen agonist in bone tissue and several lipid and coagulation markers in castrated rat models and does not show stimulation of the endometrial epithelium in preclinical studies (Ke et al. 1997). Endometrial stimulation has, however, been observed in clinical trials, which, together with the fact that as an estrogen agonist it is ten times less potent than tamoxifen in bone tissue and lipid metabolism (Hendrix et al. 2001) and that in a recent head-to-head comparison with tamoxifen droloxifene was demonstrated not to be superior in any parameter of breast cancer treatment efficacy (Buzdar et al. 2002), has resulted in cancellation of its clinical development.

Miproxifene (TAT-59) is a prodrug of 4-hydroxy-tamoxifen that has been developed for tamoxifen-resistant carcinoma, but relatively little information has been published on this drug. Compared with tamoxifen, miproxifene inhibits estradiol-stimulated proliferation of MCF-7 cells at a threefold lower dose than that of tamoxifen, and of dimethyl-benzanthracene (DMBA)-induced rat mammary tumors at a dose tenfold lower than tamoxifen (Toko et al. 1990). In any event, in preclinical castrated rat models, it shows an endometrial stimulation activity that is similar to that of tamoxifen, which means it has limited potential use in the prevention or treatment of osteoporosis or cardiovascular disease (Shibata et al. 2000). Similarly, considering the preclinical findings of endometrial stimulation reported on GW5638 (Willson et al. 1997), it is likely that this new SERM belonging to the triphenylethylene family will be limited in clinical use to the treatment of advanced tamoxifen-resistant breast cancer once its efficacy is demonstrated in human clinical trials.

More encouraging are the preliminary results of ospemifene (FC-1271a), a biologically active metabolite of toremifene (deamino-hydroxy-toremifene), which has shown a promising SERM-type pharmacological profile by preventing bone mass and bone strength loss in castrated rats and reducing cholesterol levels, without uterine wet weight gain (Qu et al. 2000). Also, it performs as a potent estrogen antagonist in ER-positive breast cancer cell lines (Taras et al. 2001), and it is now in Phase III clinical trials for the prevention and treatment of postmenopausal osteoporosis and urogenital atrophy (Gennari 2004). In Phase II trials, ospemifene had, unlike raloxifene, an estrogenic agonistic activity on the vaginal epithelium by improving symptoms of vaginal dryness (Rutanen et al. 2003). The compound also appeared to be neutral in its effects on climateric symptoms, including hot flashes and insomnia. Long-term studies will be needed to confirm the neutral effect of ospemifene on the uterus and its impact in the prevention of bone loss and osteoporotic fractures in postmenopausal women.

Fispemifene is a new triphenylethylene, closely related to ospemifene, currently going to Phase II clinical trials. It has antagonistic activity in breast tissue and acts as an estrogen agonist in bone and the vascular tissue repair response through the regulation of vascular smooth muscle cell function and reendothelialization, in a way that is very similar to that of tamoxifen, raloxifene, and ospemifene (Savolainen-Peltonen et al. 2004).

Finally, MDL 103,323 is a new SERM derived from clomiphene, originally developed as an antitumor drug for breast cancer, due to its potent inhibitor activity of breast cancer cell lines and its high affinity for ER (5–6 times higher than tamoxifen) (Baumann et al. 1998). Subsequent preclinical studies in hypogonadal osteoporosis models have demonstrated that MDL 103,323 reduces bone turnover markers and increases bone mineral density and bone biomechanical properties in castrated rats and sheep (Chavassieux et al. 2001; Bourrin et al. 2002). There are few results on its effect on lipid metabolism, showing less efficacy than other SERMs in reducing high cholesterol levels induced by ovariectomy and with no modification in triglyceride levels (Ammann et al. 1999). Similarly, there are very little data published on its uterine effects. Published data are limited to the evaluation of uterine wet weight, a subrogate parameter of endometrial stimulation, with only partial predictive value in postmenopausal women.

2.3.2 Benzothiophenes

The second group of SERMs includes drugs such as raloxifene (previously named keoxifene), arzoxifene (Fig. 2.2), and LY-117018. Raloxifene was initially designed as a drug to treat breast cancer, but its clinical development was later focused on prevention and treatment of postmenopausal osteoporosis,

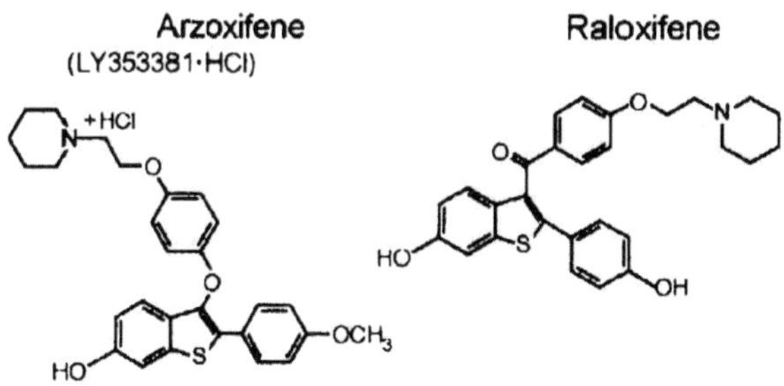

Fig. 2.2. Chemical structure of several SERMs in benzothiophene group

becoming the first SERM approved to prevent and treat this bone metabolic disorder. Raloxifene is also being investigated for the primary and secondary prevention of cardiovascular disease in postmenopausal women (Wenger et al. 2002) and in breast cancer prevention in high-risk women (Vogel et al. 2002). After tamoxifen, raloxifene is the SERM with the most information available on its pharmacological effects in postmenopausal women because of the size of its clinical program (over 40,000 women included in Phase III trials) and because of the fact that since its commercialization in 1998 it is estimated that approximately 2 million patients/year have been treated with the drug. Initial research on experimental osteoporosis models in castrated rats demonstrated raloxifene induces a bone antiresorptive effect similar to estrogens but without inducing endometrial proliferation (Black et al. 1994). In the same animal model, it has an effect on lipid metabolism very similar to estrogens (Black et al. 1994; Frolik et al. 1996). Furthermore, *in vivo* and *in vitro* studies on ER-positive breast cancer have shown raloxifene inhibits growth and tumor proliferation (Anzano et al. 1996), observations that have been confirmed in ER-positive breast cancer patients applying immunohistochemical markers of cell proliferation (Dowsett et al. 2001).

Clinical trials on postmenopausal women with osteoporosis have demonstrated that raloxifene reduces bone turnover markers by 25–35% after 1 year of treatment and reduces the relative risk of the occurrence of new vertebral fractures by 30–50% after 3 years of treatment (Ettinger et al. 1999). A *post hoc* analysis in women at high risk for cardiovascular diseases also showed a reduction of 40% in the rate of new cardiovascular events (Barrett-Connor et al. 2002), with no observed reduction in the overall study population after 4 years of treatment in the MORE trial.

The rate of invasive ER-positive breast cancer, a secondary objective in the MORE trial, showed an 84% reduction after 4 years of followup (Cauley et al. 2001); moreover, during the subsequent 4 years of followup in the so-called CORE trial (Continuous Outcomes Relevant to Evista), invasive ER-positive breast cancer, the primary objective of the study, was reduced by 66%. Over the 8 years of both trials, the incidences of invasive breast cancer and ER-positive invasive breast cancer were reduced by 66% and 76%, respectively, in the raloxifene group compared with the placebo group (Martino et al. 2004). These effects have not been associated with harmful effects on the endometrium (Cohen et al. 2000) or the pelvic floor (Goldstein et al. 2001).

Other drugs in this group are arzoxifene (LY353381-HCl), a potent benzothiophene similar to raloxifene that has demonstrated an antagonist potency 10 times greater that raloxifene in MCF-7 breast cancer and endometrial cancer cell lines (Sato et al. 1998). It is currently under research for treatment and prevention of postmenopausal osteoporosis given its favorable effects on cholesterol lowering, bone mineral density, and uterine weight in ovariectomized rats (Ma et al. 2002). LY-117018 has shown similar skeletal effects to raloxifene in osteoporotic experimental models (Li et al. 1998; Díaz Curiel et al. 1998). Phase II trials with different doses of arzoxifene in tamoxifen-sensitive and tamoxifen-resistant women with advanced or metastatic breast cancer showed positive results with reductions on the time to progression of disease (Buzdar et al. 2003) and response rates (Baselga et al. 2003).

2.3.3 Naphthalenes

The principal representative of this group of SERMs is lasofoxifene (CP-336,156) (Fig. 2.3), which is currently at Phase III of clinical research for the prevention and treatment of osteoporosis in postmenopausal women. Lasofoxifene shows excellent SERM-type properties in *in vivo* animal models, showing a binding affinity to ERα similar to estradiol, and approximately 10 times higher than other SERMs, including tamoxifen, raloxifene, and droloxifene (Ke et al. 1998). In ovariectomized rats treated with several doses of lasofoxifene for 52 weeks, there was no observation of stimulation of the endometrial epithelium, although a slight, but significant, increase in uterine weight was detected. It also was observed that bone mineral density loss and ultimate bone strength associated with ovariectomy was prevented at the lumbar spine level (Ke et al. 2004). Previous shorter studies had shown that in ovariectomized rats, lasofoxifene reduced serum cholesterol levels and fat body mass (Ke at al. 1998). Bone marrow cell cultures suggest that this bone effect may be mediated by a 15–25% increase in the number of apoptotic osteoclasts. Unlike other SERMs, lasofoxifene also has been studied in aging and orchidectomized male rat models. It has been shown that this drug prevents bone mass loss and reduction of bone biomechanical properties in these rats, which may be indicative of its potential role in the treatment of male osteoporosis secondary to hypogonadism or simply associated with old age (Ke et al. 2000, 2001).

Recently, 1-year Phase II results in postmenopausal women have been reported. Lasofoxifene significantly decreased LDL-cholesterol and biochemical

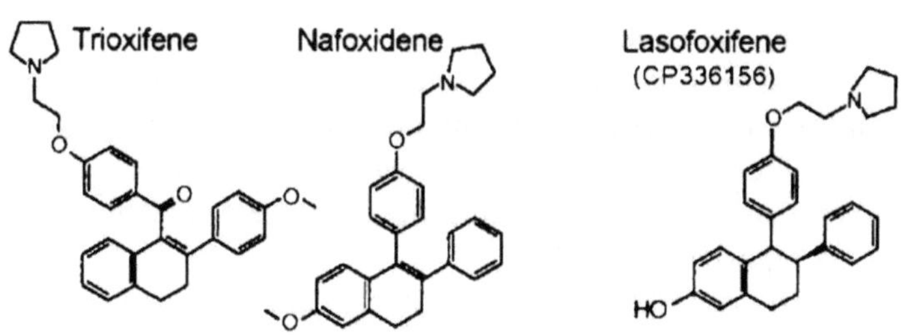

Fig. 2.3. Chemical structure of several SERMs in naphthylene group

markers of bone turnover and significantly increased lumbar spine bone mineral density in early postmenopausal women, with no adverse effects on the reproductive tract and no clinically meaningful effect on the endometrium (Moffett et al. 2004). Head-to-head studies versus raloxifene have also been reported (McClung et al. 2004a,b). After 2 years of therapy, lasofoxifene 0.25 mg and 1 mg/day was associated with greater reductions in biochemical markers of bone turnover, fibrinogen, Lp(a), and LDL-cholesterol than raloxifene 60 mg/day. Lumbar spine BMD, but not hip BMD, was higher with lasofoxifene therapy. The safety profile was relatively similar with the two SERMs having statistically significant differences versus placebo in the incidence of hot flashes and leg cramps and a significant increase in leukorrhea in the lasofoxifene arms (7%–11% versus 2% with raloxifene and 4% with placebo). No endometrial safety data were included in this preliminary report (McClung et al. 2004b).

Trioxifene is an older SERM with low estrogenic properties and a higher affinity for ER than tamoxifen. It has shown an unfavorable safety profile in clinical studies of women with breast cancer (leukopenia in 41% of patients, nausea in 31%) (Witte et al. 1986), which is why, in addition to its response rates being no better than in tamoxifen (Lee et al. 1986), its clinical development has been cancelled.

2.3.4 Indoles

The two principal representatives of this group of SERMs are pipendoxifene (ERA-923) and bazedoxifene (TSE-424, WAY-140424) (Fig. 2.4). Pipendoxifene is a potent SERM that is currently undergoing Phase II trials in women with hormone-dependent metastatic breast cancer (Sorbera et al. 2002). In preclinical studies, pipendoxifene inhibits estrogen-stimulated growth of the cell line MCF-7, at a similar rate to tamoxifen, but, unlike the latter, it also inhibits proliferation of endometrial and ovarian cancer cell lines. The most interesting aspect of pipendoxifene is that it has been shown to inhibit growth of breast cancer tumor lines that are resistant to tamoxifen, without stimulating the endometrium (Greenberger et al. 2001). Phase I trials on 50 healthy female volunteers treated for a 28-day period have not demonstrated significant effects on different bone turnover markers, on total cholesterol, HDL-cholesterol, or LDL-cholesterol, or on triglycerides (Cotreau et al. 2002); thus, its long-term effects on bone and cardiovascular disease are uncertain. About 20% of the study subjects reported hot flashes.

In addition to lasofoxifene and arzoxifene, bazedoxifene (TSE-424, WAY-140424) is one of the newer SERMs in advanced Phase III clinical development for the prevention and treatment of postmenopausal osteoporosis. In pre-

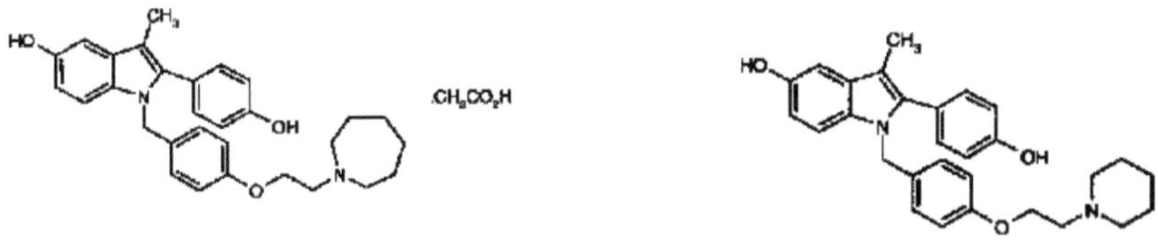

Bazedoxifene
TSE-424
WAY-140424

Pipendoxifene
ERA-923

Fig. 2.4. Chemical structure of several SERMs in indole group

clinical models, bazedoxifene has shown to fulfill the profile of a SERM: it binds with high and similar affinity to ERα and ERβ, inhibits proliferation of MCF-7 cells induced by estradiol, prevents bone mass loss in castrated rats, reduces serum cholesterol, and does not have a stimulant effect on the uterine epithelium of intact and ovariectomized rats (Miller et al. 2001). The selection of bazedoxifene in the molecular screening process to improve the SERM profile has incorporated new preclinical animal experiments especially designed to evaluate its potential secondary effects on the uterus, with the objective of avoiding problems previously encountered in the clinical development of other SERMs. Thus, bazedoxifene has not shown any agonist activity on *in vitro* models in an experiment to test the transcriptional activation of the promoter of the component of complement 3 (C3), which is a gene that requires estrogen stimulation to be expressed in the endometrial cells of rodents and has proven to be fairly reliable as a predictor of the *in vivo* endometrial response. In this model, other SERMs such as tamoxifen, idoxifene, and droloxifene do act as agonists of the C3 promoter (tamoxifen > idoxifene > droloxifene), while raloxifene stimulates it to a minimal extent (Komm et al. 2001).

Other interesting aspects that have been included in the bazedoxifene preclinical program is the evaluation of the vasomotor response in an experimental model of hot flashes, consisting of intact adult rats addicted to morphine, which develop a very marked vasomotor response when they receive a naloxone injection. This response, observed through a temperature increase of 4–5 °C in the rat's tail, may be inhibited if the animal has been treated with estrogens. However, bazedoxifene and raloxifene do not act as estrogen agonist in this model (Komm et al. 2001). The antagonist effect of bazedoxifene and raloxifene on estrogen effects, in the prevention of vasomotor crises, occurs at a dose of $\geq$ 1.0 mg/kg. Considering that the necessary dose of bazedoxifene to protect bone is 0.3 mg/kg, it appears that there is a certain therapeutic "window" to prevent the vasomotor response in these rats, and this would not be observed with raloxifene, which requires a dose of 3 mg/kg to produce beneficial effects on the bone in the castrated rat model. Published clinical data on this compound are limited. After 3 months therapy in 494 postmenopausal women, bazedoxifene (doses as low as 5 mg/d) had effects on bone turnover markers and LDL-cholesterol comparable to those seen with raloxifene. No increases in hot flashes or endometrial thickness were reported (Ronkin et al. 2001; Komm et al. 2001).

2.3.5 Benzopyrans

The SERMs that belong to the benzopyrans group form a large group of drugs (Fig. 2.5), several of which are at early stages of clinical development for the treatment of hormone-dependent breast cancer and endometrial cancer.

Ormeloxifene (centchroman) has been used since 1980 as an oral contraceptive in India using a weekly dose (Singh 2001), while its L-enantiomer (levormeloxifene) recently had its clinical program cancelled in the prevention and treatment of postmenopausal osteoporosis following the detection of uterine safety problems during Phase III clinical trials. This is probably the chemical group of SERMs that is undergoing more activity in the development of new target molecules. There has been a recent report on results in experimental models of postmenopausal osteoporosis using SP-500263 (Sutherland et al. 2003) in which has been shown a profile similar to raloxifene in the same model, also acting as an antiestrogen in *in vitro* breast cancer models.

EM-800 (SCH-57050) and its active metabolite EM-652 (acolbifene, SCH-57068), are highly potent antiestrogens in human breast and uterine cancer cells *in vitro* as well as *in vivo* in nude mice and are currently undergoing clinical trials in the treatment of hormone-dependent breast cancer and endometrial cancer (Labrie et al 1999). Acolbifene shows a higher capacity of binding to

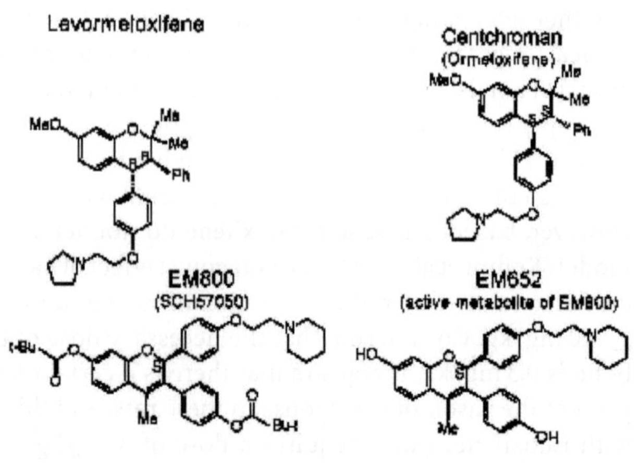

Fig. 2.5. Chemical structure of several SERMs in benzopyrans group

the estrogenic receptor than the majority of pure estrogens and SERMs, and, in fact, its affinity for ERs is 2.9 times higher than estradiol itself. It shows a 200-fold greater potency than tamoxifen in displacing [^{3}H]estradiol from ERs. In *in vitro* preclinical models on hormone-dependent breast tumors (cell lines ZR-75-1, MCF-7, and T-47D), endometrial adenocarcinoma cell lines, and also in *in vivo* tumor models (breast cancer induced by DBMA, xenografts of human breast cancer in athymic mice), acolbifene and EM-800 have been shown to inhibit tumor growth to a greater extent than pure antiestrogens such as fulvestrant (ICI 182,780) and ICI 164,384, and than 4-hydroxy-tamoxifen, toremifene, idoxifene, GW5638, droloxifene, and raloxifene (Labrie et al. 1999; Gutman et al. 2002).

Both EM-800 and acolbifene have been studied in the ovariectomized rat model, and their initial pharmacological profile (described as pure antiestrogens) has been ruled out because they also prevent bone mass loss and reduce cholesterol and triglycerides in a similar magnitude to raloxifene (Labrie et al. 1999). In a recent Phase II clinical trial in 42 patients with advanced-stage, tamoxifen-resistant breast carcinoma, EM-800 produced responses in a significant proportion of patients, results that previously had not been achieved with other SERMs, such as toremifene or raloxifene, when used as salvage therapy in tamoxifen-resistant patients (Labrie et al. 2004). The response observed was similar to fulvestrant, a pure antiestrogen, but, given the possible advantages of EM-800 and acolbifene regarding its oral bioavailability and its protective effect on bone loss, they can be considered potential alternatives once their efficacy and safety are confirmed in larger trials.

The preclinical and clinical development of levormeloxifene, a benzopyran SERM, and its final outcome present a paradigmatic experience in SERM pharmacological development because, for the first time, the data that indicated a SERM profile in animal studies were not confirmed in clinical research when the drug was subjected to Phase II–III clinical trial conditions. Thus, although levormeloxifene did not induce proliferation of the endometrial epithelium in castrated rats, postmenopausal women treated with this drug showed an increased endometrial thickness (approximately 6 mm versus placebo) after 1 year of treatment. Biopsies did not show any cellular proliferative findings (Alexandersen et al. 2001). These negative results were balanced with positive outcomes at the bone, with lumbar spine bone mineral density increases of 2.9% versus placebo, and in the lipid metabolism with 15% and 25% decreases in serum cholesterol and LDL-cholesterol in the levormeloxifene group (Alexandersen et al. 2001), respectively.

The second study, which included 2924 postmenopausal women with osteoporosis, had to be cancelled after 10 months due to a marked increase in adverse uterine effects induced by the two doses of levormeloxifene under study in comparison with the placebo arm: leukorrhea (30% versus 3%), increased endometrial thickness (19% versus 1%), increased uterine volume (17% versus 3%), uterovaginal prolapse (7% versus 2%), urinary incontinence (17% versus 4%), increased micturition frequency (9% versus 4%), and pelvic pain (17% versus 6%) (Goldstein et al. 2002). Similar findings were observed in clinical trials with idoxifene in which 1.5% of the women treated with this drug developed a uterine prolapse versus none in the placebo group (Hendrix et al. 2001). The mechanism behind these SERM-caused uterine effects is not clear, although there are several hypotheses that suggest greater elasticity of pelvic floor tissues secondary to collagen alterations, edema, or an increased uterine weight. A very recent report suggests that differences in the expression of matrix metalloproteinase 2 (MMP2) activity induced by estrogen and different SERMs in the uterus of ovariectomized rats may be relevant to collagen turnover and degradation and, hence, uterine prolapse and urinary incontinence. While estrogen, lasofoxifene, and levormeloxifene increased MMP2 activity in this model, which may result in increased proteolytic cleavage of type I and IV collagen, raloxifene did not (Helvering et al. 2004).

As a result of these findings, a scheduled standard pelvic exploration is now an obligatory procedure in clinical trials with new SERMs. It is important to note that this adverse effect has not been associated with tamoxifen or toremifene therapy (Maenpaa et al. 1997; Fisher et al. 1998), and in the case of raloxifene, a post hoc metaanalysis of 6926 nonhysterectomized postmenopausal women participating in clinical trials for 3 years or more showed a significant 50% reduction in the incidence of surgery for repairing pelvic floor relaxation, reported as an adverse event, compared with placebo (Goldstein et al. 2001).

2.4 Conclusions

The main pharmacodynamic characteristics of the SERMs that are currently available reflect their antineoplastic activity in estrogen-dependent breast cancer (tamoxifen and toremifene) and the beneficial effects on bone remodeling, bone mineral density, and reduction of osteoporotic fractures in postmenopausal women observed with raloxifene. However, one major consequence of the Women's Health Initiative findings has been an increased interest in the full therapeutic potential of SERMs – still to be explored – because of their potential to retain some of the beneficial effects of estrogen while avoiding most of its adverse effects. Given the extraordinary complexity of the different diseases that SERMs can impact, this exploration is contemplated as a major, long-term, costly task. In this respect, clinical trials that are close to being finalized with raloxifene will clarify within the next few years the potential role of this SERM in primary prevention of breast cancer and cardiovascular disease in postmenopausal women. Likewise, the encouraging preliminary results on new SERMs such as lasofoxifene, bazedoxifene, arzoxifene, ospemifene, etc. are still to be confirmed in large-scale clinical trials currently under way.

With regard to our current knowledge of these drugs, it is tempting to speculate on the ideal pharmacological characteristics of a selective estrogen receptor modulator (Fig. 2.6). Obviously, any new SERM that is intended for the treatment of breast cancer must, at a minimum, exceed tamoxifen's efficacy regarding its rates of tumor remission and relapse, without having negative effects on uterine safety in terms of hyperplasia and endometrial neoplasia or uterine prolapse. Ideally, these new SERMs must be effective against tamoxifen-resistant breast cancer, and preliminary results with some of them are encouraging (Labrie et al. 2004), although a likely shift in the gold standard endocrine therapy of hormone-responsive breast cancer is on the horizon with the introduction of aromatase inhibitors (Smith et al. 2003). New SERMs that are planned to be developed for the prevention and treatment of osteoporosis and cardiovascular disease in postmenopausal women, in addition to showing

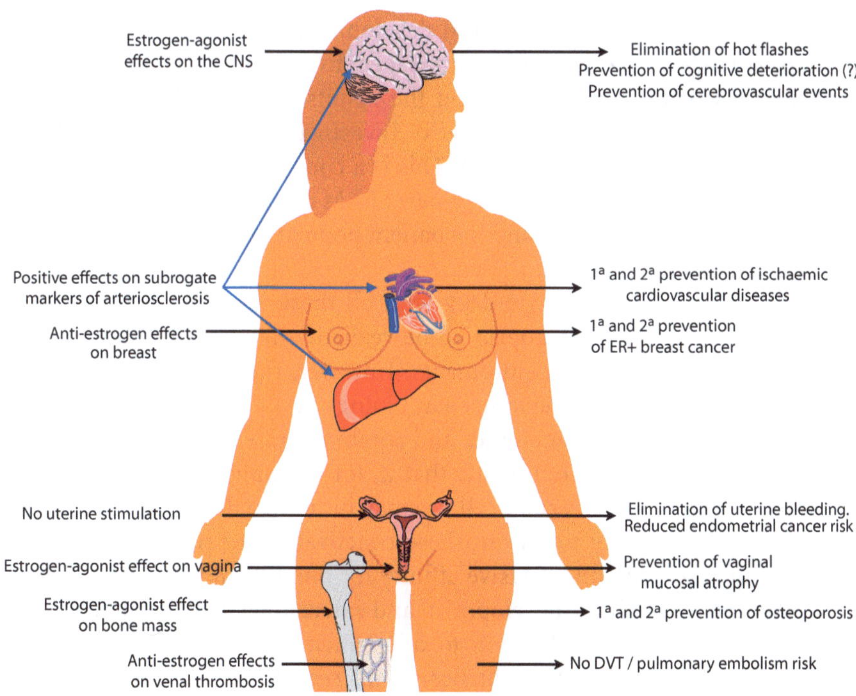

Fig. 2.6. Illustration of pharmacological characteristics of a SERM with an ideal pharmacological profile

a nonstimulant effect on the uterus and on the development of breast neoplasms, must ideally present a profile of neutral side effects with regard to the onset of hot flashes or venous thromboembolic disease, which are the principal side effects of raloxifene and tamoxifen.

It is important to note that the reported increased risk, by a factor of 1.5 to 3, observed in venous thromboembolic disease with SERMs in wide use, namely tamoxifen and raloxifene, is very similar to that reported with the use of ET/EPT and oral contraceptives. Although the in-depth molecular mechanism of this procoagulatory activity in the venous territory is as yet unknown, it would appear that it is an estrogen-agonist effect in the SERMs that should be minimized or eliminated in the development of new molecules indicated for long-term use. Considering the present uncertainty regarding the role of ET/EPT in the prevention and treatment of senile dementia, it would be risky to suggest that SERMs may play a beneficial role in this pathology, but what is considered a must is that in no way can they become harmful. Therefore, it is necessary to carry out meticulous evaluations in preclinical models and during clinical trials of the effects of these drugs on higher cognitive functions. In this respect, clinical findings with raloxifene are encouraging (Yaffe et al. 2001; Neele et al. 2001).

Finally, a major question in SERM development is whether the new compounds will behave like estrogens with respect to cardiovascular events, which would be a worthless property given the results of the WHI trial (Writing Group for the Women's Health Initiative Investigators 2002; Women's Health Initiative Steering Committee 2004). This is a complex issue that will depend on the unique profile of action of the new SERM on the different components of the atherosclerosis process and the patient population and study design and conduct that is implemented.

Is it feasible to find a single drug with all these ideal characteristics? In the short term it does not appear to be realistic that one SERM alone will be able to fulfill all these requirements. However, the great speed at which progress is being made in the molecular biology of the ER activation cascade, together with progress in genomics and combinatorial and proteomic chemistry, there is room to be optimistic that if, for example, we can identify the coactivator proteins of a certain cell, we may be able to design ligands to ERs with a selective activity to recruit these coactivators, or we may be able to design molecules with an exclusive affinity for one ER subtype. All these advances will also benefit the development and extension of the pharmacological concept of executable modulation to other members of the nuclear receptor superfamily, like selective glucocorticoid receptor modulators, selective androgen receptor modulators, selective progesterone receptor modulators, and selective peroxisome proliferator-activated receptor modulators, among others.

References

1. Alexandersen P, Riis BJ, Stakkestad JA, Delmas PD, Christiansen C (2001) Efficacy of levormeloxifene in the prevention of postmenopausal bone loss and on the lipid profile compared to low dose hormone replacement therapy. J Clin Endocrinol Metab 86:755–760
2. Ammann P, Bourrin S, Bonjour J-P, Brunner F, Meyer J-M, Rizzoli R (1999) The new selective estrogen receptor modulator MDL 103, 323 increases bone mineral density and bone strength in adult ovariectomized rats. Osteoporos Int 10:369–376
3. Anzano MA, Peer CW, Smith JM, Mullen LT, Shrader MW, Logsdon DL, et al. (1996) Chemoprevention of mammary carcinogenesis in the rat: combined use of raloxifene and 9-cis-retinoic acid. J Natl Cancer Inst 88:23–25
4. Barrett-Connor E, Grady D, Sashegyi A, Anderson PW, Cox DA, Hoszowski K, et al. (2002) Raloxifene and cardiovascular events in osteoporotic postmenopausal women: Four-year results from the MORE (Multiple Outcomes of Raloxifene Evaluation) randomized trial. J Am Med Assoc 287:847–857
5. Baselga J, Llombart-Cussac A, Bellet M, Guillem-Porta V, Enas N, Krejcy K, et al. (2003) Ann Oncol 14:1383–1390
6. Baumann RJ, Bush TL, Cross-Doersen DE, Cashman EA, Wright PS, Zwolshen JH, et al. (1998) Clomiphene analogs with activity in vitro and in vivo against human breast cancer cells. Biochem Pharmacol 55:841–851
7. Black LJ, Sato M, Rowley ER, Magee DE, Bekele A, Williams DC, et al. (1994) Raloxifene (LY139481 HCl) prevents bone loss and reduces serum cholesterol without causing uterine hypertrophy in ovariectomized rats. J Clin Invest 93:63–69
8. Bourrin S, Ammann P, Bonjour J-P, Rizzoli R (2002) Recovery of proximal tibia bone mineral density and strength but not cancellous bone architecture, after long-term bisphosphonate or selective estrogen receptor modulator in aged rats. Bone 30:195–200
9. Buzdar AU, Hortobagyi GN (1998) Tamoxifen and toremifene in breast cancer: comparison of safety and efficacy. J Clin Oncol 26:348–353
10. Buzdar A, Hayes D, El Khoudary A, Yan S, Lonning P, Lichinitser M, et al. (2002) Phase III randomized trial of droloxifene and tamoxifen as first-line endocrine treatment of ER/Pg-positive advanced breast cancer. Breast Cancer Res Treat 73:161–175
11. Buzdar A, O'Shaughnessy JA, Booser DJ, Pippen JE Jr, Jones SE, Munster PN, et al. (2003) Phase II, randomized, double-blind study of two dose levels of arzoxifene in patients with locally advanced or metastatic breast cancer. J Clin Oncol 21:1007–1014
12. Cauley JA, Norton L, Lippman ME, Eckert S, Krueger KA, Purdie DW, et al. (2001) Continued breast cancer risk reduction in postmenopausal women treated with Raloxifene: 4-year results from the MORE trial. Breast Cancer Res Treat 65:125–134
13. Chavassieux P, Garnero P, Duboeuf F, Vergnaud P, Brunner-Ferber F, Delmas PD, et al (2001) Effects of a new selective estrogen receptor modulator (MDL 103,323) on cancellous and cortical bone in ovariectomized ewes: a biochemical, histomorphometric, and densitometric study. J Bone Miner Res 16: 89–96
14. Cohen FJ, Watts S, Shah A, Akers R, Plouffe L Jr (2000) Uterine effects of 3-year raloxifene therapy in postmenopausal women younger than age 60. Obstet Gynecol 95:104–110
15. Cotreau MM, Stonis L, Dykstra KH, Gandhi T, Gutiérrez M, Xu J, et al. (2002) Multiple-dose, safety, pharmacokinetics and pharmacodynamics of a new selective estrogen

receptor modulator, ERA-923, in healthy postmenopausal women. J Clin Pharmacol 42:157–165
16. Díaz Curiel M, Calero JA, Guerrero R, Gala J, Gazapo R, de la Piedra C (1998) Effects of LY-117018 HCl on bone remodeling and mineral density in the oophorectomized rat. Am J Obstet Gynecol 178:320–325
17. Dowsett M, Bundred NJ, Decensi A, Sainsbury RC, Lu Y, Hills MJ, et al. (2001) Effect of raloxifene on breast cancer cell Ki67 and apoptosis: a double-blind, lacebo-controlled, randomized clinical trial in postmenopausal patients. Can Epidemiol Biomar Prev 10:961–966
18. Ettinger B, Black DM, Mitlak BH, Knickerbocker RK, Nickelsen T, Genant HK (1999) Reduction of vertebral fracture risk in postmenopausal women with osteoporosis treated with raloxifene. Results from a 3-year randomized clinical trial. J Am Med Assoc 282:637–645. Corrections published in J Am Med Assoc 282:2124
19. Fisher B, Costantino JP, Wickerham DL, Redmond CK, Kavanah M, Cronin, et al. (1998) Tamoxifen for prevention of breast cancer: Report of the National Surgical Adjuvant Breast and Bowel Project P-1 Study. J Natl Cancer Inst 90:1371–1388
20. Frolik CA, Bryant HU, Black EC, Magee DE, Chandrasekhar S (1996) Time dependent changes in biochemical bone markers and serum cholesterol in ovariectomized rats: effects of raloxifene HCl, tamoxifen, estrogen and alendronate. Bone 18:621–627
21. Gennari L (2004) Ospemifene. Curr Opin Invest Drugs 5:448–455
22. Goldstein SR, Nanavati N (2002) Adverse events that are associated with the selective estrogen receptor modulator levormeloxifene in an aborted phase III osteoporosis treatment study. Am J Obstet Gynecol 187:521–527
23. Goldstein SR, Neven P, Zhou L, Taylot YL, Ciaccia AV, Plouffle L (2001) Raloxifene effect on frequency of surgery for pelvic floor relaxation. Obstet Gynecol 98:91–96
24. Greenbeger LM, Annable T, Collins KI, Komm BS, Lyttle CR, Miller CP, et al. (2001) A new antiestrogen, 2-(4-hydroxy-phenyl)-3-methyl-1-[4-(2-piperidin-1-yl-ethoxy)-benzyl]-1H-indol-5-ol hydroclorhide (ERA-923), inhibits the growth of tamoxifen-sensitive and -resistant tumors and is devoid of uterotropic effects in mice and rats. Clin Cancer Res 7:3166–3177
25. Gutman M, Couillard S, Roy J, Labrie F, Candas B, Labrie C (2002) Comparison of the effects of EM-652 (SCH570068), tamoxifen, toremifene, droloxifene, idoxifene, GW-5638 and raloxifene on the growth of human ZR-75–1 breast cancer in nude. Int J Cancer 99:273–278
26. Hendrix SL, McNeeley SG (2001) Effect of selective estrogen receptor modulators on reproductive tissues other than endometrium. Ann NY Acad Sci 949:243–250
27. Helvering LM, Adrian MD, Geiser AG, Estrem ST, Wei T, Huang S, et al. (2004) Differential effects of estrogen and raloxifene on mRNA and matrix metalloproteinase 2 (MMP2) activity in the rat uterus. Biol Reprod [Epub ahead of print]. DOI:10.1095/biolreprod.104.034595
28. Hulley S, Grady D, Bush T, Furberg C, Herrington D, Riggs B, et al. (1998) Randomized trial of estrogen plus progestin for secondary prevention of coronary heart disease in postmenopausal women. J Am Med Assoc 280:605–613
29. Jordan VC, Morrow M (1999) Tamoxifen, raloxifene, and the prevention of breast cancer. Endocr Rev 20:253–78
30. Ke HZ, Chen HK, Simmons HA, Crawford DT, Pirie CM, Chidsey-Frink KL et al. (1997) Comparative effects of droloxifene, tamoxifen, and estrogen on bone, serum cholesterol, and uterine histology in the ovariectomized rat model. Bone 20:31–39

31. Ke HZ, Paralkar VM, Grasser WA, Crawford DT, Qi H, Simmons H, et al. (1998) Effects of CP-336,156, a new, nonsteroidal estrogen agonist/antagonist, on bone, serum cholesterol, uterus, and body composition in rat models. Endocrinology 139:2068–2076
32. Ke HZ, Qi H, Chidsey-Frink KL, Crawford DT, Thompson DD (2001) Lasofoxifene (CP-336,156) protects against the age-related changes in bone mass, bone strength, and total serum cholesterol in intact aged male rats. J Bone Miner Res 16:765–773
33. Ke HZ, Qi H, Crawford DT, Chidsey-Frink KL, Simmons HA, Thompson DD (2000) Lasofoxifene (CP-336,156), a selective estrogen receptor modulator, prevents bone loss induced by aging and orchidectomy in the adult rat. Endocrinology 141:1338–1344
34. Ke HZ, Foley GL, Simmons HA, Shen V, Thompson DD (2004) Long-term treatment of lasofoxifene preserves bone mass and bone strength and does not adversely affect the uterus in ovariectomized rats. Endocrinology 145:1996–2005
35. Komm BS, Lyttle CR (2001) Developing SERM: stringent preclinical selection criteria leading to an acceptable candidate (WAY-140424) for clinical evaluation. Ann NY Acad Sci 949:317–326
36. Labrie F, Labrie C, Bélanger A, Simard J, Gauthier S, Luu-The V, et al. (1999) EM-652 (SCH 57068), a third generation SERM acting as pure antiestrogen in the mammary gland and the endometrium. J Steroid Biochem Mol Biol 69:51–84
37. Labrie F, Champagne P, Labrie C, Roy J, Laverdière J, Provencher L, et al. (2004) Activity and safety of the antiestrogen EM-800, the orally active precursor of acolbifene, in tamoxifen-resistant breast cancer. J Clin Oncol 22:864–871
38. Lee RW, Buzdar AU, Blumenschein GR, Hortobagyi GN (1986) Trioxifene mesylate in the treatment of advanced breast cancer. Cancer 57:40–43
39. Li X, Takahashi M, Kushida K, Inoue T (1998) The preventive and interventional effects of raloxifene analog (LY117018 HCl) on osteopenia in ovariectomized rats. J Bone Miner Res 13:1005–1010
40. Love RR, Mazess RB, Barden HS, Epstein S, Newcomb PA, Jordan VC, et al. (1992) Effects of tamoxifen on bone mineral density in postmenopausal women with breast cancer. N Engl J Med 326:852–856
41. Ma YL, Bryant HU, Zeng Q, Palkowitz A, Jee WSS, Turner CH, et al. (2002) Long-term dosing of arzoxifene lowers cholesterol, reduces bone turnover, and preserves bone quality in ovariectomized rats. J Bone Miner Res 17:2256–2264
42. Maenpaa JU, Ala-Fossi SL (1997) Toremifene in postmenopausal breast cancer: efficacy, safety and cost. Drugs Aging 11:261–270
43. Manson JE, Martin KA (2001) Postmenopausal hormone-replacement therapy. N Engl J Med 345:34–40
44. Martino S, Cauley JA, Barrett-Connor E, Powles TJ, Mershon J, Disch D, et al. (2004) Continuing Outcomes Relevant to Evista: breast cancer incidence in postmenopausal osteoporotic women in a randomized trial of raloxifene. J Natl Cancer Inst 96:1751–1761
45. Marttunen MB, Hietanen P, Titinen A, Roth H-J, Viinikka L, Ylikorkala O (1999) Effects of tamoxifen and toremifene on urinary excretion of pyridinoline and deoxypyridinoline and bone density in postmenopausal women with breast cancer. Calcif Tissue Int 65:365–368
46. McClung M, Omizo M, Weiss S, Moffett A, Bolognese M, Civitelli R, et al. (2004a) Comparison of lasofoxifene and raloxifene for the prevention of bone loss in postmenopausal women. J Bone Miner Res 19 (Suppl 1):F424
47. McClung M, Portman D, Emkey R, McKenny J, Ettinger M, Somayaji V, et al. (2004b) Comparison of the extraskeletal effects of lasofoxifene and raloxifene. 19(Suppl 1):SA423

48. Meegan MJ, Lloyd DG (2003) Advances in the science of estrogen receptor modulation. Curr Med Chem 10:181–210
49. Miller CP, Collini MD, Tran BD, Harris HA, Kharode YP, Marzolf JT, et al. (2001) Design, synthesis, and preclinical characterization of novel, highly selective indole estrogens. J Med Chem 44:1654–1657
50. Moffett AH, Ettinger M, Bolognese M, Weiss S, Somayaji V, Brunell R, et al. (2004) Lasofoxifene, a next generation SERM, is effective in preventing loss of BMD and reducing LDL-C in postmenopausal women. J Bone Miner Res 19 (Suppl 1):F426
51. Neele SJ, Rombouts SA, Bierlaagh MA, Barkhof F, Scheltens P, Netelenbos JC (2001) Raloxifene affects brain activation patterns in postmenopausal women during visual encoding. J Clin Endocrinol Metab 86:1422–1424
52. Nuttall ME, Bradbeer JN, Stroup GB, Nadeau DP, Hoffman SJ, Zhao H, et al. (1998) Idoxifene: a novel selective estrogen receptor modulator prevents bone loss and lowers cholesterol levels in ovariectomized rats and decreases uterine weight in intact rats. Endocrinology 139:5224–5234
53. O'Regan RM, Cisneros GM, England GM, MacGregor JI, Muenzner HD, Assikis VJ, et al. (1998) Effects of the antiestrogens tamoxifen, toremifene, and ICI 182,780 on endometrial cancer growth. J Natl Cancer Inst 90:1552–1555
54. Qu Q, Zheng H, Dahllund J, Laine A, Cockcroft N, Peng Z, et al. (2000) Selective estrogen effects of a novel triphenylethylene compound, FC1271a, on bone, cholesterol level, and reproductive tissues in intact ovariectomized rats. Endocrinology 141:809–820
55. Ronkin S, Clarke L, Boudes P, Constantine G (2001) TSE-424, a novel tissue selective estrogen, reduces biochemical indices of bone metabolissm in a dose-related fashion. J Bone Miner Res 16(Suppl):S413
56. Rutanen EM, Heikkinen J, Halonen K, Komi J, Lammintausta R, Ylikorkala O (2003) Effects of ospemifene, a novel SERM, on hormones, genitl tract, climateric symptoms, and quality of life in postmenopausal women: a double-blind, randomized trial. Menopause 10:440–447
57. Sato M, Zeng GQ, Rowley E, Turner CH (1998) LY353381 HCl: an improved benzothiophe analog with bone efficacy complementary to parathyroid hormone-(1–34). Endocrinology 139:4642–4651
58. Savolainen-Peltonen H, Luoto NM, Kangas L, Häyry P (2004) Selective estrogen receptor modulators prevent neointima formation after vascular injury. Mol Cell Endocrinol 227:9–20
59. Shapiro CL, Recht A (2001) Side effects of adjuvant treatment of breast cancer. N Engl J Med 344:1997–2008
60. Shibata J, Toko T, Saito H, Fujioka A, Sato K, Hashimoto A, et al. (2000) Estrogen agonistic/antagonistic effects of miproxifene phosphate (TAT-59). Cancer Chemother Pharmacol 35:133–141
61. Shumaker SA, Legault C, Kuller L, Rapp SR, Thal L, Lane DS, et al. (2004) Conjugated equibe estrogens and incidence of probable dementia and mild cognitive impairment in postmenopausal women. Women's Health Initiative Memory Study. J Am Med Assoc 291:2947–2958
62. Singh MM (2001) Centchroman, a selective estrogen receptor modulator, as a contraceptive and for the management of hormone-related clinical disorders. Med Res Rev 21:302–347
63. Smith IE, Dowsett M (2003) Aromatase inhibitors in breast cancer. N Engl J Med 348:2431–2442
64. Sorbera LA, Castañer J, Silvestre JS (2002) Pipendoxifene. Drugs Future 27:942–947

65. Sutherland KM, Brady H, Gayo-Fung LM, Leisten J, Lipps SG, McKie JA, et al. (2003) Effects of SP500263, a novel selective estrogen receptor modulator, on bone, uterus, and serum cholesterol in the ovariectomized rat. Calcif Tissue Int 72:710–716
66. Taras TL, Wurz GT, DeGregorio MW (2001) In vitro and in vivo effects of ospemifene (FC-1271a) in breast cancer. J Steroid Biochem Mol Biol 77:271–279
67. Toko T, Sugimoto Y, Matsuo K, Yamasaki R, Takeda S, Wierzba K, et al. (1990) TAT-59, a new triphenylethylene derivative with antitumor activity against hormone-dependent tumors. Eur J Cancer 26:397–404
68. Vogel VG, Costantino JP, Wickerham DL, Cronin WM, Wolmark N (2002) The study of tamoxifen and raloxifene: preliminary enrollment data from a randomized breast cancer risk reduction trial. Clin Breast Cancer 3:153–159
69. Wenger NK, Barrett-Connor E, Collins P, Grady D, Kornitzer M, Mosca L, et al. (2002) Baseline characteristics of participants in the raloxifene use for the heart (RUTH) trial. Am J Cardiol 90:1204–1210
70. Witte RS, Pruitt B, Tormey DC, Moss S, Rose DP, Falkson G, et al. (1986) A phase I/II investigation of trioxifene mesylate in advanced breast cancer. Clinical and endocrinologic effects. Cancer 57:34–39
71. Wickerham L (2002) Tamoxifen: an update on current data and where it can now be used. Breast Cancer Res Treat 75(Suppl 1):S7–12; discussion S33-5
72. Willson TM, Norris JD, Wagner BL, Asplin I, Baer P, Brown HR, et al. (1997) Dissection of the molecular mechanism of action of GW5638, a novel estrogen receptor ligand, provides insights into the role of estrogen receptor in bone. Endocrinology 138:3901–3911
73. Women's Health Initiative Steering Committee (2004) Effects of conjugated equine estrogen in postmenopausal women with hysterectomy. The Women's Health Initiative randomized controlled trial. J Am Med Assoc 291:1701–1712
74. Writing Group for the Women's Health Initiative Investigators (2002) Risks and benefits of estrogen plus progestin in healthy postmenopausal women. J Am Med Assoc 288:321–333
75. Yaffe K, Krueger K, Sarkar S, Grady D, Barrett-Connor E, Cox DA, et al. (2001) Cognitive function in postmenopausal women treated with raloxifene. N Engl J Med 344:1207–1213

Action of Selective Estrogen Receptor Modulators (SERMs) Through the Classical Mechanism of Estrogen Action

Fernando Marín · Mª Carmen Barbancho

3.1 Introduction

The molecular mechanisms through which SERMs have an estrogen–agonist or antagonist effect, depending on the tissue in question, has been a topic of intense investigation during the last decade (Yang et al. 1996b; Shang et al. 2002; Meegan et al. 2003; Smith et al. 2004). Recent advances in the molecular biology of ERs have revealed the enormously complex nature of this process. As mentioned in Chapter XXX, estrogens regulate the activation of genes by means of a series of molecular events triggered after they bind to the estrogen receptor (ER), which is simply a transcription factor that can be activated by a ligand. The same course of events is set in motion by selective estrogen receptor modulators (SERMs). In short, the high-affinity binding to the ER, and to the ER alone, is a fundamental characteristic of SERMs. The absence of cross-binding with other members of the nuclear receptor superfamily (androgen, progesterone, glucocorticoids, mineralocorticoids, retinoic acid, vitamin D receptors, etc.) is a critical stage in the target molecule selection process. The binding of the ligand to the ER leads to a conformational change in the ligand–ER complex, causing disassociation of the stress proteins associated to the inactive receptor (heat-shock proteins). The inactive receptors, which are monomers in basal conditions, dimerize and get phosphorylated until they finally bind to a series of nuclear proteins called adaptor or coregulator proteins. This ligand–ER complex binds to one of the DNA response elements (EREs: estrogen response elements), generally located in the promoter region of estrogen target genes, and trigger the mRNA transcription and synthesis process. Depending on the cell type, coregulator protein load, ratio of coactivator and corepressor proteins, and different gene promoters, the ligand–ER dimer may activate or inhibit the gene transcription.

It is of great interest that new findings suggest that several effects of estrogen and SERMs also may be mediated by nonnuclear ER actions derived from fast activation (in a matter of minutes) of the protein–kinase cascades and other signaling processes associated to cell membrane ERs. These activation routes, described in detail in Chap. 1 by Escrich et al. are not mediated by transcription factors and nuclear ER activation. The functional effects associated with these pathways include some of the cardiovascular effects of estrogens, such as nitric oxide (NO)-dependent vasodilatation, inhibition of endothelial damage response, and reduced ischemic damage to the myocardium in experimental conditions (Ho et al. 2002; Salom et al. 2002). Raloxifene and its analog LY-117018 stimulate endothelial NO synthetase (eNOS) and lead to coronary artery relaxation and improved vasodilatation in hypertensive rats (Simoncini et al. 2002a; Wassman et al. 2002). The eNOS activation by means of protein-kinase activation (MAPKs and PI3K-Akt) has also been reported with EM-800 (Simoncini et al. 2002b). These nongenomic pathways of estrogen action have also been reported in neuronal cells (Qiu et al. 2003) and bone cells (Kousteni et al. 2003), but their contribution in the action of specific SERM compounds, and the role of different signaling pathways in tissue-specific actions, is undefined at this time.

In addition to these rapid nongenomic events, the pharmacodynamic profile of different SERMs may depend on the subtle mesh of the combined action of complex mechanisms that govern the transcription mediated by ERs. Basically, this can occur at four levels: (1) tissue amount and distribution of the different ER subtypes; (2) impact on binding capacity to promoters provoking the different 3D conformations of the SERM–ligand complex, which ultimately dictate specific coregulator interactions; (3) different content of nuclear coregulator proteins (coactivators and corepressors) in various cells; and (4) presence of different types of estrogen response elements (EREs) in the gene promoters, including the ability of ERs to affect gene expression without directly binding to target DNAs in a process known as transrepression.

3.2 Estrogen Receptor Subtypes

Until 1995, it was believed that only one gene-encoding ER existed. The description and characterization of a new ER subtype, known as ERβ, has modified the classical vision of the molecular pathways activated by estrogens (Kuiper et al. 1996). Furthermore, it is highly likely that each subtype has multiple isoforms. Although the majority of tissues express both ER subtypes (ERα and ERβ), there is a certain degree of tissue-specific distribution (Kuiper et al. 1997). For example, ERα predominates in the breast, liver, uterus, ovaries, and central nervous system. ERβ has a slightly different tissue distribution pattern, and a high expression has been reported in endothelial cells, bones, lungs, urogenital tract, ovaries, central nervous system, and prostate. While ERα acts predominantly as an activator, ERβ can down-regulate this response if it binds to ERα to form a heterodimer. Therefore, an attractive hypothesis to explain the pharmacology of SERMs is the relative content of both ER subtypes in a certain tissue, additionally considering the different relative affinities of the various SERMs to the two described ER subtypes. However, there is no clear proof to date that demonstrates that the selective action of a certain SERM is the result of its preferential binding to one of the two ER subtypes. In fact, tamoxifen and raloxifene, the two SERMs for which most data are available, show a similar degree of binding to both ER isoforms (Kuiper et al. 1997).

3.3 Conformation of Ligand–ER Complex

One of the most significant findings in this field is the demonstration that the tertiary structure of the ligand–ER complex depends on the molecular characteristics of the ligand. The ligand-binding domain (LBD) of the ER consists of a hydrophobic open pocket formed by 12 short helices. Near its carboxy-terminal end, it includes an amino acid sequence called Activating Function-2 (AF-2), which is considered essential in the activation of genes that mediate estrogenic activity in reproductive tissues, such as the uterus and breast. AF-2 is dependent on the binding of the ligand. Therefore, if AF-2 gets blocked, the transcription of these genes would be compromised. When the ER-LBD binds to 4-hydroxy-tamoxifen, the active metabolite of tamoxifen, the change in the alignment of helix 12 prevents the interaction between the ligand–ER complex and a coactivator protein. In contrast, if the ligand is estradiol, helix 12 goes over the ligand, snuggling it in a tight fitting pocket that permits the coactivator proteins to bind to this region (Shiau et al. 1998). Similar findings have been reported with X-ray protein crystallization techniques that have analyzed the 3D structure of the ERα and raloxifene complex. The basic side chain of the raloxifene molecule is very rigid and does not fit in the pocket formed by the ligand-binding domain of the ERα. Therefore, helix 12 cannot fit properly over the ligand and remains outside the "pocket", preventing AF-2 from interacting with the coregulator protein in order for the transcription to take place (Brzozowski et al. 1997). The different SERMs give rise to different 3D conformations of the SERM–ligand complex, forming a continuum of different intermediary forms, from the binding of estradiol at one end to the binding of a pure antiestrogen at the other (McDonnell et al. 2002).

3.4 Coregulator Protein Cell Content and Coactivators/Corepressors Ratio

In order for estrogen-mediated genomic activation to occur, the ligand–ER complex must bind to other nuclear proteins (coregulator proteins) that can either act as coactivators (stimulators of gene transcription) or corepressors (inhibitors of gene transcription) for access of the complex to the EREs (for a review see Rosenfeld et al. 2001) (Fig. 3.1). The discovery and cloning of these coregulator proteins has been another key milestone in our understanding of gene expression pathways mediated by transcription factors (Smith et al. 2004). Several coregulator proteins are known to be capable of binding to ERs and modulating their function. Major ER coactivators fall into three groups of proteins: steroid receptor coactivator-1 (SRC-1), SRC-2, and SRC-3. In addition, proteins such as cyclic AMP response element binding protein (CBP/p300) act as coactivators for multiple transcription factors. Some of the corepressors associated with raloxifene and 4-hydroxy-tamoxifen antiestrogenic actions are the silencing mediator of retinoic acid and thyroid hormone receptor (SMRT) and the nuclear receptor corepressor (NcoR). Whether the coregulator protein that binds to the ligand–ER complex is a coactivator or corepressor protein depends on the conformational alteration that the ER undergoes, which in turn depends on the type of ligand to which it is bound. Furthermore, the amount of coregulator proteins, in both absolute and relative terms, varies according to the different cells that respond to estrogens. An extraordinary example of this fact was described recently by Shang et al. (2002). These authors demonstrated that the estrogen–antagonist action of tamoxifen and raloxifene on breast cells is mediated by the action of corepressor proteins present in these cells. However,

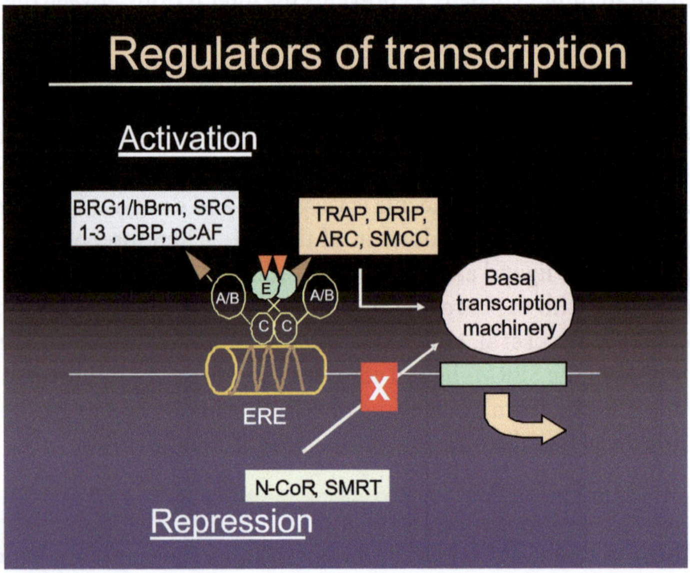

Fig. 3.1. Coregulator proteins and gene transcription. The DNA-bound receptor can either positively or negatively regulate target gene transcription. Agonist-bound ERs can recruit transcriptional adaptors, proteins that permit the receptor to transmit its regulatory information to the cellular transcriptional apparatus. Among those adaptors are coactivators (stimulators of gene transcription) and correpresors (inhibitors of gene transcription)

the opposite action of these two SERMs on the endometrium is explained by the capacity that tamoxifen shows in facilitating the recruitment of coactivator proteins of a group of genes in endometrial cells. In short, the agonist effect of tamoxifen on the endometrium is based on the induction in this tissue of a high expression of coactivator SRC-1. This effect is not observed with raloxifene. Therefore, differences in cell type and ratio of different coregulator proteins in such cells may determine the response to different types of SERMs (Shang et al. 2002).

3.5 Transrepression: Regulation of Gene Expression by an ERE-Independent Mechanism

One last mechanism that has been put forward to explain the tissue selectivity of SERMs, or even gene-specific regulation within the same cell, derives from the existence of estrogen-dependent genes containing not the classic ERE sequence in the gene promoter region but other alternative response sequences, in such a way that only the genes that contain these non-ERE sequences are transcribed when the tamoxifen–ERα or raloxifene–ERα complexes interact with

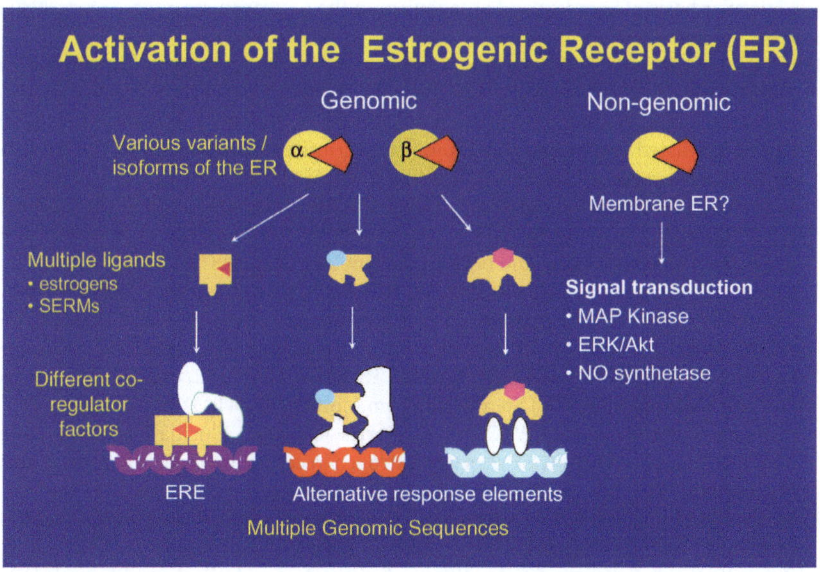

Fig. 3.2. Potential genomic and nongenomic activation routes that may be induced by natural or synthetic ER ligands. The hypotheses that explain the tissue-selective action of SERMs include (a) selective activation of ER subtypes, (b) different changes in the 3D configuration of the ligand–ER complex, (c) recruitment of coactivator and corepressor proteins, and (d) activation of alternative response elements in certain inducible genes

the gene promoter (Paech et al. 1997; Yang et al. 1996b). The gene expression in this ERE-independent mechanism involves other DNA-bound transcription factors (Kushner et al. 2000; Abdelrahim et al. 2002). It should be noted that in many estrogen-responsive genes a direct DNA binding of ER is not required for ER-mediated activation of transcription. ER, through protein-to-protein contacts with other transcription factors, such as AP-1 and Sp-1, allows increased efficiency of transcription mediated by these factors (Kushner et al. 2000). This is the case of the Transforming Growth Factor β_3 (TGF-β_3) gene, a highly abundant growth factor in the bone matrix with a highly potent antiresorptive activity whose expression has been reported with raloxifene and other SERMs but not with 17-β-estradiol through a nonclassical ERE-independent mechanism (Yang et al. 1996a,b).

Figure 3.2 provides a summary of the different mechanisms that have been hypothesized to explain the selective tissue action of SERMs.

References

1. Abdelrahim M, Samudio I, Smith R, Burghart R, Safe S (2002) Small inhibitory RNA duplexes for Sp! MRNA block basal and estrogen-induced gene expression and cell cycle progression in MCF-7 breast cancer cells. J Biol Chem 77:28815–28822
2. Brzozowski AM, Pike ACW, Dauter Z, Hubbard RE, Bonn T, Engström O, et al. (1997) Molecular basis of agonism and antagonism in the oestrogen receptor. Nature 89:753–758
3. Ho KJ, Liao JK (2002) Non-nuclear actions of estrogen. Arterioscler Throm Vas Biol 2:1952–1961
4. Kousteni S, Han L, Chen JR, Almeida M, Plotkin LI, Bellido T, Manolagas SC (2003) Kinase-mediated regulation of common transcription factors accounts for the bone-protective effects of sex steroids. J Clin Invest 11:1651–1664
5. Kuiper GG, Carlsson B, Grandien K, Enmark E, Haggblad J, Nilsson S, Gustafsson JA (1997) Comparison of the ligand binding specificity and transcript tissue distribution of estrogen receptors alpha and beta. Endocrinology 38:863–870
6. Kuiper GG, Enmark E, Pelto-Huikko M, Nilsson S, Gustafsson JA (1996) Cloning of a novel estrogen receptor expressed in rat prostate and ovary. Proc Natl Acad Sci USA 3:5925–5930
7. Kushner PJ, Agard DA, Greene GL, Scanlan TS, Shiau AK, Uth R, et al. (2000) Estrogen receptor pathways to AP-1. J Steroid Biochem Mol Biol 74:311–317
8. McDonnell DP, Wijayarate A, Chang C, Norris JD (2002) Elucidation of the molecular mechanism of action of selective estrogen receptor modulators. Am J Cardiol 0(suppl):35F-43F
9. Meegan MJ, Lloyd DG (2003) Advances in the science of estrogen receptor modulation. Curr Med Chem 0:181–210
10. Paech K, Webb P, Kuiper GGJM, Nilsson S, Gustafsson JA, Kushner PJ, et al. (1997) Differential ligand activation of estrogen receptors ERα and ERβ at AP1 sites. Science 77:1508–1510
11. Qui J, Bosch MA, Tobias SC, Grandy DK, Scanlan TS, Ronnekleiv OK, et al. (2003) Rapid signaling of estrogen in hypothalamic neurons involves a novel G-protein-coupled estrogen receptor that activates protein kinase C. J Neurosci 3:9529–9540

12. Rosenfeld MG, Glass CK (2001) Coregulator codes of transcriptional regulation by nuclear receptors. J Biol Chem 276:36865–36868
13. Salom JB, Burguete MC, Pérez-Asensio FJ, Centeno JM, Torregrosa G, Alborch E (2002) Acure relaxant effects of 17-β-estradiol through non-genomic mechanisms in rabbit carotid artery. Steroids 7:339–346
14. Shang Y, Brown M (2002) Molecular determinants for the tissue specificity of SERMs. Science 295:2465–2468
15. Shiau AK, Barstad D, Loria PM, Cheng L, Kushner PJ, Agard A, Greene GL (1998) The structural basis of estrogen receptor/co-activator recognition and the antagonism of this interaction with tamoxifen. Cell 5:927–937
16. Simoncini T, Genazzani AR, Liao JK (2002a) Nongenomic mechanisms of endothelial nitric oxide synthetase activation by the selective estrogen receptor modulator raloxifene. Circulation 105:1368–1373
17. Simoncini T, Varone G, Fornari L, Mannella P, Luisi M, Labrie F, et al (2002b) Genomic and nongenomic mechanisms of nitric oxide synthesis induction in human endothelial cells by a fourth-generation selective estrogen receptor modulator. Endocrinology 43:2052–2061
18. Smith CL, O'Malley BW (2004) Co-regulator function: a key to understanding tissue specificity of selective receptor modulators. Endocr Rev 25:45–71
19. Wassmann S, Laufs U, Stamenkovic D, Linz W, Stasch JP, Ahlbory K, Rosen R, Bohm M, Nickening G (2002) Raloxifene improves endothelial dysfunction in hypertension by reduced oxidative stress and enhanced nitric oxide production. Circulation 105:2083–2091
20. Yang NN, Bryant HU, Hardikar S, Sato M, Galvin RJS, Glasebrook AL, et al. (1996a) Estrogen and raloxifene stimulate transforming growth factor-β_3 expression in rat bone: a potent mechanism for estrogen- or raloxifene-mediated bone maintenance. Endocrinology 37:2075–2084
21. Yang NN, Venugopalan M, Hardikar S, Glasebrook AL (1996b) Identification of an estrogen response element activated by metabolites of 17-β-estradiol and raloxifene. Science 73:1222–1225. [Letter. Published errata: Science 275:1249, 1997 Feb 28]

Chapter 4

Cellular and Molecular Basis for Acute Nongenomically Mediated Actions of SERMs

Mario Díaz · Jorge Marrero-Alonso · Benito García Marrero · Raquel Marín · Tomás Gomez · Rafael Alonso

4.1 Introduction

Compelling evidence accumulated over the past three decades have demonstrated that, besides their ability to antagonize estrogen binding to their intracellular specific estrogen receptors (ER), selective estrogen receptor modulators (SERMs) can affect a number of biochemical processes in eukaryotic cells. Experimental data from in vivo and in vitro studies have revealed that SERMs and estrogens are surprisingly pleiotropic molecules affecting molecular targets in both estrogen receptor positive (ER+) and negative (ER–) cells. Such "alternative" actions of SERMs and estrogens are typically independent of canonical ERs and do not involve transcriptional or translational events, thereby mediated nongenomically, and usually initiated (and accomplished) within seconds to minutes after presentation of the molecule (Falkestein et al. 2000; Nadal el al. 2001). The spectrum of SERM-induced acute actions includes a wide set of molecular targets, from modulation of ion channels and signaling molecules to alteration of membrane fluidity. In the following sections we review data from different laboratories, including ours, in the context of cellular and molecular evidences for acute nongenomic effects of SERMs observed at pharmacological circulating concentrations. Special emphasis will be placed on actions that might underlie clinically relevant beneficial effects as well as undesirable side effects.

4.2 Cellular and Molecular Targets for Rapid Actions

4.2.1 Interaction with Ion Channels

4.2.1.1 *Sodium and Potassium Channels*

Electrophysiological studies on primary cultures of hypothalamic neurons and C1300 neuroblastoma cells have shown that the triphenylethylene SERMs tamoxifen and toremifene are able to rapidly inhibit macroscopic voltage-gated tetradotoxin-sensitive Na^+ currents (TTX-sensitive I_{Na}, $IC_{50} \approx 1-2\,\mu M$) and delayed rectifier K^+ currents (I_{DR}) ($IC_{50} \approx 2-3\,\mu M$), while only toremifene exhibits a significant inhibition of transient outward (I_{to}) currents ($IC_{50} \approx 3\,\mu M$) (Hardy et al. 1998). Similar results have been reported in rat cortical glial cells for voltage-gated TTX-sensitive I_{Na} and I_{DR} (Smitherman and Sontheimer 2001). Moreover, in isolated cardiac myocytes, tamoxifen inhibits voltage-gated delayed rectifier K^+ in a time-, concentration-, and voltage-dependent fashion (Liu et al. 1998) and, more importantly, inhibits the inward rectifier (I_{K1} and I_{to}). Inhibition of I_{K1} and I_{to} is especially noticeable since it markedly prolongs the action potential duration, decreases the maximal rate of depolarization, and decreases the resting membrane potential in cardiac myocytes (He et al. 2003). The results of these studies suggest that inhibition of I_{to}, I_{DR}, and I_{K1} by tamoxifen may contribute to prolonged QT interval of the electrocardiogram observed in some patients receiving tamoxifen treatment,

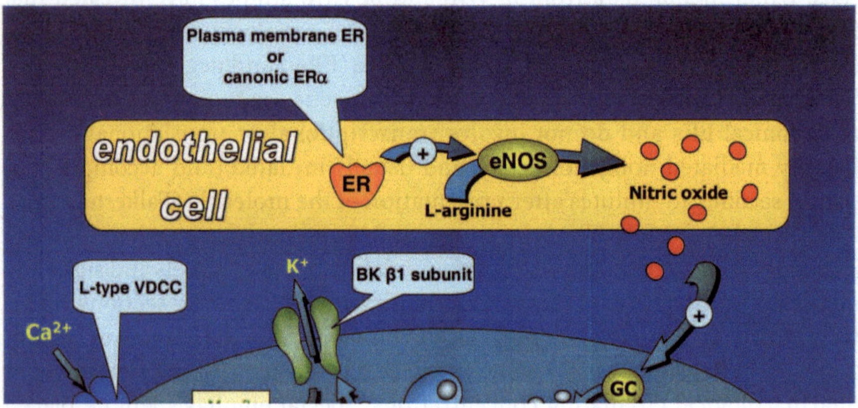

Fig. 4.1. Cellular model illustrating cell types in vascular wall involved in vasorelaxation induced by SERMs. Putative targets of SERMs are indicated within *cyan* tags. SERMs directly affect L-type VDCC, BK $\beta 1$ subunit in smooth muscle cells, and ER in endothelial cells. *L-type VDCC*: L-type voltage-dependent calcium channel; *BK*: calcium-activated large conductance K^+ channel; *PKG*: protein kinase G; *eNOS*: endothelial nitric oxide synthase; *GC*: soluble guanylate cyclase; *cGMP*: cyclic GMP; V_M: electrochemical membrane potential; *ER*: estrogen receptor. See text for further details

thereby potentially causing untoward life-threatening polymorphic ventricular arrhythmias (De Ponti et al. 2000; Pollack et al. 1997).

Tamoxifen also modulates a different set of K^+ channels, namely large-conductance calcium-activated potassium channels (BK), by directly interacting with the regulatory $\beta 1$ subunit of the channel protein (Dick et al. 2001). Interaction of tamoxifen, as well as 4-OH-tamoxifen and the impermeant analog ethylbromide tamoxifen (EBTx), with the $\beta 1$ subunit dramatically alters the Ca^{2+}/voltage sensitivity of BK, increasing the channel open probability ($EC_{50} = 0.65-0.96\ \mu M$) and decreasing the unitary conductance of the channel pore (Dick et al. 2001, 2002). Interestingly, the stimulatory effect of tamoxifen on $\beta 1$ is mimicked by 17β-estradiol (Valverde et al. 1999), though tamoxifen is nearly fivefold more effective than 17β-estradiol (Dick et al. 2001). These results are clinically relevant since BK channels play a key role in maintaining the dynamic equilibrium between vasoconstriction and vasodilation in vascular smooth muscle, thereby controlling blood pressure. Activation of BK channels leads to hyperpolarization of the cell membrane, which causes deactivation of voltage-dependent calcium channels and subsequent vasodilation (reviewed in Patterson et al. 2002). Positive modulation of large-conductance potassium channels by tamoxifen and 17β-estradiol likely underlie the acute endothelium-independent relaxing effect of these compounds on vasculature (Patterson et al. 2002; Valverde et al. 1999) (Fig. 4.1).

4.2.1.2
Calcium Channels

The ability of estrogens and nonsteroidal SERMs to modify calcium channel activity in smooth muscle cells was initially inferred from competition binding studies. Thus, it has been shown that tamoxifen and clomiphene compete with dihydropyridine calcium channel antagonists (^{3}H-nitrendipine) in binding in membrane fractions of human and rabbit urinary bladder and myometrium (Batra 1990). On the other hand, functional studies in different preparations of vascular and visceral smooth muscle have revealed that estrogens, xenoestrogens, and SERMs induce relaxation through ER-independent mechanisms. Thus, in vitro studies on isolated uterine, vascular, detrusor, and intestinal smooth muscles from different species, including humans, have shown that tamoxifen rapidly inhibits spontaneous and agonist-induced contractile activity by interfering with transmembrane calcium influx (Cantabrana and Hidalgo 1992; Díaz 2002; Fernández et al. 1993; Lipton 1987; Lipton et al. 1984; Ratz et al. 1999; Song et al. 1996). Reported IC_{50} values for triphenylethylene SERMs in these preparations were in the submicromolar range, i.e., for tamoxifen and ethylbromide tamoxifen in mouse duodenal muscle values were 0.85 and 0.37 μM, respectively (Díaz 2002; J. Marrero-Alonso et al. in press), and for uterine muscles values were 0.70 and 0.58 μM, respectively (J. Marrero-Alonso et al. in press) (Fig. 4.2). In addition, direct electrophysiological evidence has demonstrated that tamoxifen inhibits calcium entry through L-type calcium channels in A7r5 and aortic smooth muscle cells (Song et al. 1996), isolated colonic myocytes (Dick et al. 1999), and other nonmuscle cells, like clonal pituitary cells (Sartor et al. 1988) and PC12 neurosecretory cells (Greenberg et al. 1987). Recently, similar effects on vascular voltage-dependent L-type calcium channels and contractile response of cerebral arteries (Tsang et al. 2004) and pulmonary vessels (Chan et al. 2004) have been reported for the more recent benzotiophene SERM raloxifene.

Obviously, the effects of tamoxifen and derivatives and of raloxifene on L-type calcium channels from aortic and other blood vessels would reduce vascular smooth muscle contractility. This action, in synergy with the aforementioned effect on BK channels, would reduce blood peripheral resistance and blood pressure, which may partially account for the reduction in cardiovascular risk (Da Costa et al. 2004; Trump et al. 1992) (Fig. 4.1).

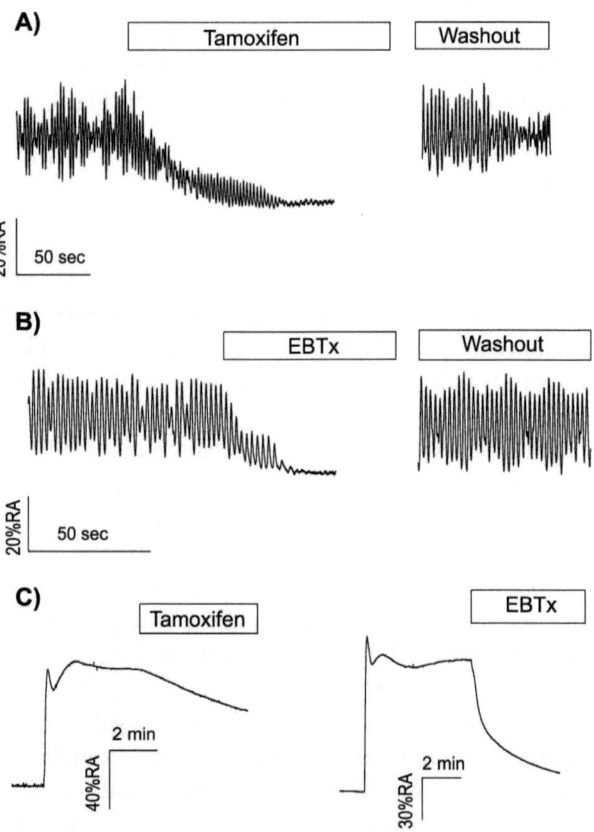

Fig. 4.2. Effects of triphenylethylene SERMs on spontaneous and depolarization-induced contractions in visceral smooth muscle. Tamoxifen (**a**) and ethylbromide tamoxifen (EBTx, **b**) rapidly and reversibly inhibit spontaneous peristaltic activity in duodenal muscle. Both compounds also inhibit depolarization-induced tonic contraction of uterine muscle (**c**). The inhibition of L-type voltage-dependent calcium channels underlies the relaxing effects illustrated here. Drugs concentrations were 10 μM in all cases. *%RA*: percent of activity related to maximal activity

On the other hand, we have shown that 4-OH-tamoxifen is as effective as tamoxifen in relaxing duodenal and ileal smooth muscle through inhibition of L-type calcium channels (Díaz 2002). Since tamoxifen is metabolized in the liver to produce the active circulating metabolite 4-OH-tamoxifen, the existence of effects induced by this metabolite provides a critical indication of an in vivo pharmacological action. Indeed, levels of tamoxifen and 4-OH-tamoxifen shown in intestinal preparations to cause a significant reduction of calcium channels are well within the range of tamoxifen concentrations clinically observed in humans and might provide a clue to explaining the occurrence of gastrointestinal disorders in patients receiving high-dose tamoxifen therapies.

4.2.1.3
Chloride Channels

Maxi-Cl^- channels are large conductance voltage-dependent anion channels with widespread distribution in eukaryotic cells, yet they have rarely been recorded in intact cells. We have reported that Maxi-Cl^- channels are activated in intact neuroblastoma C1300, vascular A7r5 myocytes, and NIH3T3 cells by low micromolar concentrations of the extracellular triphenylethylene SERMs tamoxifen and toremifene, as well as by the nonpermeant analog ethylbromide tamoxifen (Díaz 1999; Díaz et al. 2001; Hardy and Valverde 1994; Valverde et al. 2002), which suggests the involvement of membrane antiestrogen binding sites for these compounds (Fig. 4.3). The fact that Maxi-Cl^- channels are generally inactive in whole cells but activate upon membrane-patch excision has suggested the existence of regulatory mechanisms that keep Maxi-Cl^- channels closed under nonstimulatory conditions, probably due to either basal phosphorylation of the channel protein or putative regulatory subunits. In this sense, our observations on neuroblastoma C1300 and NIH3T3 fibroblasts revealed that activation of Maxi-Cl^- channels by antiestrogens is triggered upon activation of an okadaic acid-sensitive PP2A-like phosphatase in response to tamoxifen and its derivatives, which dephosphorylates Maxi-Cl^- channels and switches them to a voltage-sensitive active state (Díaz et al. 2001). Interestingly, activation of Maxi-Cl^- channels can be prevented by preincubation with 17β-estradiol via activation of protein kinase A (PKA), which likely keeps the channels in their phosphorylated inactive state (Díaz et al. 2001). The physiological significance of the modulation of Maxi-Cl^- channels by estrogens and triphenylethylene SERMs remains unresolved, but a number of studies have emphasized their role in transmembrane electrolyte transport and setting of the membrane potential (Gelband et al. 1996).

Volume-sensitive chloride channels are also sensitive to triphenylethylene SERMs. Thus, tamoxifen, 4-OH-tamoxifen, and toremifene were all found to

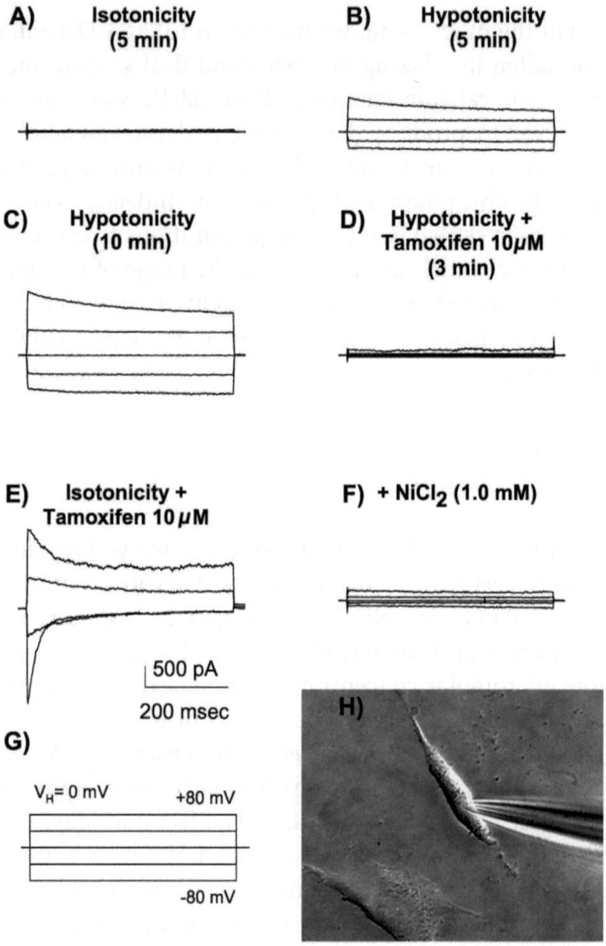

Fig. 4.3. Modulation of different types of chloride currents by tamoxifen in a single rat aortic A7r5 cell (shown in **H**). Currents were elicited under voltage-clamp conditions in response to the voltage protocol depicted in *G*, in symmetrical *N*-methyl-D-glucamine chloride. The cell was initially recorded under isotonic conditions (**A**) and afterwards exposed to hypotonicity for different times (**B**, **C**). Volume-activated chloride currents activated by hypotonicity were completely blocked by tamoxifen (**D**). Under isotonic conditions, tamoxifen also activates Maxi-Cl^- currents in the same cell (**E**), which were inhibited by niquel chloride (**F**). V_H: holding potential

be high-potency fast blockers of volume-sensitive chloride channels in nearly all cell types analyzed so far (Díaz 1996; Valverde et al. 1993; Zhang et al. 1994) by mechanisms independent of estrogen receptor activation that involve direct interaction with the channel protein (Fig. 4.3). Furthermore, the IC_{50} for tamoxifen-induced inhibition of volume-sensitive channels ($\approx 0.3\ \mu M$) is, by far, lower than for any other blocker of this type of chloride channels identified to date (Zhang et al. 1994). Interestingly, lens fibers express volume-sensitive chloride channels that play a crucial role in maintaining the hydroelectrolytic equilibrium for normal lens clarity. It is known that one of the side effects of tamoxifen therapies is cataracts (Gerner 1992; Jordan and Murphy 1990). The fact that tamoxifen readily blocks volume-sensitive chloride channels in isolated patches of lens fibers, and that tamoxifen reduces lens transmittance in lens organ cultures at similar concentrations (Zhang et al. 1994), has raised the hypothesis that tamoxifen induces opacity and cataract formation through its effect on channel function.

4.2.1.4
Neurotransmitter Receptors

Tamoxifen can compete with the binding of histamine and antihistaminergic compounds such as DPPE (*N*,*N*-Diethyl-2-[(4-phenylmethyl)-phenoxy]ethanamine hydrochloride) in rat brain microsomes and can antagonize histaminergic contraction of canine tracheal smooth muscle preparations (Brandes et al. 1987; Kroeger and Brandes 1985). Comparison of relative binding affinities of tamoxifen with those of histamine agonists and antagonists revealed a common binding entity that is neither H_1 nor H_2 (Kroeger and Brandes 1985). Similarly, tamoxifen competes with high affinity the binding of ^{3}H-domperidone (Kd=0.62 nM) to the D_2 dopaminergic receptor in membrane preparations of rat brain (Hiemke and Ghraf 1984). The Ki for tamoxifen in this system ($\approx$ 12 μM) was one order of magnitude larger than the Ki for dopamine ($\approx$ 1 μM), but much smaller than for 17β-estradiol (Hiemke and Ghraf 1984). These interactions of tamoxifen with dopaminergic systems may be clinically relevant since they could explain the emetic effects of antiestrogens, which are among the most common mild side effects of adjuvant therapies (Hiemke and Ghraf 1984).

Other neurotransmitter receptors are equally susceptible to modulation by SERMs. For instance, Ben-Baruch and coworkers (1982) have investigated the possible interaction between the triphenylethylene drug clomiphene citrate and muscarinic receptors in homogenates from various regions of rat brain. Binding analyses and dissociation kinetics studies using the highly specific antagonist ^{3}H-*N*-methyl-4-piperidyl benzilate (4-NMPB) have shown that clomiphene binds in a positively cooperative pattern to muscarinic receptors (Ben-Baruch et al. 1982). More recently, both tamoxifen and clomiphene have been shown to compete with quinuclidinyl benzilate (QNB) for their binding to muscarinic receptors in membrane fractions of human and rabbit urinary bladder and myometrium, with IC_{50} values ranging from 5.0 to 13.6 μM (Batra 1990). In addition, electrophysiological studies on adult-type human muscle nicotinic receptors expressed in *Xenopus* oocytes have shown that tamoxifen and toremifene inhibit inward cationic currents with IC_{50} values of 1.2 μM (Allen et al. 1998). Interestingly, tamoxifen (and also the impermeant analog ethylbromide tamoxifen) was also able to non-competitively block another member of the nicotinic receptor family, the ionotropic 5-HT3 receptor channel, in neuroblastoma x glioma NG108-15 hybrid cells with high affinity (IC_{50} = 0.22 μM for EBTx) (Allen et al. 2000).

4.2.2 Multidrug Resistance and P-glycoprotein

Clinical success in the treatment of tumors with chemotherapy has significantly improved over the past several years, though treatment failure due to drug resistance of cancer cells has remained a major problem. The classical form of multiple drug resistance (MDR) is perhaps the most common type of drug resistance and represents the overexpression of a transmembrane glycoprotein pump (P-170 or Pgp) that mediates an energy-dependent active efflux of a spectrum of structurally and functionally unrelated drugs (reviewed in Mansouri et al. 1992; Ling 1997). Drug transport by P-170 is stoichiometrically coupled to ATPase hydrolysis in a high chemical-potential coupling transition state, where two ATP molecules are bound before the drug is moved to the external side of the membrane (Al-Shawi et al. 2003). The strict dependence of the Pgp ATPase activity on the presence of transport substrates indicates that the drug-stimulated ATPase activity is a direct reflection of the drug transport function of the Pgp. A number of studies in cellular models of drug resistance have shown that the triphenylethylene SERMs tamoxifen, its metabolites (4-OH-tamoxifen and *N*-desmethyltamoxifen), droloxifen, and toremifene all stimulate Pgp ATPase activity and reverse drug resistance (Berman et al. 1994; Chatterjee and Harris 1990; Li et al. 2001; Rao et al. 1994), often equalling the maximal stimulation obtained by verapamil, the best known MDR chemosensitizer (Rao et al. 1994). Interestingly, a single report on adriamycin-resistant MCF-7 cells showed that triphenylethylene SERMs were effective inhibitors of ceramide-induced toxicity, while the raloxifene analog LY117,018 was without influence (Lucci et al. 1999). These results suggest that triphenylethylene SERMs, but not benzotiophene derivatives, reverse the multidrug-resistant phenotype by directly interacting with Pgp, thus interfering with its anticancer-drug-extruding activity (Rao et al. 1994).

The use of triphenylethylene SERMs as Pgp inhibitors for clinical application has been hampered by unacceptable toxicity at doses required to achieve adequate cellular concentration, which is likely due to the involvement of proteins with the ability to bind these compounds. For instance, toremifene is able to reverse MDR and to sensitize human renal cancer cells to vinblastine in vitro. However, in vivo toremifene is tightly bound to serum proteins, in particular α1-acid glycoprotein (AAG), which may limit its tissue availability (Braybrooke et al. 2000). In agreement with this, Chatterjee and Harris (1990) have shown that tamoxifen and 4-OH-tamoxifen were similarly potent in reversing MDR in Chinese hamster ovary (CHO) cells with acquired resistance to adriamycin. However, the addition of AAG (0.5 to 2 mg/ml, the range found in vivo) to cell cultures decreased the effect of tamoxifen on reversing MDR, and at the highest AAG concentration there was a complete reversal of the effects of both tamoxifen and 4-OH-tamoxifen (Braybrooke et al. 2000). Furthermore, AAG has been found to bind ^{3}H-tamoxifen in a nonsaturable and nonspecific manner, in contrast to the binding of tamoxifen to albumin (Chatterjee and Harris 1990). Thus, the use of tamoxifen as a reversal agent for MDR in vivo might be impaired by high binding to AAG.

4.2.3
Signalling Transducers

4.2.3.1
Calcium Signalling

Tamoxifen also affects Ca^{2+} signalling independently of conventional ERs. This compound binds calmodulin (CaM) in a Ca^{2+}-dependent manner and thus inhibits the many functions that are activated by this Ca^{2+}-binding protein, including control of cell proliferation (Kahl and Means 2003; Lam 1984; Lopes et al. 1990). Some studies have hypothesized that CaM inhibition might be responsible for the ER-independent tamoxifen cytotoxicity (Borras et al. 1994; Li et al. 2001). In isolated mammalian brain membranes, tamoxifen interacts with two different binding sites of CaM, with an apparent dissociation constant of about 6 nM and 9 μM, respectively (Lopes et al. 1990). In the micromolar range, there exists cooperativity for tamoxifen inhibition that is competed for by the CaM antagonist trifluoperazine (Lopes et al. 1990). Interestingly, tamoxifen interacts with CaM in its cation-activated form, which induces exposure of a hydrophobic domain of the C-terminal region of CaM. This domain serves the acceptor site for CaM-modulated enzymes or for CaM-antagonist drugs (La Porte et al. 1980). Molecular modeling of tamoxifen and its derivatives' interaction with CaM has revealed that the benzene rings of the triphenylethylene moiety and ethyl group (Fig. 4.4) fit in hydrophobic pockets of the protein, while the aminoethoxy side chain extends toward a region of acidic residues close to the hydrophobic cavity (Hardcastle et al. 1995).

Because of its ability to bind CaM, tamoxifen can increase cyclic AMP surges by inhibiting cyclic AMP hydrolysis by the Ca^{2+}-calmodulin-dependent cyclic nucleotide phosphodiesterase (Fanidi et al. 1989; Rowlands et al. 1990). In bovine brain preparations, tamoxifen appears to act as a competitive inhibitor of calmodulin-activated phosphodiesterase with an IC_{50} of 2 μM, similar to the value reported for trifluoperazine under the same experimental conditions (Lam 1984).

Nonsteroidal SERMs can also amplify signal-induced Ca^{2+} surges by inhibiting Ca^{2+}-calmodulin-dependent membrane (Ca^{2+} + Mg^{2+})-ATPase. For instance, in synaptic plasma membranes and red cell membrane ghosts, tamoxifen and other triphenylethylene compounds (but not estradiol) have been

Fig. 4.4. Structure of tamoxifen molecule showing some substructures (modified from De Medina et al. 2004a)

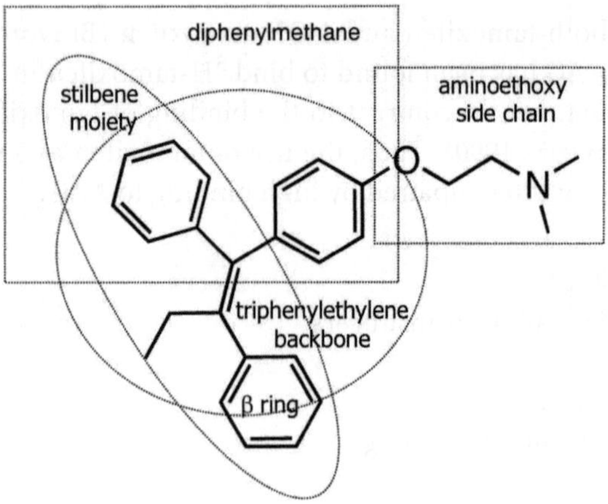

shown to inhibit (Ca^{2+} + Mg^{2+})-ATPase in a calmodulin-dependent fashion that was mimicked by trifluoperazine (Malva et al. 1990). In addition, tamoxifen decreases the calcium affinity of (Ca^{2+} + Mg^{2+})-ATPase, as does trifluoperazine in heart sarcolemma (Ca^{2+} + Mg^{2+})-ATPase. This reduction of the enzyme sensitivity for calcium is probably due to an impairment of calmodulin-induced transition from a low to a high Ca^{2+} affinity form (Caroni and Carafoli 1981). Moreover, tamoxifen greatly reduces trifluoperazine-insensitive calmodulin-independent microsomal (Ca^{2+} + Mg^{2+})-ATPase isolated from brain cortex (Malva et al. 1990), a finding that has been interpreted as the result of a direct interaction of this compound with the enzyme at the endoplasmic reticulum. All these evidences suggest that triphenylethylenes could affect cell proliferation through its ability to modulate CaM, a finding that might explain, at least in part, its cytostatic and cytocidal effects on ER(−) tumors and cell lines (Brandt et al. 2004; Fisher et al. 1983).

4.2.3.2
Protein Kinase C (PKC)

One of the most relevant targets for tamoxifen is PKC. These enzymes belong to a family of proteins that play crucial roles in signal transduction and cell growth control (Nishizuka 1992), and numerous studies have demonstrated that PKCs are involved in carcinogenesis and malignant transformations (Caponigro et al. 1997). Recently, in mammary carcinoma, PKC activity was found to be more than twice that found in normal breast tissue from the same patients (Boyan et al. 2003). Moreover, a high positive correlation between PKC activity and tumor severity has been demonstrated in breast cancer specimens, with the relationship being even greater in ER(−) tumors (Boyan et al. 2003). In fact, several PKC inhibitors, in combination with cytotoxic drugs, are being used in clinical trials for cancer treatment (Chen et al. 2003), though the precise role of the different PKC isoforms is not fully understood. Tamoxifen, its 4-OH or *N*-desmethyl metabolites, and clomiphene have been shown to reduce the activity of partially purified PKC and to inhibit the growth of several cell types in culture (O'Brian et al. 1986, 1988).

Tamoxifen has also been reported to inhibit classical PKC isoforms (α, $\beta 1$, $\beta 2$, and γ, which need calcium, phospholipids, and diacylglycerol (DG) for catalytic activity) in different preparations, both in vitro and in vivo (Horgan et al. 1986; O'Brian et al. 1986), and to induce the translocation of different PKC isoforms from the cytosol to the plasma membrane (Ahn et al. 2003; Cabot et al. 1997). The IC_{50} values for the inhibition of Ca^{2+}- and phospholipid-dependent PKC by 4-OH-tamoxifen and *N*-desmethyl-tamoxifen, the two main metabolites of tamoxifen, were 2 and 8 μM, respectively (O'Brian et al. 1986), which are well within the range of concentrations detected in plasma. The inhibitory effect of tamoxifen and its derivatives on PKC activity has been demonstrated in both ER(+) MCF-7 cells and ER(-) HCC38 cells, which is an indication that the blocking effect is ER independent. In agreement with this, triphenylethylenes have been shown to inhibit phorbol ester (PDBu) binding and it is competed for by MgATP. This provides strong evidence that triphenylethylenes can inhibit PKC by binding directly to the enzyme, likely to the ATP-binding region of the active site of the enzyme (O'Brian et al. 1986, 1988), though other reports are consistent with modulation of the catalytic site. Indeed, recent structure–activity studies have shown that the loss of a side chain in tamoxifen molecules triggers the ability of compounds to inhibit the catalytic site of PKC, whereas the absence of both the aminoethoxy side chain and the β-ring makes compounds activators of PKC (De Medina et al. 2004a) (Fig. 4.4).

4.2.3.3
Phospholipases and Lipid Signalling

Hyperactivation of phospholipase D (PLD) in certain tumor-derived cell lines have been reported, and recent findings suggest a role for PLD in transformation and metastasis. Elevated levels of PLD have been demonstrated in human breast cancer tissues (Noh et al. 2000) and human gastric carcinoma cells (Uchida et al. 1999). Furthermore, elevated PLD activity, specifically by the isoform PLD_2, was reported in human colon adenocarcinoma cells, human breast adenocarcinoma cells (Fiucci et al. 2000), and human renal cancers (Zhao et al. 2000). PLD catalyzes the hydrolysis of phosphatidylcholine (PC) to choline and phosphatidic acid (PA), which has been implicated in signalling cascades that regulate cell growth and metastasis (reviewed in Foster and Xu 2003). Hydrolysis of PA by phospholipase A2 generates the potent mitogen lysophosphatidic acid, whose serum levels have been shown to increase in correlation with the malignancy degree in ovarian cancer patients (Westermann et al. 1998). Interestingly, it has been shown that tamoxifen can stimulate cellular PLD activity through an ER-independent mechanism (Kiss 1994).

In CCD986SK human mammary fibroblasts, incubation with tamoxifen results in dose- and time-dependent increases in the cellular second messengers PA and diacylglycerol (DG) and activates PLD and phospholipase C (PLC) (Cabot et al. 1997). Moreover, the addition of tamoxifen to cultures elicits selective membrane association of PKCε (Cabot et al. 1997), indicating that tamoxifen exerts considerable extranuclear influence at the transmembrane signalling level. The proposed mechanism of this tamoxifen stimulation involves the PLD activator PKC. Using the ER+ mammary epithelial cell line MCF-12A and the ER highly tumorigenic mammary carcinoma cell line MDA-MB-23, it was recently demonstrated that tamoxifen and raloxifene have differential effects on PLD catalytic activity. Thus, tamoxifen stimulates PLD in both ER-positive and ER-negative cells in vivo and in vitro, whereas raloxifene inhibits PLD activity in these same cell types (Eisen and Brown 2002).

Other laboratories have reported that tamoxifen causes ER-independent stimulation of phosphatidylinositol kinase and phosphatidylinositol-4-phosphate kinase activities in GH4C1 cells, a rat pituitary adenoma cell line (Friedman 1994). These enzymes are normally product inhibited by the polyphosphoinositides. It has been suggested that tamoxifen binds to polyphosphoinositides, which thereby releases the kinases from product inhibition. Binding of tamoxifen to the polyphosphoinositides also leads to inhibition of phospholipase C (PLC) activity. Tamoxifen causes inhibition of inositol phosphate accumulation and phosphoinositide breakdown in whole GH4C1 cells in culture. No other enzymes of the phosphoinositide breakdown cascade are inhibited by this drug (Friedman 1994). These findings are interesting since increased concentrations of inositol triphosphate (IP_3) have been detected in hepatomas and numerous human carcinomas in both clinical samples and tissue culture cells, where the elevated signal transduction activity, as measured by the IP_3 concentration, was downregulated in a time- and dose-dependent fashion by tamoxifen (Weber et al. 1999).

Tamoxifen also releases arachidonic acid (AA) and stimulates prostacyclin (PGF1α) production from rat liver cells at micromolar concentrations (Levine 2003a). This ability of tamoxifen to release AA is rapid and not affected by preincubation with either actinomycin or the estrogen antagonist ICI182780, indicating its nongenomic nature (Levine 2003b). Since AA and tamoxifen have been associated with the induction of apoptosis (even in ER-negative cells), the induction of AA release by tamoxifen suggests a mechanism for cancer chemoprevention that does not require metabolism by cyclooxygenase (Levine 2003a).

4.2.3.4
Nitric Oxide

In the vascular system, nitric oxide (NO) is synthesized in the endothelium from L-arginine by endothelial nitric oxide synthase (eNOS) (Palmer et al. 1988). NO can diffuse rapidly to smooth muscles, causing relaxation via stimulation of soluble guanylate cyclase, followed by an increase in cyclic GMP (Rapoport et al. 1983) (Fig. 4.1). Subsequent activation of protein kinase G leads to phosphorylation of BK channels, which increases BK open probability and causes vasorelaxation (Patterson et al. 2002). A number of in vitro studies have demonstrated a direct relationship between SERMs (and estrogens) and acute activation of endothelial NO production (Kim et al. 1999; Simoncini and Genazzani 2000). Tamoxifen induces significant endothelium-dependent rapid relaxation in precontracted rabbit coronary arteries (Fig. 4.1). This relaxation is inhibited by the NO synthase inhibitor N^{ω}-nitro-L-arginine methyl ester (L-NAME) and also by the estrogen receptor antagonist ICI 182,780 (Figtree et al. 2000). Similar L-NAME-sensitive acute effects caused by toremifene on thoracic aorta (Gonzalez-Pérez and Crespo 2003) and by the novel tryphenylethylene SERM idoxifene have been observed in aortic and mesenteric tromboxane A_2-precontracted vessels (Christopher et al. 2002).

Benzothiphene SERMs have also been demonstrated to have an endothelium-dependent relaxing effect. In cultured human umbilical vein endothelial cells, clinically effective concentrations of raloxifene triggered a rapid and dose-dependent release of NO from endothelial cells (Simoncini and Genazzani 2000). Interestingly, raloxifene-induced NO production was abolished by the pure ER antagonist ICI 182,780, though it was not associated with changes in eNOS messenger RNA (Simoncini and Genazzani 2000). Indeed, raloxifene-induced NO production is due to an ER-dependent acute stimulation of eNOS enzymatic activity via a phosphatidylinositol 3-kinase (PI3K) pathway (Simoncini et al. 2002a). Similar ER- and NO-dependent vasodilation has been observed for raloxifene in coronary arteries (Figtree et al. 1999). These studies strongly argue in favor of raloxifene exerting a potentially important direct vasculoprotective effect by stimulating endothelial NO production.

Recently, it was found that EM-652 (acolbifene), a fourth-generation SERM exerting complete antiestrogenic effects on the breast and uterus, potently stimulates endothelial NO production in vitro and in vivo (Simoncini et al. 2002b). EM-652 triggers NO release by human umbilical vein endothelial cells through nongenomic mechanisms, rapidly activating eNOS via an ER-dependent sequential activation of MAPKs and PI3K/Akt pathways independently from gene transcription or protein synthesis. Moreover, EM-652 increases eNOS protein levels during prolonged treatment. Upon pharmacological comparison, EM-652 has been demonstrated to be markedly more potent than the SERMs raloxifene and tamoxifen in increasing NO synthesis from endothelial cells (Simoncini et al. 2002b).

4.2.4 Lipids, Membrane Lipids, and Fluidity

Triphenylethylene SERMs, like most anticancer drugs, are amphiphilic molecules of highly lipophilic character and likely to accumulate in membrane lipids and protein moieties. Experimental studies performed on artificial and biological membranes show that tamoxifen is enriched in lipid bilayers and affects both physical properties and composition (Custodio et al. 1993; Engelke et al. 2002; Wiseman et al. 1993). Thus, tamoxifen, 4-OH-tamoxifen, droloxifene (3-OH-tamoxifen), and other related compounds (such as 17-β-estradiol and cholesterol) inhibit metal-ion-dependent lipid peroxidation in liver microsomes and brain liposomes in vitro (Wiseman et al. 1992b). Nonetheless, the chemical structure of tamoxifen indicates that it is unlikely to act as a chain-breaking antioxidant because it does not possess easily donatable hydrogen atoms (Wiseman et al. 1992a). Instead, the beneficial antioxidant action of tamoxifen seems to be related to its role as membrane stabilizer against lipid peroxidation, via decreased membrane fluidity. Direct evidence exists that tamoxifen decreases membrane fluidity and increases the physical order of pure phospholipid liposomes, human cancer breast cells, and retinal epithelium (Custodio et al. 1993; Engelke et al. 2002; Wiseman et al. 1993). In addition, a good correlation has been found between decreased membrane fluidity and the antioxidant ability of tamoxifen (Wiseman et al. 1993). Computer molecular modeling indicates that this property of tamoxifen is shared by cholesterol, which stabilizes membranes via interactions between the rigid hydrophobic structure of cholesterol and the saturated, monounsaturated, and polyunsaturated fatty acid chain of phospholipids (Wiseman et al. 1992a).

These effects on cell membrane physicochemical properties could also explain some side effects of tamoxifen. For instance, there is clear evidence that tamoxifen, prescribed for long-term low-dose therapy of breast cancer, induces retinopathy (Pavlidis et al. 1992), although the underlying mechanisms are largely unknown. Recently, studies performed on human retinal pigment epithelial cell line D407 have provided evidence for the involvement of cellular membranes in the cytotoxic action mechanism (Engelke et al. 2002). Tamoxifen increases the physical order of the lipid bilayer in D407 cells, which is accompanied by a compensatory decrease in the cholesterol content of the plasma membrane. In intracellular membranes, phosphatidylcholine content is reduced to 50% of the controls, and this reduction may be related to the sustained activation of protein kinase C via the phospholipase C pathway. Since increased plasma membrane fluidity, as well as sustained activation of protein kinase C, influences the rod outer segment binding and/or ingestion by retinal pigment epithelial cells, these membrane-mediated pathways might contribute to the tamoxifen-induced retinopathy (Engelke et al. 2002).

The compensatory effect of cholesterol observed in D407 cells have also been demonstrated in other cell lines (Cho et al. 1998; Holleran et al. 1998) and may well be a consequence of tamoxifen-induced severe inhibition of lanosterol (to cholesterol)-converting enzymes. In rat liver preparations and CHO cells, sterol $\Delta 8$-isomerase ($IC_{50} \approx 0.21-0.15\,\mu M$) was the most sensitive lanosterol-converting enzymes to inhibition (which is noncompetitive) by tamoxifen. In these cells, inhibition of $\Delta 8$-isomerase activity was paralleled by a decreased rate of $[^{14}C]$-mevalonate incorporation into cholesterol (Cho et al. 1998). These findings might explain the fact that administration of tamoxifen to either humans or laboratory animals results in both a marked accumulation of sterol metabolites in serum and a drastic reduction in cholesterol. Clearly, these results provide important insights into the underlying mechanism(s) of tamoxifen's cardioprotective role by interfering with cholesterol biosynthesis by lanosterol in mammals.

Paralleling the acute effect of tamoxifen and metabolites on cholesterol biosynthesis, triphenylethylenes have been reported to protect against the progression of coronary artery diseases in human and different atherosclerosis animal models by blocking the appearance of the atheromatous plaque, though the precise molecular mechanisms of cardioprotective remain unknown. Recently, evidence for Acyl–CoA:cholesterol acyl transferase (ACAT) being a putative target for tamoxifen has been provided. ACAT catalyzes the biosynthesis of cholesteryl esters, which are the major lipids found in atheromatous plaque, using both long-chain coenzyme-A-activated fatty acids and cholesterol as substrates (Chang et al. 1997). Tamoxifen inhibits ACAT in a concentration-dependent manner on rat liver microsomal extract (De Medina et al. 2004b). More importantly, tamoxifen is able to inhibit ACAT on intact macrophages stimulated with acetylated low-density lipoproteins and block the formation of foam cells, a step that precedes the formation of the atheromatous plaque (De Medina et al. 2004b). Molecular modeling reveals that tamoxifen displays three-dimensional structural homology with Sah 58-035, a prototypical inhibitor of ACAT, and that the major structural element of tamoxifen responsible for this effect is the stilbene moiety present in the triphenylethylene backbone (De Medina et al. 2004a) (Fig. 4.4). This work constitutes the first evidence that tamoxifen is an inhibitor of ACAT and foam cell formation at therapeutic doses, and that this may account for its atheroprotective action.

The antioxidant effect of tamoxifen has also been postulated to underlie some beneficial cardiovascular effect of this and other SERMs. Oxidative damage of LDL plays an important role in the development of atherosclerosis, and it has been postulated that these highly lipophilic molecules stabilize LDL against lipid peroxidation by interaction between its hydrophobic rings and the polyunsaturated residues of the phospholipid layer of LDL (Resch et al. 2004; Wiseman 1994). In fact, tamoxifen (and more potently 4-OH-tamoxifen) and raloxifene can protect human LDL against Cu^{2+}-dependent lipid peroxidation (Resch et al. 2004; Wiseman 1994). Recent studies have demonstrated that the in vitro antioxidant activity of raloxifene on LDL in postmenopausal women is substantially more potent than that of tamoxifen or 17-β-estradiol (Arteaga et al. 2003).

4.2.5 Specific Antiestrogen-Binding Sites (AEBS)

The existence of specific antiestrogen binding sites was initially reported by Sutherland and coworkers in 1980 in the microsomal fraction of human mammary and endometrial carcinomas (Sutherland et al. 1980). Since then, AEBS have been found in microsomes from most normal and tumorigenic tissues and cells investigated (Jordan and Murphy 1990; Lazier and Bapat 1988) including ER(–) cells (Mehta and DasGupta 1987). Such AEBS correspond to high-affinity (Kd $\approx$ 1 nM for tamoxifen in rat uterus), saturable binding sites that do not bind estradiol or ICI182,780 or ICI164,384 but compounds that retain both a basic aminoether side chain and a di- or tricyclic aromatic ring structure (De Medina et al. 2004a; Watts and Sutherland 1987) (Fig. 4.4). This shows that the important feature for tamoxifen binding to the AEBS is the presence of a dimethylmethano moiety linked to the aminoethoxy side chain (De Medina et al. 2004a) (Fig. 4.4). Such structure–activity relationship outcomes have prompted the development of selective AEBS ligands such as 1-Benzyl-4-(*N*-2-pyrrolidinylethoxy)benzene · HCl (PBPE) or 4-(2-morpholinoethoxy) benzophenone (MBoPE), which has been used to demonstrate that these binding sites are membranous multiproteic complexes that require phospholipids to bind tamoxifen (Kedjouar et al. 2004; Mesange et al. 2002). These studies provide strong evidence that AEBSs are hetero-oligomeric complexes including, among others, carboxylesterase ES-10, liver fatty acid binding protein (FABP), epoxide hydrolase mEH, 3β-hydroxysterol-Δ^8-Δ^7-isomerase, and the 3β-hydroxysterol-Δ^7-reductase as subunits (reviewed in De Medina et al. 2004a). The latter two proteins are necessary and sufficient for tamoxifen binding in mammary cells (Kedjouar et al. 2004). Altogether, these data indicate that AEBSs are enzymatically linked to cholesterol metabolism at a postlanosterol step under acute regulation by triphenylethylene antiestrogens. Furthermore, because selective AEBS ligands are antitumoral compounds, these data suggest a link between cholesterol metabolism and tumor growth control (De Medina et al. 2004b).

4.3
Final Considerations

Since the introduction in the early 1980s of tamoxifen, the first SERM used in clinical therapeutics, evidence has steadily grown that this compound is able to affect biochemical processes other than interacting, either in an agonistic or antagonistic manner, with intracellular ERs. Similarly, tamoxifen metabolites (4-OH-tamoxifen and *N*-desmethyltamoxifen), as well as other triphenylethylene derivatives, share many of the pleiotropic actions of tamoxifen. It seems now that benzothiphene derivatives led by raloxifene or LY156,758, as representatives of another class chemically different from SERMs, can also trigger acute effects in different molecular models. In general, these acute actions are non-ER-mediated and nongenomically transduced and take place with a short delay after exposure to SERMs. More importantly, we have emphasized the fact that these nongenomic actions take place at concentrations that fall within the low micromolar and submicromolar ranges, as indicated by the EC_{50} or IC_{50} values reported by different laboratories.

Continual administration of therapeutic doses of tamoxifen (about 40 mg daily as adjuvant for breast cancer) gives serum concentrations that increase linearly with tamoxifen intake, averaging 4–6 μM at the higher dose levels (Trump et al. 1992). Moreover, tamoxifen is a lipophilic compound, meaning its concentration in plasma membranes may be even higher than in serum. In fact, tissue concentration of tamoxifen is approximately 10- to 60-fold higher than in serum (Lien et al. 1991). These observations strengthen the notion that acute nongenomic effects of triphenylethylene and benzothiphene SERMS reviewed here are therapeutically and clinically relevant. Indeed, as we have discussed, some of these demonstrated effects account satisfactorily for both beneficial (i.e., vasorelaxation) and undesirable side effects (i.e., ocular toxicity) reported in individuals receiving different pharmacological therapies based on SERMs. Undoubtedly, these experimental and epidemiological observations will support the rationale for the design and development of new function- and tissue-specific SERMs.

In this sense, we have observed that, unlike tamoxifen, the quaternary derivative ethylbromide tamoxifen fails to block volume-sensitive chloride channels (as those found in lens fibers) in HeLa and C1300 neuroblastoma cells (unpublished data). Likewise, ethylbromide tamoxifen is totally ineffective on delayed rectifier K^+ channels in NG108-15 cells, while tamoxifen is a potent reversible blocker (Allen et al. 2000). From this point of view, nonpermeant SERM derivatives are useful pharmacological tools for investigating whether binding sites in membrane targets are located in the extracellular domains of membrane proteins or, because they can partition into the membrane, interact at some level within the lipid bilayers.

As a final remark, though the spectrum of acute actions induced by SERMs from in vitro assays is considerable, it is widely assumed, and has been clinically proven, that tamoxifen toxicity is generally low. Several reasons can be advanced to account for the apparent discrepancy between in vivo and in vitro data. The concentrations of an unbound drug are likely to be different, and insufficient, in tissues and cells that, like nerve cells, have limited access to circulating plasma molecules. This observation could explain the low incidence of neurological disorders in patients under tamoxifen treatments, in spite of proven inhibitory in vitro effects found in critical voltage-dependent Na^+ and K^+ channels as well as neurotransmitter receptor cationic channels (see above). Furthermore, SERMs are protein bound in serum, and even in vitro the presence of serum proteins (like albumin and AAG) reduces the effectiveness of SERMs. Nevertheless, accumulation will occur after time, especially in long-term therapies, and therefore appropriate concentrations are likely to be reached.

Acknowledgements

Work from the authors' laboratories has been supported by Grants SAF2001-3614-C03-01, SAF2001-3614-C03-02, and SAF2004-08316-C02-01 (Ministerio de Ciencia y Tecnología, Spain), PI2003/098 and PI2003/153 (Gobierno de Canarias, Spain), PI042640 (Instituto de Salud Carlos III, Spain), and from the Spanish Network of Neurological Research (CIEN, ISCIII-C03/06). R.M. is a fellow of the "Ramon y Cajal" Programme (Ministerio de Ciencia y Tecnología, Spain).

References

1. Ahn SJ, Yoon MS, Hyuk S, Han W, Yoon YD, Han JS, Noh DY (2003) Phospholipase C-protein kinase C mediated phospholipase D activation pathway is involved in tamoxifen induced apoptosis. J Cell Biochem 89(3):520–528
2. Allen MC, Gale PA, Hunter AC, Lloyd A, Hardy SP (2000) Membrane impermeant antioestrogens discriminate between ligand- and voltage-gated cation channels in NG108–15 cells. Biochim Biophys Acta 1509(1–2):229–236
3. Allen MC, Newland C, Valverde MA, Hardy SP (1998) Inhibition of ligand-gated cation-selective channels by tamoxifen. Eur J Pharmacol 354(2–3):261–269
4. Al-Shawi MK, Polar MK, Omote H, Figler RA (2003) Transition state analysis of the coupling of drug transport to ATP hydrolysis by P-glycoprotein. J Biol Chem 278(52):52629–52640
5. Arteaga E, Villaseca P, Bianchi M, Rojas A, Marshall G (2003) Raloxifene is a better antioxidant of low-density lipoprotein than estradiol or tamoxifen in postmenopausal women in vitro. Menopause 10(2):142–146
6. Batra S (1990) Interaction of antiestrogens with binding sites for muscarinic cholinergic drugs and calcium channel blockers in cell membranes. Cancer Chemother Pharmacol 26:310–312

7. Ben-Baruch G, Schreiber G, Sokolovsky M (1982) Cooperativity pattern in the interaction of the antiestrogen drug clomiphene with the muscarinic receptors. Mol Pharmacol 21:287–293
8. Berman E, McBride M, Tong W (1994) Comparative activity of tamoxifen and *N*-desmethyltamoxifen in human multidrug resistant leukemia cell lines. Leukemia 8(7):1191–1196
9. Borras M, Jin L, Bouhoute A, Legros N, Leclerck G (1994) Evaluation of estrogen receptor, antiestrogen binding sites and calmodulin for antiestrogen resistance of two clones derived from the MCF-7 breast cancer cell line. Biochem Pharmacol 48:2015–2024
10. Boyan BD, Sylvia VL, Frambach T, Lohmann CH, Dietl J, Dean DD, Schwartz Z (2003) Estrogen-dependent rapid activation of protein kinase C in estrogen receptor-positive MCF-7 breast cancer cells and estrogen receptor-negative HCC38 cells is membrane-mediated and inhibited by tamoxifen. Endocrinology 144(5):1812–1824
11. Brandes LJ, Bogdanovic RP, Cawker MD, LaBella FS (1987) Histamine and growth: interaction of antiestrogen binding site ligands with a novel histamine site that may be associated with calcium channels. Cancer Res 47(15):4025–4031
12. Brandt S, Heller H, Schuster KD, Grote J (2004) Tamoxifen induces suppression of cell viability and apoptosis in the human hepatoblastoma cell line HepG2 via down-regulation of telomerase activity. Liver Int 24(1):46–54
13. Braybrooke JP, Vallis KA, Houlbrook S, Rockett H, Ellmen J, Anttila M, Ganesan TS, Harris AL, Talbot DC (2000) Evaluation of toremifene for reversal of multidrug resistance in renal cell cancer patients treated with vinblastine. Cancer Chemother Pharmacol 46(1):27–34
14. Cabot MC, Zhang Z, Cao H, Lavie Y, Giuliano AE, Han TY, Jones RC (1997) Tamoxifen activates cellular phospholipase C and D and elicits protein kinase C translocation. Int J Cancer 70(5):567–574
15. Cantabrana B, Hidalgo A (1992) Effects of nonsteroidal antiestrogens in the in vitro rat uterus. Pharmacology 45:329–337
16. Caponigro F, French RC, Kaye SB (1997) Protein kinase C: a worthwhile target for anticancer drugs? Anticancer drugs 8:26–33
17. Caroni P, Carafoli E (1981) Regulation of Ca^{2+}-pumping ATPase of heart sarcolemma by a phosphorylation-dephosphorylation process. J Biol Chem 256:3262–3270
18. Chan Y, Leung F, Yao X, Lau C, Vanhoutte PM, Huang Y (2004) Raloxifene relaxes rat pulmonary arteries and veins: roles of gender, endothelium and antagonism of Ca^{2+} influx. J Pharmacol Exp Therap
19. Chatterjee M, Harris AL (1990) Reversal of acquired resistance to adriamycin in CHO cells by tamoxifen and 4-hydroxy tamoxifen: role of drug interaction with alpha 1 acid glycoprotein. Br J Cancer 62(5):712–717
20. Cho SY, Kim JH, Paik YK (1998) Cholesterol biosynthesis from lanosterol: differential inhibition of sterol delta 8-isomerase and other lanosterol-converting enzymes by tamoxifen. Mol Cells 8(2):233–239
21. Christopher TA, Lopez BL, Stillwagon JC, Gao F, Gao E, Ma XL, Ohlstein EH, Yue TL (2002) Idoxifene causes endothelium-dependent, nitric oxide-mediated vasorelaxation in male rats. Eur J Pharmacol 446(1–3):139–143
22. Custodio JB, Almeida LM, Madeira VM (1993) The active metabolite hydroxytamoxifen of the anticancer drug tamoxifen induces structural changes in membranes. Biochim Biophys Acta 1153(2):308–314
23. Da Costa LS, de Oliveira MA, Rubim VS, Wajngarten M, Aldrighi JM, Rosano GM, Neto CD, Gebara OC (2004) Effects of hormone replacement therapy or raloxifene on am-

bulatory blood pressure and arterial stiffness in treated hypertensive postmenopausal women. Am J Cardiol 94(11):1453–1456
24. De Medina P, Favre G, Poirot M (2004a) Multiple targeting by the antitumor drug tamoxifen: a structure-activity study. Curr Med Chem Anti-Cancer Agents 4(6):491–508
25. De Medina P, Payré BL, Bernad J, Bosser I, Pipy B, Silvente-Poirot S, Favre G, Faye JC, Poirot M (2004b) Tamoxifen is a potent inhibitor of cholesterol esterification and prevents the formation of foam cells. J Pharmacol Exp Ther 308:1165–1173
26. De Ponti F, Poluzzi E, Montanaro N (2000) QT-interval prolongation by non-cardiac drugs: lessons to be learned from recent experience. Eur J Clin Pharmacol 56:1–18
27. Díaz M (1996) Volume-activated chloride channels in neuroblastoma cells are blocked by the antiestrogen toremifene. Cell Mol Neurobiol 16(3):403–409
28. Díaz M (1999) Modulation of Maxi Cl^- channels by oestrogens and antioestrogens. J Physiol 517P:7S
29. Díaz M, Bahamonde MI, Lock H, Muñoz F, Hardy SP, Posas F, Valverde MA (2001) Okadaic acid-sensitive activation of Maxi Cl^- channels by triphenylethylene antiestrogens in C1300 neuroblastoma cells. J Physiol 536(1):79–88
30. Díaz M (2002) Triphenylethylene antiestrogen-induced acute relaxation of mouse duodenal muscle. Possible involvement of calcium channels. Eur J Pharmacol 445:257–266
31. Dick GM, Hunter AC, Sanders KM (2002) Ethylbromide tamoxifen, a membrane-impermeant antiestrogen, activates smooth muscle calcium-activated large-conductance potassium channels from the extracellular side. Mol Pharmacol 61(5):1105–1113
32. Dick GM, Kong ID, Sanders KM (1999) Effects of anion channel antagonists in canine colonic myocytes: comparative pharmacology of Cl^-, Ca^{2+} and K^+ currents. Br J Pharmacol 127:1819–1831
33. Dick GM, Rossow CF, Smirnov S, Horowitz B, Sanders KM (2001) Tamoxifen activates smooth muscle BK channels through the regulatory beta 1 subunit. J Biol Chem 276:34594–34599
34. Eisen SF, Brown HA (2002) Selective estrogen receptor (ER) modulators differentially regulate phospholipase D catalytic activity in ER-negative breast cancer cells. Mol Pharmacol 62(4):911–920
35. Engelke M, Tykhonova S, Zorn-Kruppa M, Diehl H (2002) Tamoxifen induces changes in the lipid composition of the retinal pigment epithelium cell line D407. Pharmacol Toxicol 91(1):13–21
36. Falkenstein E, Tillmann HC, Christ M, Feuring M, Wehling M (2000) Multiple actions of steroid hormones-a focus on rapid, nongenomic effects. Pharmacol Rev 52:513–556
37. Fanidi A, Courion-Guichardaz C, Fayard JM, Pageaux JF, Laugier C (1989) Effects of tamoxifen, tamoxifen metabolites, and nafoxidine on adenosine 3′,5′-monophosphate phosphodiesterase: correlations with growth inhibitory activities but not estrogen receptor affinities. Endocrinology 125:1187–1193
38. Fernández A, Cantabrana B, Hidalgo A (1993) Estrogen and antiestrogen non-genomic effect in rat uterus contraction in calcium-free solution. Gen Pharmacol 24(2):391–395
39. Figtree G, Webb C, Collins P (1999) Raloxifene acutely relaxes rabbit coronary arteries in vitro by an estrogen receptor-dependent and nitric oxide-dependent mechanism. Circulation 100:1095–1101
40. Figtree G, Webb C, Collins P (2000) Tamoxifen acutely relaxes coronary arteries by an endothelium, nitric oxide and estrogen receptor-dependent mechanism. J Pharmacol Exp Ther 295:519–523

41. Fisher B, Redmond C, Brown A, Wickerham DL, Wolmark N, Allegra J, Escher G, Lippman M, Savlov E, Wittliff J, et al. (1983) Influence of tumor estrogen and progesterone receptor levels on the response to tamoxifen and chemotherapy in primary breast cancer. J Clin Oncol 1(4):227–241
42. Fiucci G, Czarny M, Lavie Y, Zhao D, Berse B, Blusztajn JK, Liscovitch M (2000) Changes in phospholipase D isoform activity and expression in multidrug-resistant human cancer cells. Int J Cancer 85:882–888
43. Foster DA, Xu L (2003) Phospholipase D in cell proliferation and cancer. Mol Cancer Res 1(11):789–800
44. Friedman ZY (1994) The antitumor agent tamoxifen inhibits breakdown of polyphosphoinositides in GH4C1 cells. J Pharmacol Exp Ther 271(1):238–245
45. Gelband CH, Greco PG, Martens JR (1996) Voltage-dependent chloride channels: invertebrates to man. J Exp Zool 275(4):277–282
46. Gerner EW (1992) Ocular toxicity of tamoxifen. Ann Ophthalmol 21:420–423
47. Gonzalez-Perez J, Crespo MJ (2003) Acute effects of toremifene on the vasculature of intact and menopause-induced rats. Vascul Pharmacol 40(4):205–211
48. Greenberg DA, Carpenter CL, Messing RO (1987) Calcium channel antagonist properties of the antineoplastic antiestrogen tamoxifen in the PC12 neurosecretory cells. Cancer Res 47:70–74
49. Hardcastle IR, Rowlands MG, Houghton J, Parr IB, Potter GA, Jarman M, Edwards KJ, Laughton CA, Trent JO, Neidle S (1995) Rationally designed analogues of tamoxifen with improved calmodulin antagonism. J Med Chem 38:241–248
50. Hardy SP, Valverde MA (1994) Novel plasma membrane action of estrogen and antiestrogens revealed by their regulation of a large conductance chloride channel. FASEB J 8(10):760–765
51. Hardy SP, deFelipe C, Valverde MA (1998) Inhibition of voltage-gated cationic channels in rat embryonic hypothalamic neurones and C1300 neuroblastoma cells by triphenylethylene antioestrogens. FEBS Lett 434(3):236–240
52. He J, Kargacin ME, Kargacin GJ, Ward CA (2003) Tamoxifen inhibits Na^+ and K^+ currents in rat ventricular myocytes. Am J Physiol 285(2):H661–H668
53. Hiemke C, Ghraf R (1984) Interaction of non-steroidal antiestrogens with dopamine receptor binding. J Steroid Biochem 21:663–667
54. Holleran AL, Lindenthal B, Aldaghlas TA, Kelleher JK (1998) Effect of tamoxifen on cholesterol synthesis in HepG2 cells and cultured rat hepatocytes. Metabolism 47(12):1504–1513
55. Horgan K, Cooke E, Hallett MB, Mansel RE (1986) Inhibition of protein kinase C mediated signal transduction by tamoxifen: importance for antitumour activity. Biochem Pharmacol 35(24):4463–4465
56. Jordan VC, Murphy CS (1990) Endocrine pharmacology of antiestrogens as antitumor agents. Endocr Rev 11(4):578–610
57. Kahl CR, Means AR (2003) Regulation of cell cycle progression by calcium/calmodulin-dependent pathways. Endocr Rev 24:719–736
58. Kedjouar B, de Medina P, Oulad-Abdelghani M, Payre B, Silvente-Poirot S, Favre G, Faye JC, Poirot M (2004) Molecular characterization of the microsomal tamoxifen binding site. J Biol Chem 279(32):34048–34061
59. Kim HP, Lee JY, Jeong JK, Bae SW, Lee HK, Jo I (1999) Nongenomic stimulation of nitric oxide release by estrogen is mediated by estrogen receptor alpha localized in caveolae. Biochem Biophys Res Commun 263(1):257–262
60. Kiss Z (1994) Tamoxifen stimulates phospholipase D activity by an estrogen receptor-independent mechanism. FEBS Lett 355:173–177

61. Kroeger EA, Brandes LJ (1985) Evidence that tamoxifen is a histamine antagonist. Biochem Biophys Res Commun 131(2):750–755
62. Lam HY (1984) Tamoxifen is a calmodulin antagonist in the activation of cAMP phosphodiesterase. Biochem Biophys Res Commun 118:27–32
63. La Porte DC, Wierman BM, Store DR (1980) Calcium-induced exposure of a hydrophobic surface on calmodulin. Biochemistry 19:3814–3819
64. Lazier CB, Bapat BV (1988) Antiestrogen binding sites: general and comparative properties. J Steroid Biochem 4B:665–669
65. Levine L (2003a) Does the release of arachidonic acid from cells play a role in cancer chemoprevention? FASEB J 17(8):800–802
66. Levine L (2003b) Tamoxifen stimulates arachidonic acid release from rat liver cells by an estrogen receptor-independent, non-genomic mechanism. BMC Cancer 3(1):24
67. Li J, Xu LZ, Yao JJ, Guo WJ, Xia P, Chen Y (2001a) Reversal effects of droloxifene on multidrug resistance in adriamycin-resistant K562 cell line. Acta Pharmacol Sin 22(11):1023–1027
68. Li Z, Joyal JL, Sacks BD (2001b) Calmodulin enhances the stability of the estrogen receptor. J Biol Chem 276:17354–17360
69. Lien EA, Solheim E, Ueland PM (1991) Distribution of tamoxifen and its metabolites in rat and human tissues during steady-state treatment. Cancer Res 51:4837–4844
70. Ling V (1997) Multidrug resistance: molecular mechanisms and clinical relevance. Cancer Chemother Pharmacol 40(Suppl):S3–S8
71. Lipton A, Vinijsanun A, Martin L (1984) Acute inhibition of rat myometrial responses to oxytocin by tamoxifen stereoisomers and oestradiol. J Endocrinol 103(3):383–388
72. Lipton A (1987) The anti-oestrogen tamoxifen is a calcium antagonist in perfused rat mesentery. Cancer Chemother Pharmacol 20:125–127
73. Liu XK, Katchman A, Ebert SN, Woosley RL (1998) The antiestrogen tamoxifen blocks the delayed rectifier potassium current, IKr, in rabbit ventricular myocytes. J Pharmacol Exp Ther 287:877–883
74. Lopes MCF, Vale MGP, Carvalho AP (1990) Ca^{2+}-dependent binding of tamoxifen to calmoduline isolated from bovine brain. Cancer Res 50:2753–2758
75. Lucci A, Giuliano AE, Han TY, Dinur T, Liu YY, Senchenkov A, Cabot MC (1999) Ceramide toxicity and metabolism differ in wild-type and multidrug-resistant cancer cells. Int J Oncol 15(3):535–540
76. Malva JO, Lopes MCF, Vale MGP, Carvalho AP (1990) Actions of antiestrogens on the (Ca^{2+} + Mg^{2+})-ATPase and Na^{+}/Ca2 + exchange of brain cortex membranes. Biochem Pharmacol 40:1877–1884
77. Mansouri A, Henle KJ, Nagle WA (1992) Multidrug resistance: prospects for clinical management. SAAS Bull Biochem Biotechnol 5:48–52
78. Marrero-Alonso J, García Marrero B, Gomez T, Diaz M (2005) Functional inhibition of intestinal and uterine muscles by non-permeant triphenylethylene derivatives. Eur J Pharmacol (in press)
79. Mehta RR, DasGupta TK (1987) Antiestrogen binding sites in microsomal fractions of malignant and nonmalignant human breast tissues. Breast Cancer Res Treat 9(1):61–67
80. Mesange F, Sebbar M, Capdevielle J, Guillemot JC, Ferrara P, Bayard F, Poirot M, Faye JC (2002) Identification of two tamoxifen target proteins by photolabeling with 4-(2-morpholinoethoxy)benzophenone. Bioconjug Chem 13(4):766–772
81. Nadal A, Díaz M, Valverde MA (2001) The estrogen trinity: membrane, cytosolic, and nuclear effects. News Physiol Sci 16:251–255
82. Nishizuka Y (1992) Intracellular signaling by hydrolysis of phospholipids and activation of protein kinase C. Science 258:607–614

83. Noh DY, Ahn SJ, Lee RA, Park IA, Kim JH, Suh PG, Ryu SH, Lee KH, Han JS (2000) Overexpression of phospholipase D1 in human breast cancer tissues. Cancer Lett 161:207–214
84. O'Brian CA, Liskamp RM, Solomon DH, Weinstein IB (1986) Inhibition of protein kinase C by tamoxifen. Cancer Res 45:2462–2465
85. O'Brian CA, Ward NE, Anderson BW (1988) Role of specific interactions between protein kinase C and triphenylethylenes in inhibition of the enzyme. J Natl Cancer Inst 80(20):1628–1633
86. Palmer RMJ, Ashton DS, Moncada S (1988) Vascular endothelial cells synthesize nitric oxide from L-arginine. Nature 333:664–666
87. Patterson AJ, Henrie-Olson J, Brenner R (2002) Vasoregulation at the molecular level: a role for the beta1 subunit of the calcium-activated potassium (BK) channel. Trends Cardiovascul Med 12(2):78–82
88. Pavlidis NA, Petris C, Briassoulis E, Klouvas G, Psilas C, Rempapis J, Petroutsos G (1992) Clear evidence that long-term, low-dose tamoxifen treatment can induce ocular toxicity: a prospective study of 63 patients. Cancer 69(12):2961–2964
89. Pollack IF, DaRosso RC, Robertson PL, Jakacki RL, Mirro JR, Blatt J, Nicholson S, Packer RJ, Allen JC, Cisneros A, Jordan VC (1997) A phase I study of high-dose tamoxifen for the treatment of refractory malignant gliomas of childhood. Clin Cancer Res 3:1109–1115
90. Rao US, Fine RL, Scarborough GA (1994) Antiestrogens and steroid hormones: substrates of the human P-glycoprotein. Biochem Pharmacol 48(2):287–292
91. Rapoport RM, Draznin MB, Murad F (1983) Endothelium-dependent relaxation in rat aorta may be mediated through cyclic GMP-dependent protein phosphorylation. Nature 306:174–176
92. Ratz PH, MacCammon KA, Altstatt D, Blackmore PF, Shenfeld OZ, Schlossberg SM (1999) Differential effects of sex hormones and phystoestrogens on peak and steady state contractions in isolated rabbit detrusor. J Urol 162:1821–1828
93. Rowlands MG, Parr IB, McCague R, Jarman M, Goddard PM (1990) Variation of the inhibition of calmodulin dependent cyclic AMP phosphodiesterase amongst analogues of tamoxifen: correlations with cytotoxicity. Biochem Pharmacol 40:283–289
94. Sartor P, Vacher P, Mollard P, Dufy B (1988) Tamoxifen reduces calcium currents in a clonal pituitary cell line. Endocrinology 123:534–540
95. Simoncini T, Genazzani AR (2000) Raloxifene acutely stimulates nitric oxide release from human endothelial cells via an activation of endothelial nitric oxide synthase. J Clin Endocrinol Metab 85(8):2966–2969
96. Simoncini T, Genazzani AR, Liao JK (2002a) Nongenomic mechanisms of endothelial nitric oxide synthase activation by the selective estrogen receptor modulator raloxifene. Circulation 105:1368–1373
97. Simoncini T, Varone G, Fornari L, Mannella P, Luisi M, Labrie F, Genazzani AR (2002b) Genomic and nongenomic mechanisms of nitric oxide synthesis induction in human endothelial cells by a fourth-generation selective estrogen receptor modulator. Endocrinology 143(6):2052–2061
98. Smitherman KA, Sontheimer H (2001) Inhibition of glial Na^+ and K^+ currents by tamoxifen. J Memb Biol 181:125–135
99. Song J, Standley PR, Zhang F, Joshi D, Gappy S, Sowers JR, Ram JL (1996) Tamoxifen (estrogen antagonist) inhibits voltage-gated calcium current and contractility in vascular smooth muscle from rats. J Pharmacol Exp Ther 277:1444–1453

100. Sutherland RL, Murphy LC, San Foo M, Green MD, Whybourne AM, Krozowski ZS (1980) High-affinity anti-oestrogen binding site distinct from the oestrogen receptor. Nature 288(5788):273–275
101. Chen TC, Su S, Fry D, Liebes L (2003) Combination therapy with irinotecan and protein kinase C inhibitors in malignant glioma. Cancer 97:2363–2373
102. Trump DL, Smith DC, Ellis PG, Rogers MP, Schold SC, Winer EP, Panella TJ, Jordan VC, Fine RL (1992) High-dose oral tamoxifen, a potential multidrug-resistance-reversal agent: Phase I trial in combination with vinblastine. J Natl Cancer Inst 84:1811–1816
103. Tsang SY, Yao X, Essin K, Wong CM, Chan FL, Gollasch M, Huang Y (2004) Raloxifene relaxes rat cerebral arteries in vitro and inhibits L-type voltage-sensitive Ca^{2+} channels. Stroke 35(7):1709–1714
104. Uchida N, Okamura S, Kuwano H (1999) Phospholipase D activity in human gastric carcinoma. Anticancer Res 19:671–675
105. Valverde MA, Hardy SP, Diaz M (2002) Activation of Maxi Cl^- channels by antiestrogens and phenothiazines in NIH3T3 fibroblasts. Steroids 67(6):439–445
106. Valverde MA, Mintenig GM, Sepulveda FV (1993) Differential effects of tamoxifen and I- on three distinguishable chloride currents activated in T84 intestinal cells. Pflügers Arch 425(5–6):552–554
107. Valverde MA, Rojas P, Amigo J, Cosmelli D, Orio P, Bahamonde MI, Mann G, Vergara C, Latorre R (1999) Acute activation of Maxi-K channels (Hslo) by estradiol binding to the β subunit. Science 285:1929–1931
108. Watts CK, Sutherland RL (1987) Studies on the ligand specificity and potential identity of microsomal antiestrogen-binding sites. Mol Pharmacol 31:541–551
109. Weber G, Shen F, Yang H, Prajda N, Li W (1999) Regulation of signal transduction activity in normal and cancer cells. Anticancer Res 19(5A):3703–3709
110. Westermann AM, Havik E, Postma FR, Beijnen JH, Dalesio O, Moolenaar WH, Rodenhuis S (1998) Malignant effusions contain lysophosphatidic acid (LPA)-like activity. Ann Oncol 9:437–442
111. Wiseman H, Cannon M, Arnstein HR, Barlow DJ (1992a) The structural mimicry of membrane sterols by tamoxifen: evidence from cholesterol coefficients and molecular-modelling for its action as a membrane anti-oxidant and an anti-cancer agent. Biochim Biophys Acta 1138(3):197–202
112. Wiseman H, Quinn P, Halliwell B (1993) Tamoxifen and related compounds decrease membrane fluidity in liposomes: mechanism for the antioxidant action of tamoxifen and relevance to its anticancer and cardioprotective actions? FEBS Lett 330(1):53–56
113. Wiseman H, Smith C, Halliwell B, Cannon M, Arnstein HR, Lennard MS (1992b) Droloxifene (3-hydroxytamoxifen) has membrane antioxidant ability: potential relevance to its mechanism of therapeutic action in breast cancer. Cancer Lett 66(1):61–68
114. Wiseman H (1994) Tamoxifen: new membrane-mediated mechanisms of action and therapeutic advances. Trends Pharmacol Sci 15(3):83–89
115. Zhang JJ, Jacob TJC, Valverde MA, Hardy SP, Mintenig GM, Sepúlveda FV, Gill DR, Hyde SC, Trezise AEO, Higgins CF (1994) Tamoxifen blocks chloride channels: a possible mechanism for cataract formation. J Clin Invest 94:1690–1697
116. Zhao Y, Ehara H, Akao Y, Shamoto M, Nakagawa Y, Banno Y, Deguchi T, Ohishi N, Yagi K, Nozawa Y (2000) Increased activity and intranuclear expression of phospholipase D2 in human renal cancer. Biochem Biophys Res Commun 278:140–143
117. Resch U, Mellauner V, Budinsky A, Sinzinger H (2004) Inhibition of low-density lipoprotein and high-density lipoprotein oxidation by raloxifene. J Womens Health (Larchmt) 13(4):404–11

The Hypothalamus-Pituitary-Ovarian Axis as a Model System for the Study of SERM Effects: An Overview of Experimental and Clinical Studies

R. Alonso · F. Marín · M. González · P. Guelmes · C. Bellido ·
G. Hernández · R. Marín · M. Díaz · J.E. Sánchez-Criado

5.1 Introduction

Female reproductive function depends on the coordinated activity of different brain areas and peripheral organs, finally leading to pregnancy and delivery. These include the hypothalamus, the anterior pituitary, the ovaries, and the uterus. During reproductive age, oocytes mature and are released from the ovaries in a cyclic manner in response to a neural signal. Central in the control of female reproduction is the feedback action of the ovarian hormones estradiol and progesterone, which act at different levels of the reproductive system through specific receptors and modulate the activity of a wide variety of cell types. Therefore, although the primary control of female reproductive cycles arises from the brain, it is actually the ovary that controls its own function by cyclically secreting estradiol and progesterone, which in turn feed back at different levels of the system (Freeman 1994; Hotchkiss and Knobill 1994).

In all sex-steroid-responding tissues, the magnitude and type of response are determined by the relative population of specific steroid hormone receptors and their space-temporal expression pattern (Conneely 2001). In the classical model of steroid hormone action, cell response to a particular hormone depends upon different receptor subtypes and the presence of a constellation of proteins that act in complexes as coactivators, corepressors, and coregulators and whose interactions after hormone-receptor binding induce either an increment or an inhibition of gene transcription (Tsai and O'Malley 1994; McKenna et al. 1999; Glass and Rosenfeld 2000; Smith and O'Malley 2004). In the case of estrogen receptors (ERs), two main subtypes, ERα and ERβ, encoded by two different genes have been identified (Kuiper et al. 1996; Couse and Korach 1999).

During the last decade, the development of animal models with selective ablation of specific genes has allowed the identification of physiological responses associated with each receptor subtype, as well as their complementarity in the regulation of reproductive function (Lubahn et al. 1993; Krege et al. 1998; Dupont et al. 2000). In addition, a large number of recent reports have shown that in a variety of tissue and cell types sex steroids are also able to interact with specific binding sites at the plasma membrane to activate different, highly coordinated signaling pathways (Nadal et al. 2001; Morales et al. 2003; Guerra et al. 2004; Marín et al. 2005). To add more complexity, ERs can be activated either by the cognate ligand or, in some tissues, in a ligand-independent manner (Demay et al. 2001; Blaustein 2004). These findings explain the wide spectrum of estrogen physiological actions, as well as the diverse repertoire of responses to either endogenously or exogenously administered steroid molecules in a given organism (Conneely 2001; McDonnell 2003). Furthermore, the variety of estrogen actions and the potential beneficial effects of this sex hormone on a number of tissues, in addition to the reproductive system, has opened a fascinating field of pharmacological development (McDonnell 2003). As described in other parts of this book, selective estrogen receptor modulators (SERMs) are compounds that can interact with ERs and act either as estrogen agonists or antagonists, depending on the tissue and the cellular environment (McDonnell 1999; McDonnell et al. 2002; Smith and O'Malley 2004). Due to the development of SERMs, pharmacology is now growing up in the context of modern hormone therapy (Turgeon et al. 2004), and there is a need to analyze the potential effects of these compounds on different levels of the female reproductive system. In this chapter we attempt to discuss results from our and other laboratories regarding the effects of SERMs on the hypothalamus-pituitary system of female rats or tissue explants. In addition, we have reviewed most relevant clinical findings in women treated with different SERMs. Because of the complexity of this subject and to avoid undesirable confusion, we have focused on the functional unit formed by gonadotropin releasing hormone (GnRH) secreted by hypothalamic neurons and gonadotropins secreted by the anterior pituitary.

5.2 Hypothalamus-Pituitary-Ovarian Axis of Mammals

5.2.1 General Aspects

During follicular development and while circulating levels of ovarian hormones are reduced, basal secretion of gonadotropins, follicle stimulating hormone (FSH), and luteinizing hormone (LH) determine both maturation of granulose cells and production of steroid hormones. A gradual rise in ovarian hormone levels exerts several coordinated actions at different levels of the reproductive axis (Fink 1988). On one hand, estrogen exerts a negative feedback effect on gonadotropin secretion by acting both at the hypothalamus and the anterior pituitary, which partially prevents the development of additional follicles during a cycle. At the same time, estrogen stimulates its own secretion by granulose cells, which allows continuous follicular steroid hormone secretion even at a low gonadotropin secretory rate. When circulating estrogen reaches a critical concentration, it switches to a positive feedback mode of action, at both the hypothalamic and pituitary levels (Fink 1995, 2000). This is potentiated by rising levels of progesterone released from granulose cells of dominant follicles. These synergistic influences induce a dramatic increase in the synthesis and secretion of GnRH from a subset of hypothalamic neurons (Kimura and Fumabashi 1998) as well as an enhancement of pituitary responsiveness to this peptide (de Koning et al. 2001).

GnRH has the capacity to enhance pituitary responsiveness to itself, a unique phenomenon known as GnRH self-priming (Fink 1995, 2000; de Koning et al. 2001). In addition, the stimulatory action of GnRH is facilitated by a decreased bioactivity of the putative ovarian protein gonadotropin surge-attenuating/inhibiting factor (GnSAF/IF, attenuin) (Fowler and Templeton 1996), a 60–66 Kda protein that is presently being isolated and characterized (Fowler et al. 2002, 2003; Fowler and Spears 2004). The secretion of GnSAF/IF is dependent on FSH action on granulose cells, and it has been suggested that its inhibitory action on pituitary sensitivity to GnRH might be exerted through interactions with estrogen-dependent PR activation (Byrne et al. 1996; Tebar et al. 1998). The overall consequence of all these convergent inputs is a surge of LH – the preovulatory peak – and, to a lesser extent, of FSH.

5.2.2 Functional Organization

In the majority of mammals, functional relationships between the hypothalamus and the anterior pituitary are mediated by similar mechanisms (Levine et al. 1985; Moenter et al. 1991; Freeman 1994; Hotchkiss and Knobil 1994). Since most information on SERM effects in experimental animals comes from the female rat, we will refer to this model in the following description. As mentioned above, gonadotropin secretion exhibits two patterns: a tonic pattern, which is responsible for follicular growth, and a phasic pattern, which is characterized by the preovulatory surge of LH and FSH (Fink 1988, 2000). Both secretory patterns are under the control of GnRH, which is released episodically from nerve terminals at the median eminence into the hypophyseal portal system (Levine et al. 1991; Terasawa 2001). GnRH secretion also shows two patterns of secretory activity, one characterized by pulses of low amplitude and high frequency and one characterized by pulses of high amplitude and low frequency (Levine et al. 1995). A neuronal subset of GnRH neurons localized at the arcuate and ventromedial nucleus of the mediobasal hypothalamus (MBH) seems to be responsible for the tonic pattern of GnRH secretion ("pulse generator"), while another group of neurons at the preoptic area (POA) is responsible for the GnRH surge ("surge generator") (Kimura and Funabashi 1998).

As described below, GnRH neurons receive several synaptic afferents from both hypothalamic and extrahypothalamic regions (for a review see Herbison 1998; Herbison and Pape 2001). Some of these influences are excitatory in nature and probably mediated by excitatory aminoacids (López et al. 1990; van den Pol et al. 1990; Ping et al. 1994), while others are inhibitory and exerted through a variety of interneurons that use γ-aminobutyric acid (GABA) (Jarry et al. 1991; Herbison et al. 1991; Mitsushima et al. 1997) or opioid peptides (Weisner et al. 1984; Lustig et al. 1988; Mallory and Gallo 1990). In addition, many other synaptic contacts, including different monoaminergic and peptidergic terminals, may modulate the activity of GnRH neurons (Herbison 1998; Herbison and Pape 2001). Thus, the activity of different subsets of GnRH neurons may be the consequence of a complex interplay between their intrinsic oscillatory activity and the overall synaptic input (Suter et al. 2000; Nunemaker et al. 2002). The combination of cyclic fluctuations in the secretory pattern of GnRH neurons with changes in the synthetic and secretory capacity of pituitary gonadotropes generates the dramatic changes in gonadotropin secretory profiles observed during the ovarian cycle in all mammals (Freeman 1994; Hotchkiss and Knobil 1994).

5.2.3 Estrogen Feedback Regulation of Hypothalamus-Pituitary Axis

In both males and females during the luteal phase of the ovarian cycle estrogen restrains LH secretion through what has been called its "negative feedback". This effect is due to a combined inhibitory action on GnRH secretion by hypothalamic GnRH neurons (Sarkar and Fink 1980; Chongthammakun and Teresawa 1993; Evans et al. 1994) and, although less documented, on pituitary gonadotropes (Shupnik 1996). In addition, in the female of most mammalian species, estrogen also exerts a "positive feedback" action on GnRH neurons (Sarkar et al. 1976; Moenter et al. 1990; Rosie et al. 1990; Xia et al. 1992) and sensitizes anterior pituitary cells to GnRH (Speight et al. 1981). However, specific cellular mechanisms responsible for these estrogen actions remain partially understood.

5.2.3.1 *Estrogen Receptors in GnRH Neurons*

Up until the last few years, it was thought that hypothalamic GnRH neurons did not contain ERs, as they were not able to either concentrate estradiol within the nucleus (Shivers et al. 1983) or present immunoreactivity corresponding to the classical ER (Watson et al. 1992; Herbison et al. 1993; Sullivan et al. 1995).

However, the finding of a second subtype of ER (Kuiper et al. 1996), ERβ, completely changed this point of view. With the use of highly sensitive techniques of *in situ* hybridization and immunocytochemistry, it has been recently shown that certain populations of GnRH neurons from rats and mice express both the mRNA encoding ERβ (Skynner et al. 1999; Hrabovsky et al. 2000; Sharifi et al. 2002) and the protein (Hrabovsky et al. 2001; Kallo et al. 2001; Legan and Tsai 2003) (Table 5.1). On the other hand, studies from immortalized cell lines producing GnRH (Mellon et al. 1990) have allowed the combination of immunocytochemical identification of ERs with the characterization of signaling pathways. Thus, GnRH-releasing GT1-7 cells appear to express ERα and ERβ transcripts and proteins (Butler et al. 1999; Roy et al. 1999; Martínez-Morales et al. 2001; Navarro et al. 2003), as well as plasma membrane estrogen binding sites. Nevertheless, while GT1-7 cells clearly express ERα, with the exception of one study in rats treated with colchicine (Butler et al. 1999), this protein has not been detected in vivo. Since GT1-7 cells may represent immature GnRH neurons, developmental studies must be performed in different species in order to clarify this point.

Table 5.1. Detection of ERα and ERβ protein and/or mRNA in hypothalamic GnRH neurons of rats and mice

Hypothalamus			
ERα	**ERβ**	**Technique**	**Reference**
Low levels		Dual immunolabeling	Butler et al. 1999
High levels	Low levels	RT-PCR	Skynner et al. 1999
Not detected	High levels	Dual-label in situ hybridization	Hrabovszky et al. 2000
Not detected	High levels	Dual immunolabeling	Hrabovszky et al. 2001
Not detected	High levels	Dual immunolabeling	Kallo et al. 2001
Not detected	High levels	Immunohistochemistry	Legan and Tsai 2003

5.2.3.2
Estrogen Receptors in Anterior Pituitary Cells

In rats and mice both ER transcripts and proteins have been identified in 60–70% of anterior pituitary cells (Kuiper et al. 1997; Wilson et al. 1998; Wilson et al. 1998; Nishihara et al. 2000; Pelletier et al. 2000). While ERα is the predominant subtype in adult rats, in anterior pituitaries from fetal and prepubertal animals ERβ appears to be expressed in greater abundance (Nishihara et al. 2000). In addition, differential developmental and estrogen-dependent expression of pituitary ERs has been reported (Pasqualini et al. 1999). Approximately

8–10% of anterior pituitary cells express both ER subtypes, suggesting that interaction between them through heterodimers may have functional significance (Mitchner et al. 1998). With respect to cell types expressing each ER subtype, ERα is expressed at high levels in lactotropes and, to a lesser extent, in gonadotropes, while ERβ is expressed at low levels in all anterior pituitary cells (Mitchner et al. 1998; Nishihara e al. 2000; Childs et al. 2001; Sánchez-Criado et al. 2004) (Fig. 5.1; Table 5.2). Two isoforms of truncated estrogen receptor products (TERP), TERP1 and TERP2, are also expressed in the rat pituitary and are capable of forming heterodimers with ERα and ERβ (Schreihofer et al. 2002; Vaillant et al. 2002). In addition, several reports have indicated the presence of ERα associated with the plasma membrane of rat pituitary cell lines (Pappas et al. 1994; Norfleet et al. 1999), which might be related to rapid estrogen actions on prolactin (PRL) secretion (Christian and Morris 2002).

Table 5.2. Detection of ERα and/or ERβ in different cell types of rat anterior pituitary

Anterior pituitary gland			
ERα	**ERβ**	**Technique**	**Reference**
Lactotropes, folicullostellate cells, corticotropes, and gonadotropes	Lactotropes, folicullostellate cells, corticotropes, and gonadotropes	Combined in situ hybridization and immunohistochemistry	Mitchner et al. 1998
	Lactotropes and gonadotropes	Immunohistochemistry	Nishihara et al. 2000
Gonadotropes	Gonadotropes	Dual immunolabeling	Childs et al. 2001
Gonadotropes	Gonadotropes	Dual immunolabeling	Sánchez-Criado et al. 2005
Lactotropes, somatotropes, thyrotropes, and gonadotropes	Lactotropes, somatotropes, and gonadotropes	Dual immunolabeling	González et al. unpublished

5.2.3.3
Estrogen Negative Feedback on GnRH Neurons

Estradiol represses GnRH gene expression in immortalized GT1 cells (Roy et al. 1999; Bowe et al. 2003) and may exert either stimulatory or inhibitory effects

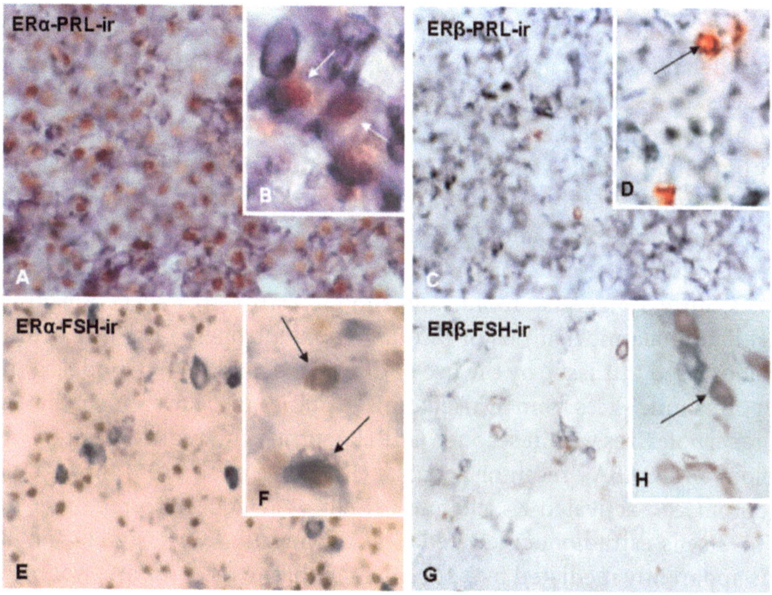

Fig. 5.1. Comparison between ERα and ERβ immunoreactivities in lactotropes (PRL-ir) and gonadotropes (FSH-ir) of the female rat anterior pituitary. The *left* panel shows anterior pituitary sections of double-label immunostaining for ERα and PRL (**A, B**) or FSH (**E, F**). The *right* panel shows anterior pituitary sections double-label immunostaining for ERβ and PRL (**C, D**) or FSH (**G, H**). Numerous ERα-positive nuclei are seen in many lactotrope (**A**) and several gonadotrope (**E**) cells, whereas scarce ERβ-positive cytoplasms are detected in isolated lactotrope (**C**) and gonadotrope (**G**) cells. Cellular details with double labels are depicted in the *upper-right* sections (**B, D, F, H**). *Arrows* indicate double-labeled cells. Magnifications are 270× (**C, G**), 320× (**E**), 340× (**A**), 430× (**D, H**), and 650× (**B, F**). Briefly, anterior pituitaries were fixed with 4% paraformaldehyde in phosphate buffer saline (PBS, 0.1 M, pH 7.4) and frozen. The indirect immunocytochemical procedure was carried out by incubating pituitary sections with MC20 rabbit antimouse ERα (1/250, Santa Cruz Biotechnology) or with Y-19 goat antimouse ERβ (1/250, Santa Cruz Biotechnology). This first immunostaining was revealed by the streptavidin-biotin-peroxidase method (1:1000 and 1:1500, respectively) using diethyl-carbazol (red product). The same pituitary sections were also incubated in rabbit anti-PRL (1:1000, Chemicon International) or in rabbit anti-FSH (1:1000, Chemicon International), and 4-chloro-1-naftol was used for the subsequent labeling (blue product)

in transfected nonneural cells through ERα (Wierman et al. 1992; Dong et al. 1996; Chen et al. 2001). In addition, estrogen inhibitory effects on GnRH gene expression have been found after in vivo treatment in experimental animals (El Majdoubi et al. 1998; Pelletier et al. 2001) as well as in brain tissue from menopausal women (Rance and Uswandi 1996). On the other hand, in mice lacking ERα, but not ERβ, the inhibitory effects of estrogen on either hypothalamic GnRH mRNA levels or LH secretion are absent (Wersinger et al. 1999;

Dorling et al. 2003). However, direct estrogen actions on GnRH gene expression of hypothalamic GnRH neurons have not been demonstrated. Therefore, since these cells do not express ERα in large amounts, it is reasonable to think that classical ER-mediated negative feedback is not exerted on GnRH neurons directly but rather through modulation of excitatory or inhibitory interneurons.

Results from experimental animals have shown that estrogen administration to ovariectomized mammals reduces GnRH (Sharkar and Fink 1980) and LH levels (Condon et al. 1988) in portal blood and peripheral plasma within minutes. Since it suggests a rapid, nongenomic, estrogen direct action on either GnRH hypothalamic neurons or pituitary gonadotropes, a number of studies have addressed this issue by the use of different experimental models. Studies in hypothalamic slices from ovariectomized guinea pigs have shown that estradiol hyperpolarizes within seconds GnRH neurons and reduces the potency of μ-opioid and $GABA_B$ receptor agonists (Lagrange et al. 1995) through modulation of Ca^{2+}-activated K^+-channels (Kelly et al. 2002). On the other hand, in GT1-7 cells estradiol acutely reduces ACh-induced Ca^{2+} signals, an effect that is apparently mediated by a specific membrane receptor and not blocked by the antiestrogen ICI 182,780 (Morales et al. 2003). In addition, estradiol could exert part of its negative feedback effect indirectly by modulating the activity of some presynaptic inputs. Thus, in hypothalamic slices from guinea pigs and mice, estradiol increases the inhibitory tone of both GABAergic and β-endorphin neurons by interaction with specific membrane receptors coupled to Gαq-protein and activation of PKC (Qiu et al. 2003). Therefore, although the identity of receptor proteins and the second messenger cascades that are activated remain to be clarified, all these findings indicate that estradiol may exert a critical part of its negative feedback effects on GnRH neurons through specific membrane sites, either directly or transynaptically.

5.2.3.4
Estrogen Positive Feedback on GnRH Neurons

Clear experimental evidence supporting direct estrogen action on GnRH neurons in its positive feedback mode is lacking at the present time. Nevertheless, recent studies have shown that estradiol can exert rapid stimulatory effects (less than 30 min) on mice GnRH neurons, both in vivo (Ábrahám et al. 2003) and in nasal explants (Temple et al. 2004). Apparently, these estrogen effects are exerted through intracellular ERβ and may be related to phosphorylation of cAMP response element binding protein (CREB) (Ábrahám et al. 2003) and changes in transcriptional activity (Temple et al. 2004). However, neither the downstream signals activated by estradiol nor their relation to GnRH synthesis or secretion is presently known. On the other hand, in GT1-7 cells expressing both ERα and ERβ, biphasic, dose-dependent effects of estradiol on cAMP signaling have been demonstrated; these effects are apparently exerted through membrane receptors and coupled to changes in pulsatile GnRH secretion (Navarro et al. 2003). Unfortunately, given the difficulty of generalizing results from immortalized cell lines, the interpretation of these findings should await further experimentation.

In contrast, most available evidence suggests that estrogen positive feedback effects on GnRH neurons are exerted via indirect, transynaptic mechanisms (Herbison and Pape 2001). Thus, ERα and ERβ containing neurons at the anteroventral periventricular region of rats (AVPV) appear to be critical for estrogen positive feedback since they are coactivated with GnRH neurons at the time of LH surge (Le et al. 1999). In addition, electrolytic lesions of this region impair the LH surge (Wiegand et al. 1982), and antiestrogen microimplants block both the estrogen-induced LH surge and the phasic increase in GnRH gene expression (Petersen et al. 1995). Even though the identity of these neuronal inputs on GnRH neurons remains to be clarified, most experimental evidence indicates that they are mainly GABAergic and glutamatergic (for review see Herbison and Pape 2001; Petersen et al. 2003). Thus, estrogen-sensitive neurons projecting to the location of GnRH neurons contain and release GABA (Ondo et al. 1982; Flugge et al. 1986) or glutamate (Ping et al. 1994; Jarry et al. 1995), and receptors for these neurotransmitters have been found in GnRH neurons (Eyigor and Jennes 1997; Spergel et al. 1999). In addition, estrogen-dependent progesterone receptor (PR) on AVPV neurons (Chappel and Levine 2000) as well as several paracrine factors released from glial cells (Prevot et al. 2000) also appear to be critical components of events leading to the preovulatory GnRH surge.

5.2.3.5
Estrogen Feedback Actions on Anterior Pituitary

It has been known for years that estrogen regulation of the hypothalamus–pituitary axis in females is the result of a combined action on hypothalamic neurons releasing GnRH (as described above) and on the responsiveness of anterior pituitary to GnRH (Fink 1995, 2000; de Koning et al. 2001). Since both gonadotropes and lactotropes contain ERs, anterior pituitary cells are potential targets for estrogen action in the regulation of the female reproductive cycle. However, even though estrogen seems to contribute to the negative feedback on LH secretion by direct actions on gonadotropes (Henderson et al. 1977), most evidence indicates that the major site for estrogen action is the hypothalamus rather than the pituitary (Leipheimer et al. 1983). By contrast, in the case of the positive feedback, there is little doubt that estrogen acts directly on gonadotropes to enhance their responsiveness to GnRH (Dronin and Labrie 1981). In addition, estradiol elicits GnRH self-priming by inducing pituitary

PR receptor expression in the gonadotrope (Szabo et al. 2000; Scott et al. 2002), a phenomenon that is determinant in the expression of the preovulatory LH surge (Levine 1997; Fink 2000). Although the intracellular signals and downstream cascades activated by estradiol remain to be clarified, most positive estrogen effects on gonadotropin and PRL synthesis and secretion at the level of anterior pituitary cells seem to be dependent on ERα (Scully et al. 1997; Sánchez-Criado et al. 2004). Studies from pituitary cell lines and rat pituitary cells have demonstrated that estrogen differentially regulates gene expression of different ER subtypes, a mechanism that may serve to modulate estrogen responsiveness (Mitchner et al. 1998; Schreihofer et al. 2000). Also, ERs in anterior pituitary cells can be activated in a ligand-independent manner through several signal cascades that include PKA, PKC, or MAPK activation (Schreihofer et al. 2001). Furthermore, in gonadotrope α-T3-1 cells, GnRH triggers signaling pathways that result in estrogen-independent transactivation of ERα and potentiate estrogen-dependent ERα transactivation (Demay et al. 2001).

5.2.4 Overview of Hypothalamic-Pituitary Function at Time of Gonadotropin Surge

In summary, even though the evidence concerning GnRH neurons is still fragmentary, regulatory estrogen effects on the activity of the GnRH neuronal system and the secretion of GnRH to the hypophyseal-portal system have been demonstrated in most species. In addition, estrogen modulates the expression of its own receptors in anterior pituitary cells and thereby regulates their responsiveness to GnRH. Some estrogen effects may be exerted directly on GnRH neurons through intracellular estrogen receptors (probably ERβ) and/or putative membrane receptors. Also, a variety of estrogen actions on GnRH neurons are exerted transynaptically through interactions on different estrogen-sensitive interneurons that send a complex synaptic input to GnRH neurons.

Although the precise cellular mechanisms underlying estrogen feedback actions on the GnRH neuronal system and, as a consequence, GnRH secretion remain to be clarified, a rather speculative working model can be provided (Fig. 5.2). In rats and other mammals, low estrogen concentrations during most of the cycle exert a direct negative feedback action on a population of GnRH neurons at MBH ("pulse generator") through ERβ and, perhaps, several potential estrogen-sensitive membrane sites. This low activity of GnRH neurons is probably reinforced or maintained by a variety of inhibitory afferents from different interneurons. A rise in estrogen levels prior to ovulation would reclute several estrogen-sensitive presynaptic neurons through ERα and ERβ, which in turn modulate the activity of another subgroup of GnRH neurons

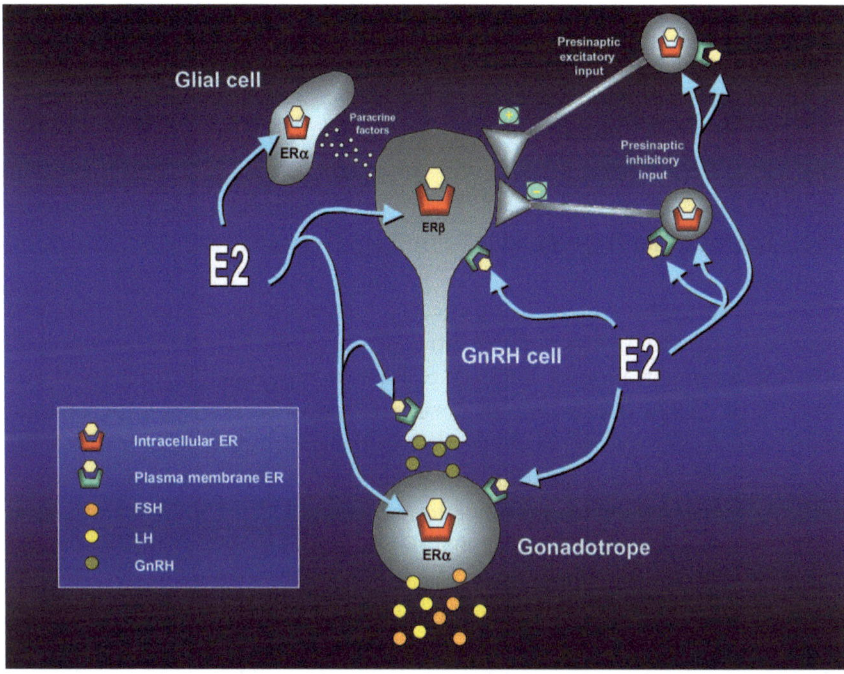

Fig. 5.2. Schematic representation of estrogen feedback actions on GnRH-gonadotrope system in mammals. As described in the text, estrogen may modulate the activity of hypothalamic GnRH neurons either directly or transynaptically. In rats and mice, direct estrogen interactions with GnRH neurons seem to be exerted via genomic mechanisms through nuclear ERβ. In addition, acute estrogen effects on GnRH neurons may also be exerted directly through potential membrane binding sites, which remain to be characterized. On the other hand, estrogen also interacts with several interneurons and glial cells, which in turn exert either excitatory or inhibitory actions on GnRH neurons. Thus, low estrogen concentrations during most of the ovarian cycle exert a direct negative feedback action on GnRH neurons and thereby maintain the tonic pattern of GnRH secretion. This low rate of GnRH secretion is probably reinforced by a variety of inhibitory afferents from different interneurons. A rise in estrogen levels prior to ovulation would reclute several estrogen-sensitive presynaptic neurons through ERα and ERβ to further modulate, transynaptically, the activity of other subgroups of GnRH neurons. The overall predominance of afferent excitatory inputs and/or the reduction of inhibitory inputs would allow GnRH neurons to increase their firing rate and the magnitude of GnRH secretion in the hypophyseal-portal system. In addition, the concurrent action of estrogen and GnRH on gonadotrope cells in the anterior pituitary elicits GnRH self-priming and increases gonadotrope responsiveness, which is further increased by progesterone

at POA ("surge generator"). The overall predominance of afferent excitatory inputs and/or the reduction of inhibitory inputs would allow GnRH neurons to increase their firing rate and the magnitude of GnRH secretion in the hypophyseal-portal system. In addition, the concurrent action of estrogen and GnRH on gonadotrope cells in the anterior pituitary elicits GnRH self-priming and increases gonadotrope responsiveness, which is further increased by progesterone. Thus, estrogen appears to coordinate the surge of GnRH and the gonadotrope responsiveness to it in such a way that both events reach a peak at the same time and provoke the preovulatory surge of LH.

5.3 Effects of SERMs on Hypothalamus-Pituitary-Ovarian Axis

Since, as described above, estrogen exerts a complex constellation of effects on the female reproductive axis, differential effects of SERMs would be expected. Thus, the administration of different SERMs to experimental animals shows a variety of results depending on dose, method of treatment, experimental model, and tissue-specific response. While the use of cycling rats allows the observation of the hypothalamus-pituitary-ovarian axis as a whole, ovariectomized animals permit the modification of estrogen status as an experimental controlled variable (Bellido et al. 2003; Hernández et al. 2003; Sánchez-Criado et al. 2002). In addition, studies on tissue explants, dispersed pituitary cells, or immortalized cell lines give the possibility of detailed analysis of signaling pathways involved in a particular estrogen response. Nevertheless, all this information must be integrated in order to understand the relative effect of a particular compound on different levels of the female reproductive axis.

In the case of clinical studies, although pharmacological effects of SERMs have been extensively analyzed in several reproductive and nonreproductive tissues of menopausal women, the influence of these compounds upon regulation of the hypothalamus-pituitary-ovarian axis has not been fully clarified, and conflicting results are frequently published. Whereas high physiological concentrations of estradiol in postmenopausal women inhibit GnRH secretion and reduce plasma LH and FSH levels, exogenous pharmacological estrogen concentrations sensitize the anterior pituitary to GnRH and lead to increased gonadotropin levels. As a consequence, the net estrogenic or antiestrogenic activity of a given SERM will depend upon the balance between these opposite actions (Ravdin et al. 1988; Jordan et al. 1991; Számel et al. 1998). On the other hand, the effect of SERMs on the human hypothalamus-pituitary-gonadal axis may also depend on a combination of clinical variables. Thus, diverse and conflicting results have been reported depending on gender, ovarian function status (pre- or postmenopausal), dose and duration of treatment, coexistence of diseases, and use of concomitant medications that can alter the hypothalamus-pituitary axis, like the frequent case of adjuvant chemotherapy in advanced breast cancer patients (Jordan et al. 1987a,b; Kostoglou-Athanassiou et al. 1997; Ellmen et al. 2003). Moreover, several of the published reports included small sample sizes or heterogeneous patient populations which may account for nonsignificant results.

In the following sections, we will first review recent experimental findings from our and other laboratories on the effects of different SERMs on the hypothalamus-pituitary-ovarian axis in the cyclic female rat, as well as from anterior pituitary explants from ovariectomized rats subjected to different estrogen environments. We will next review most of the relevant published data on the effects of SERMs on the hypothalamus-pituitary-ovarian axis in humans, with special emphasis to gonadotropin and sex hormones in postmenopausal women. Given the extensive current use of these drugs in both the prevention and treatment of breast cancer and postmenopausal osteoporosis, as well as the continuous flow of new SERMs in late-phase clinical development, it is interesting to know whether these compounds differ in terms of their effects on gonadotropin secretion. Moreover, the analysis of pharmacological effects of SERMs on the hypothalamus-pituitary-ovarian axis of both humans and experimental animals may help to understand the complex mechanisms that control the regulation of reproductive function.

5.3.1 Experimental Studies in the Rat

5.3.1.1 *Trifenilethylene Derivatives*

Clomiphen is a racemic mixture of two molecules with different estrogen agonist and antagonist activity, which induces ovulation in rats, probably acting at all levels of the hypothalamus-pituitary axis (Adashi 1984). In perifusion experiments of MBH and pituitary, this compound induces GnRH and LH release, both effects being potentiated by estrogen in the incubation medium (Miyake et al. 1983). However, when implanted into the MPA of ovariectomized rats, clomiphen has been shown to inhibit both negative and positive estrogen feedback actions on LH secretion (Docke et al. 1989, 1990). At the level of the anterior pituitary, clomiphen blocks nuclear translocation of ERs (Terakawa et al. 1985) and inhibits estrogen-induced PR in ovariectomized rats (Terakawa et al. 1986). However, both in cyclic (Kilic-Okman et al. 2003) and ovariectomized rats (Schuiling et al. 1985) clomiphen stimulates gonadotropin release by enhancing pituitary responsiveness to GnRH (Adashi et al. 1981; Engel et al. 2002), probably through an increase in the number of pituitary GnRH receptors (Shimizu et al. 1986).

Tamoxifen was the first SERM described and has been used for the treatment of breast cancer for decades (Jordan et al. 1987, 1991; Jordan and Morrow 1999). It exhibits either estrogen agonist or antagonist activities on several reproductive parameters in the female rat. Tamoxifen inhibits ovulation both in adult (Donath and Nisshino 1998) and in prepubertal rats given exogenous gonadotropins to induce follicular development (Gao et al. 2002), and it reduces estrogen and progesterone levels at proestrus (Donath and Nishino 1998). These effects are mainly due to an impairment of the preovulatory surges of LH and FSH since the anovulatory action was reversed by treatment with human chorionic gonadotropin (Gao et al. 2002). Furthermore, tamoxifen treatment of cyclic rats at proestrus reduces both basal and GnRH-stimulated LH secretion, either in vivo or in vitro (Sánchez-Criado et al. 2002). In addition, tamoxifen reverses estrogen facilitation of high K^+-induced GnRH release from rat hypothalamic explants (Drouva et al. 1988) and antagonizes the stimulatory effect of estradiol and E-BSA on nitric oxide (NO) release from the rat median eminence (Prevot et al. 1999). With respect to other brain areas that are involved in reproductive behavior, chronic tamoxifen treatment increases oxytocin receptor binding and ERβ gene expression either in the ventromedial nucleus (VMN) (Pautisaul et al. 2003) or in the total hypothalamus (Zhou et al. 2002) by itself, without antagonizing the effects of estradiol on this parameter, and inhibits estrogen-dependent PR gene expression and PR immunoreactivity in the medial preoptic nucleus (MPN) and the VMN (Shugrue et al. 1997; Yin et al. 2002; Patisaul et al. 2003).

While the above-mentioned results indicate that this compound may act mainly as an overall estrogen antagonist on the estrogen positive feedback, their effects on gonadotropin secretion suggest a more complex behavior. Thus, tamoxifen elevates GnRH-induced LH release and PRL release in anterior pituitaries from proestrous rats (González et al. 2000) and increases GnRH self-priming (Sánchez-Criado et al. 2002). Interestingly, while tamoxifen induces GnRH self-priming by itself, it reduces the estrogen-sensitizing effect on GnRH-stimulated LH secretion and abolishes estrogen-dependent GnRH self-priming (see discussion below). On the other hand, treatment of ovariectomized rats with tamoxifen enhances PR-B mRNA levels in a similar extent to that of estradiol and increases the number of anterior pituitary cells expressing immunoreactive PR (Sánchez-Criado et al. 2003). Moreover, pretreatment with the "pure" antiestrogen RU58668 reduces tamoxifen-induced PR expression and GnRH self-priming, while pretreatment with the antiprogestin RU38486 blocks tamoxifen-induced GnRH self-priming (Sánchez-Criado et al. 2003). In addition, treatment of ovariectomized rats with tamoxifen increases the number of LH-positive cells expressing ERα to an extent similar to that of of cycling proestrous rats (Sánchez-Criado et al. 2005a). Therefore, at the rat gonadotrope level, tamoxifen behaves either as an estrogen agonist or antagonist, its estrogen agonistic activity being related to a direct induction of PR expression in the gonadotrope through ERα (Tena-Sempere et al. 2004). With respect to PRL secretion, tamoxifen shows also a mixed agonist/antagonist activity depending on the estrogen status of the animal. Thus, this compound increases PRL levels in both ovariectomized (González et al. 2000) and prepubertal rats (Toney and Katzenellenbogen 1986), whereas it inhibits estrogen-induced PRL elevations (Donath and Nishino 1998; Toney and Katzenellenbogen 1986).

5.3.1.2
Benzotiophene Derivatives

In the female rat, raloxifene acts as a complete antiestrogen on the hypothalamus-pituitary-gonadal axis and displays clear anovulatory effects under chronic treatment (Long et al. 2001). Although there are few studies at hypothalamic level, this compound apparently lacks estrogen agonist activity on the expression of ERs or PR in all brain areas (Zhou et al. 2002), and reduces estrogen-induced PR expression in the MPN (Shughrue et al. 1997). With respect to the anterior pituitary, raloxifene inhibits the expression of ERα in cyclic rats to the same extent of "pure" antiestrogens and completely abolishes nuclear localization of ERα in gonadotropes at proestrus (Sánchez-Criado et al. 2002). In addition, in ovariectomized rats, raloxifene exhibits rather deleterious effects on pituitary ERs since it decreases the proportion of LH-positive cells staining for ERα and shows no evidence of estrogen agonist activity on ERβ or PR expression (Sánchez-Criado et al. 2004). These effects are consistent with an overall antiestrogenic activity on basal and GnRH-stimulated LH release or estrogen-induced GnRH self-priming (González et al. 2000; Sánchez-Criado et al. 2002). On the other hand, raloxifene treatment of ovariectomized rats reduces estrogen-induced PRL release (Buelke-Sam et al. 1998), whereas it has either no effect (González et al. 2000) or a stimulatory action (Pinilla et al. 2001) on PRL secretion.

We have used a pyrroliding analog of raloxifene, LY117018, to study SERM effects at different levels of the reproductive system of normal cycling rats. In the anterior pituitary, LY117018 inhibits the expression of ERα and blocks the proestrus-induced nuclear localization of this protein to the same extent as raloxifene (Sánchez-Criado et al. 2002). In addition, treatment with LY117018 inhibits ovulation in a dose-dependent manner and reduces both negative and positive estrogen feedback actions on gonadotropin secretion in ovariectomized rats (Hernández et al. 2003), without significantly affecting the release of GnRH into the hypophyseal system at proestrus, and reduces estrogen-induced GnRH self-priming (Sánchez-Criado et al. 2002). Therefore, LY117018 anovulatory actions seem to be due mainly to the inhibitory effect of this compound on the preovulatory surge of LH, probably by reducing the pituitary responsiveness to GnRH (Fig. 5.3) (Guelmes et al. 2003; Hernández et al. 2003).

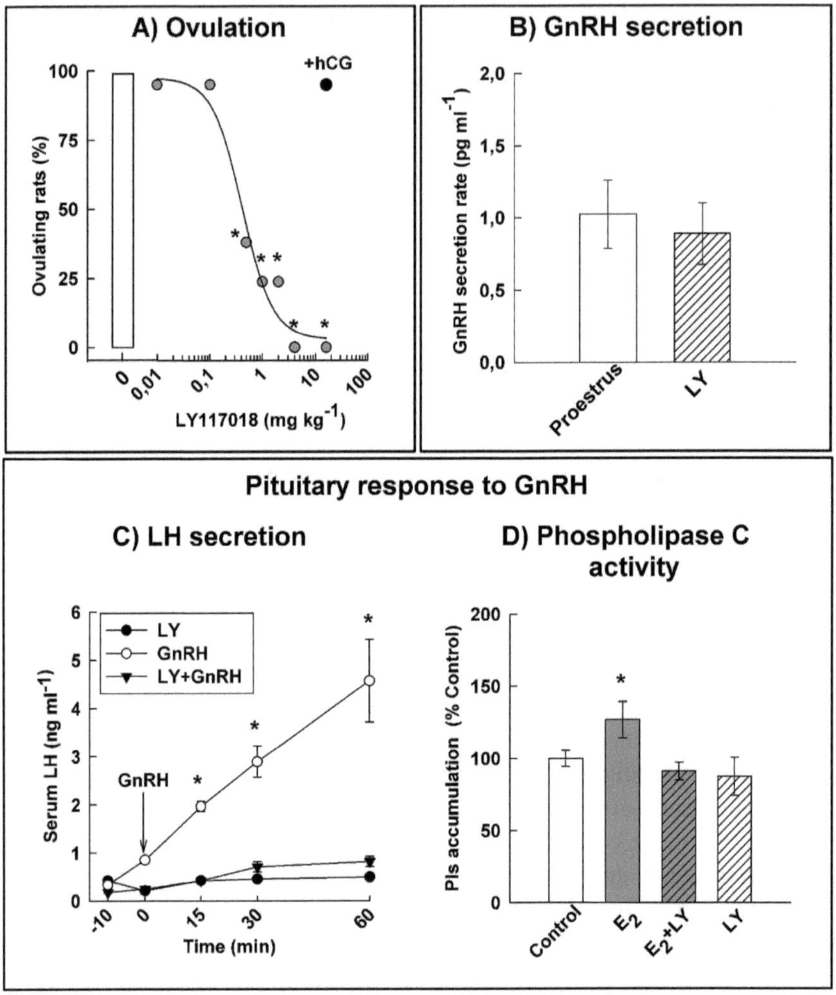

Fig. 5.3. Effect of benzothiophen derivative LY117018 on various reproductive parameters in female rats (modified from Hernández et al. Reproduction 125:597–606, 2003). In this and other similar figures, values are mean ± SEM of the corresponding variable. (**A**) Different doses of LY117018 were administered s.c. to female rats at diestrus, and ovulation was assessed at estrus by inspection of the ampullary region. (**A**) • represents the percentage of ovulating rats after treatment with high doses of LY117018 plus human chorionic gonadotropin (hCG). $^*P < 0.01$ by two-tailed Fisher's exact probability test versus controls (*bar*). (**B**) Effect of administration of LY117018 (16 mg/Kg) to cyclic female rats at proestrus on GnRH secretion rate from hypophyseal portal system. (**C**) Time course of effect of LY117018 (16 mg/Kg) on pituitary sensitivity to GnRH (50 nG/100 g) in cyclic female rats. Blood samples were collected during proestrus at the time of expected endogenous surge of LH. $^*P < 0.01$ versus controls. (**D**) Effect of estradiol (40 μg/day, 2 d) and LY117018 (16 mg/Kg) on GnRH-induced (10 nM during 40 min) phospholipase activity in hemipituitaries from ovariectomized rats. $^*P < 0.05$ versus controls

5.3.2 Lessons in SERM Behavior from Effects of Tamoxifen on Rat Pituitary Function

In 1994, we found that endogenous estradiol decreased serum LH concentrations in tamoxifen-treated cyclic rats, and we explained this paradoxical effect as an "inappropriate feedback of endogenous estradiol" (Tebar et al. 1994). More recently, our laboratories have routinely used anterior pituitary glands harvested from ovariectomized rats treated with different ER ligands. Thereafter, these pituitaries were incubated with the corresponding ligand and LH secretion was measured (González et al. 2000; Sánchez-Criado et al. 2002; Bellido et al. 2003; Sánchez Criado et al. 2004, 2005a,b). More by accident than on purpose, it was observed that 2-h incubation with 10^{-8} M estradiol of pituitaries from ovariectomized rats treated with 3 mg tamoxifen blocks the agonist effect of this SERM on GnRH self-priming (Fig. 5.4). GnRH self-priming is a phenomenon different from the GnRH-releasing action in which, under endogenous estrogen levels, the magnitude of LH release after a first

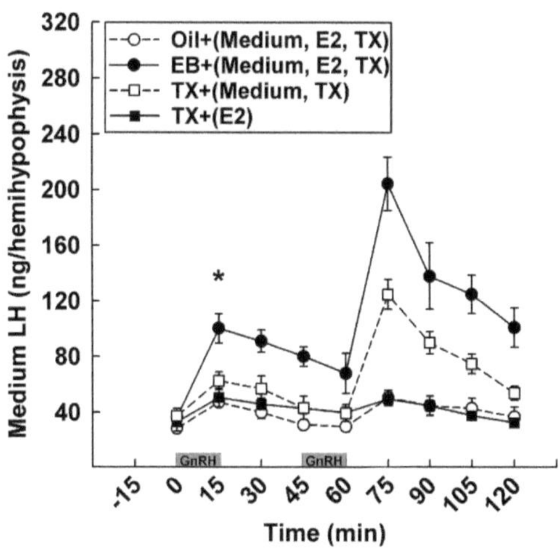

Fig. 5.4. LH secretion from hemipituitaries from ovariectomized rats treated during 3 d with oil (0.2 ml), estradiol benzoate (EB, 25 μg), or tamoxifen (TX, 3 mg) and incubated for 3 h with medium alone, 17β-estradiol (E_2, 10^{-8} M), or TX (10^{-7} M), in response to two consecutive GnRH challenges (10^{-8} M, for 15 min) at indicated time periods. Values of LH secretion from hemipituitaries of oil- and EB-injected ovariectomized rats incubated with medium alone, E_2, or TX (24 hemipituitaries), and from hemipituitaries of TX-injected rats incubated with medium alone or TX (16 hemipituitaries) are represented together, as no effect of the incubation conditions was observed. Values of LH secretion from hemipituitaries of TX-injected ovariectomized rats incubated with E_2 are the mean of 8 half glands. $^*P < 0.01$ versus non-EB-treated rats (modified from Sánchez-Criado et al. J Endocrinol 186:43–49, 2005)

exposure to GnRH ("umprimed response") sensitizes pituitary gonadotropes to a second GnRH pulse given 60 min later ("primed response") (Fink 1995; 2000; de Koning et al. 2001). Therefore, as described above, although tamoxifen treatment has no effect on LH secretion in ovariectomized rats, it induces PR expression in the gonadotrope (Sánchez-Criado et al. 2004), as well as a robust GnRH self-priming (Bellido et al. 2003) that is abolished by incubation with estradiol (Fig. 5.5). Moreover, whereas coincubation with ICI 182,780, a "pure" type-II antiestrogen, reverses the inhibitory effect of estradiol on tamoxifen-induced GnRH self-priming, tamoxifen by itself (a type-I antiestrogen) has no effect (Sánchez-Criado et al. 2005b). These findings indicate that the inhibitory effect of estradiol on tamoxifen-induced GnRH self-priming is probably exerted at the level of an unknown ER with extremely low affinity for tamoxifen, which is different from classical ERs. Additional preliminary data have shown that both the ERα agonist PPT (Sánchez-Criado et al. 2004) and the membrane impermeant estradiol analog E-BSA also inhibit tamoxifen-induced GnRH self-priming (Sánchez-Criado et al. 2005b). Taken together, these findings lead us to the conclusion that tamoxifen may evoke GnRH self-priming in the anterior pituitary of ovariectomized rats by acting on ERα. This interpretation would imply that, under physiological conditions, a cross-talk between nuclear and membrane ERs may exist in the gonadotrope to modulate estrogen action on GnRH self-priming and, hence, on LH release.

Furthermore, using the new selective ER agonists PPT and DPN (Sun et al. 1999; Stauffer et al. 2000; Meyers et al. 2001), we have found that ERα, which is

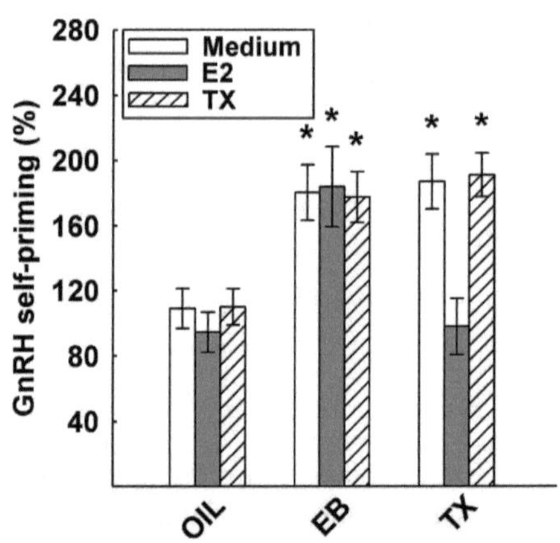

Fig. 5.5. Percentage of GnRH self-priming in hemipituitaries from ovariectomized rats treated for 3 d with oil, B, or TX and incubated for 3 h with medium alone, E_2, or TX. GnRH self-priming was calculated as the peak response to the second GnRH pulse $\times$ 100/peak response to the first GnRH pulse. A value of 100% or less indicates absence of GnRH self-priming. *$P < 0.05$ versus oil (modified from Sánchez-Criado et al. J Endocrinol 186:43–49, 2005)

predominant in the anterior pituitary (Scully et al. 1997; Nishihara et al. 2000), mediates all actions of estradiol on the gonadotrope (Sánchez-Criado et al. 2004; Tena-Sempere et al. 2004). However, in the absence of ERα activation, the ERβ isoform can replace the effect of ERα on the synthesis, but not on the release, of gonadotropins (Sánchez-Criado et al. 2004). In addition, our recent results indicate that, whereas selective ERα activation by PPT restores the estrogen negative feedback on LH secretion, sensitizes the gonadotrope to GnRH, and induces PR expression and GnRH self-priming (Sánchez-Criado et al. 2004), selective ERβ activation by DPN stimulates all steps leading to LH secretion except exocytosis (Sánchez-Criado et al. 2005b). Therefore, this suggests that, in the gonadotrope, ERα and ERβ are not mere components of a redundant regulatory system but rather complementary players involved in the regulation of gonadotropin synthesis in a "ying-yang" relationship.

We are now tempted to speculate that estrogen action on gonadotropin secretion, which includes both synthesis and release, not only involves the two ER isoforms identified so far, but also plasma membrane ERs working in an integrated manner (Fig. 5.6). Whereas the predominant action of nuclear ERα on gonadotropin synthesis, but not release, is probably modulated by nuclear ERβ, plasma membrane ER may inhibit gonadotropin release elicited by nuclear ERα by acting specifically on PR-dependent GnRH self-priming (Waring and Turgeon 1992; Sánchez-Criado et al. 2004). Whether these as yet

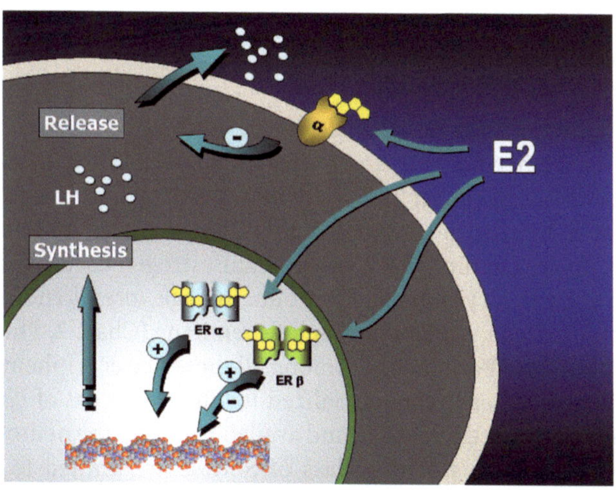

Fig. 5.6. Schematic diagram of estrogen (E2) actions on LH secretion in rat gonadotropes. Activation of nuclear ERα stimulates LH secretion (synthesis + release), whereas activation of nuclear ERβ modulates the effect of ERα on the synthesis, but not the release, of LH in a sort of ying-yang relationship. In addition, activation of putative membrane ERα by the cognate ligand would blunt the releasing effects of nuclear ERα activation by a potential, and as yet uncharacterized, cross-talk interaction

unidentified plasma membrane ERs in the anterior pituitary are structurally related to ERα, as has been suggested for other cellular functions (Marín et al. 2003), and how signaling pathways activated after estrogen binding to membrane ERs are coordinated with those dependent on nuclear ER activation is just starting to be understood (Valverde and Parker 2002; Azuma et al. 2004; Razandi et al. 2004; Marín et al. 2005). The finding that particular SERMs, like tamoxifen, may differentially interact with different ER-dependent pathways within the same cell and modulate a particular cell function, as occurs in the rat gonadotrope, may be extremely useful in both cell biology and estrogen pharmacology (McDonnell 2003). On one hand, the discovery of the action mechanisms of different SERMs is a key factor for their proper clinical use. On the other hand, the combination of SERMs with ERα and ERβ selective analogs will surely provide investigators with tools needed to dissect the biology of classical nuclear ERα and ERβ isoforms and novel, membrane-related ERs. Most probably, a "new" estrogen biology will be discovered in the near future using these compounds to isolate ER isoforms and plasma membrane estrogen actions that had been masked by the simultaneous activation of the complete orchestra of ERs by the cognate ligand.

5.3.3 Clinical Studies

5.3.3.1 *Trifenilethylene Derivatives*

Tamoxifen has been used for over 30 years, and the clinical experience from over 10 million women per year is a proof of its beneficial effect in the treatment of disseminated breast cancer and as an adjuvant drug in primary prevention in women at high risk of developing this disease. Other members of this chemical group are clomiphene, a classical antiestrogen used for initiation of ovulation in anovulatory women of reproductive age, toremifene, droloxifene, idoxifene, miproxifene, ospemifene, and fispemifene (Chap. 2, Pharmacology of SERMs, Marín and Barbancho). Among all these newer triphenylethylenes, only toremifene has been commercialized for the treatment of disseminated hormone-responsive breast cancer, and available data on the neuroendocrinological effects in humans of this class of SERMs are limited to tamoxifen, toremifene, and droloxifene. It should be noted that many of these results originated in women with advanced breast carcinoma who were receiving adjuvant chemotherapy, which likely influenced the hormonal results, mainly in premenopausal women (Jordan et al. 1987a; Ravdin et al. 1988; Jordan et al. 1991; Ellmen et al. 2003).

Administration of tamoxifen to postmenopausal women reduces plasma gonadotropin levels, probably due to a partial estrogen agonist activity at both the hypothalamus and the anterior pituitary, and increases plasma levels of sex hormone binding globulin (SHBG) by an estrogen agonist action on the liver (Kostoglou-Athanassiou et al. 1997). In a recent series of 32 postmenopausal women with breast cancer, plasma FSH and LH fell by a mean of 45% and 48%, respectively, after approximately 12 months of treatment, with increases in SHBG of 65% and slight decreases in plasma estradiol and testosterone (Lønning et al. 1995). This magnitude of gonadotropin suppression is similar to previous reports in postmenopausal women receiving tamoxifen and adjuvant chemotherapy (Jordan et al. 1987b) or to the suppression of basal and GnRH-induced gonadotropin secretion observed in estrogen-deprived postmenopausal women receiving clomiphene, the first SERM used in humans (Messinis and Templeton 1990; Garas et al. 2004). The modest decrease in plasma estradiol observed by Lønning et al. (1995) may be due to the drop in plasma testosterone, as aromatization indexes are not influenced by tamoxifen. Overall, the moderate but significant reduction in plasma estradiol concentrations during tamoxifen therapy, combined with an increase in plasma SHBG, indicates a reduced plasma level of its free fraction. The influence of these effects on estradiol delivery to breast cancer tumor cells is unknown. However, it should be noted that the effects of tamoxifen on serum estradiol levels are not a uniform finding in postmenopausal women, as some reports show either no significant changes in this sex hormone during treatment (Ellmen et al. 2003) or a slight increase (Kostoglou-Athanassiou et al. 1997).

Data on hypothalamic-pituitary and ovarian hormonal parameters in premenopausal women treated with tamoxifen are rather scarce and limited to short series of subjects receiving this drug as adjuvant therapy after mastectomy (Jordan et al. 1991). These women continue having menstrual cycles, unaffected SHBG levels, and normal circulating levels of FSH and LH, including LH surges and subsequent increases in progesterone, which indicates that ovulation has occurred and patients remain at risk of pregnancy. Overall, the results in women with circulating estrogen levels in the normal premenopausal range indicate that the activity of tamoxifen at the hypothalamus-pituitary axis is negligible when used at therapeutic doses. These results are in contrast with the estrogen antagonistic effects of tamoxifen and clomiphene in anovulatory or oligo-ovulatory women at reproductive age, where both drugs initiate or augment ovulation by blocking endogenous estrogen negative feedback and promote FSH and LH release (Messini and Nillius 1982; Adashi 1984).

In contrast with the partial estrogen agonist effect of tamoxifen on gonadotropins, several studies have consistently shown that PRL levels are suppressed by 30–50% in pre- and postmenopausal women taking the drug (Jordan et al. 1987b, 1991; Kostoglou-Athanassiou et al. 1997), which indicates a partial estrogen antagonistic effect on lactotropes in humans. This antiestrogenic action has also been observed with toremifene (chlorotamoxifen) on both basal and thyrotropin-releasing hormone (TRH)-induced PRL release (Számel et al. 1994). In addition, an increase in SHBG and a reduction in serum estradiol concentrations have also been shown, thereby confirming similar effects of toremifene and tamoxifen on both the anterior pituitary and the liver. The effects of toremifene (60 and 200 mg daily) and tamoxifen (20 mg daily) on FSH and LH levels were also studied in another recent phase II trial in a large series of postmenopausal women with advanced breast cancer (Ellmen et al. 2003). Serum FSH and LH declined during the 10 months of treatment with both drugs, reaching premenopausal values after 8 weeks (Fig. 5.7), whereas SHBG increased in all treated groups by approximately 100%. Similar results have been reported in postmenopausal women with breast cancer in shorter phase I trials with droloxifene (3-hydroxy-tamoxifen) and idoxifene (4-iodo-pirrolidine-tamoxifen). After 3 months of droloxifene therapy, plasma levels of SHBG increased in a dose-dependent manner by 17–74%, while FSH and LH levels decreased by approximately 16–20%, which suggests a less potent estrogen agonistic effect of this drug on the liver and on the hypothalamus–pituitary axis as compared with tamoxifen (Geisler et al. 1995a,b). In addition, two weeks of idoxifene treatment at several doses was also associated with significant reductions in FSH and LH levels, with no differences in serum estradiol or SHBG concentrations in postmenopausal women with advanced breast cancer (Coombes et al. 1995).

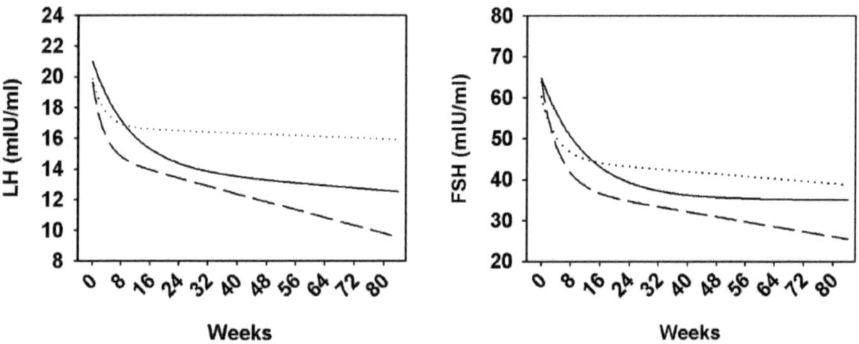

Fig. 5.7. Effect of daily treatment with 20 mg tamoxifen (*solid line*), 60 mg toremifene (*dotted line*), or 200 mg toremifene (*dashed line*) on mean LH and FSH serum concentrations of postmenopausal breast cancer patients for at least 8 weeks (modified from Ellmen et al. Breast Cancer Res Treat 82:103–111, 2003)

5.3.3.2
Benzotiophene Derivatives

The effects of raloxifene on the human hypothalamus-pituitary-gonadal axis have been studied primarily in postmenopausal women (Lasco et al. 2002; Reindollar et al. 2002; Cheng et al. 2004; Garas et al. 2004), although results in normal premenopausal women (Baker et al. 1998) and healthy men (Blum et al. 2000; Doran et al. 2001; Ueberlhart et al. 2004) have also been reported. The analysis of results from these studies reveals clear differences based on gender, hormonal *milieu*, and ovarian functional status that are incompletely understood at the present time and await further investigations. Regarding the gonadal axis, the reported results on the effects of raloxifene on basal gonadotropin levels in postmenopausal women are not uniform. While treatment with 60 mg daily of raloxifene, the approved dose in humans, induced a significant decrease in FSH levels after 3 months (Reindollar et al. 2002), and of FSH and LH after 12 months of therapy (Cheng et al. 2004), other studies have reported no changes (Lasco et al. 2002; Garas et al. 2004). Although the reasons for these discrepancies are unclear, they may be due to the small sample size and the variety of doses used. Nevertheless, the reported decreases in gonadotropin levels after raloxifene treatment are of smaller magnitude than those described for tamoxifen, which suggests a less potent estrogen agonist effect of the former compound on the hypothalamus-pituitary-gonadotrope axis.

Like tamoxifen and toremifene, raloxifene induces a decrease in both baseline and TRH-induced PRL levels (Lasco et al. 2002; Cheng et al. 2004), which may indicate a direct antiestrogenic effect on the lactotrope or, alternatively, an increase in β-endorphin (Florio et al. 2001; Genazzani et al. 2003). The effects of raloxifene on sex hormones and SHBG in healthy or osteoporotic postmenopausal women are also similar to those of tamoxifen or toremifene. Thus, raloxifene increases SHBG by 21% (Coombes et al. 1995), without significant changes (Geisler et al. 1995a) or even producing small decreases (Doran et al. 2001) in serum estradiol levels.

The effects of raloxifene in premenopausal women have been analyzed in subjects with normal ovarian function treated with high doses (100 to 400 mg daily) at either different time points of their menstrual cycle or continuously for 4 weeks (Baker et al. 1998). Raloxifene did not prevent ovulation, nor did it alter the length of the menstrual cycle or the day of the LH surge. However, it did stimulate FSH secretion, increase serum estradiol levels, and decrease serum PRL. These results are also similar to those reported for premenopausal women taking tamoxifen (Jordan et al. 1991) and are indicative of some antiestrogenic action at either the hypothalamic and/or pituitary level.

The effects of arzoxifene, a third-generation SERM similar to raloxifene but with improved estrogen antagonistic activity in the breast and the uterus, has been recently investigated in two short-term phase I studies in pre- and postmenopausal women (Fabian et al. 2004). As observed for other SERMs, arzoxifene increased SHBG levels after 2 weeks of treatment and induced a slight reduction in serum LH levels, without affecting estradiol, estrone, or FSH serum concentrations. This probably indicates certain estrogenic properties on the gonadotrope axis and the liver similar to other SERMs clinically tested.

Finally, although it is beyond the scope of this review, the effects of raloxifene on the hypothalamus-pituitary axis of human males have been analyzed in few clinical trials. Even though different doses and treatment duration have been used, in contrast with the findings in postmenopausal women, raloxifene appears to increase serum gonadotropin levels in adult eugonadal men (Doran et al. 2001; Uebelhart et al. 2004) and either elevate or not affect serum estradiol and testosterone levels (Blum et al. 2000; Doran et al. 2001; Uebelhart et al. 2004). Since those subjects with low baseline estrogen levels displayed a higher response to both gonadotropin and sex hormones, it is possible that sex hormonal status may influence overall SERM actions in men. Further studies must be conducted before a clear relationship between gender and hormonal status could be established for the differential effects of SERMs in humans.

5.4 Summary and Conclusions

Ovarian hormones control female reproductive function by acting at different levels of the hypothalamus-pituitary-gonadal axis throughout the synergistic activation of several receptor subtypes. In most mammalian species, including the human, the activity of this highly coordinated system is aimed at maintaining reproductive cycles, leading to eventual pregnancy, and at promoting body adaptations to maternal metabolism. In the case of women, given the beneficial effects of sex steroid hormones on a variety of reproductive and nonreproductive tissues, the development of specific molecules capable of reproducing steroid hormone action after cessation of ovarian function with aging has been a main objective of modern pharmacology. As described in different parts of this book, SERMs are compounds that may act either as estrogen agonists or antagonists in a tissue- or cell-specific manner and therefore have the capacity to influence hypothalamus-pituitary function in a complex manner. In this chapter, we have analyzed the available evidence from both experimental and clinical studies in order to understand the impact of SERM treatment on gonadotropin secretion. Recent findings indicate that particular SERMs may interact with several ER-dependent pathways within the same cell, thereby inducing a variety of responses that are highly dependent on estrogen and progesterone status. This fact partially explains why treatment with different SERMs in human subjects frequently gives conflicting results depending on dose, age, gender, reproductive status, duration of treatment, and coadjuvant medication. Therefore, the use of newer SERMs in whole animal and cell studies not only will provide basic investigators with tools to dissect the biology of classical and alternative ERs but also will surely help to design specific and selective approaches in hormone therapy. In addition, the analysis of clinical trials with steroid hormone analogs from the consideration of integrated estrogen and progesterone molecular interactions will provide critical insight for drug development in this promising field.

Acknowledgments

Work from the authors' laboratories has been supported by Grants BFI2002-00485, 1FD97-1065-C03-01/03, SAF2001-3614-C03-01/02, and SAF2004-08316-C02/01 (Ministerio de Ciencia y Tecnología, Spain), PI2003/98 and PI2003/154 (Consejería de Educacion, Gobierno de Canarias), and PI042640 (ISCIII, Ministerio de Sanidad y Consumo, Spain). The authors also thank Lilly S.A. and AstraZeneca for financial support. M.G. holds a fellowship from the Spanish Network of Neurological Research (CIEN, ISCIII-C03/06), and R.M. is a fellow of the Ramón y Cajal Programme (Ministerio de Ciencia y Tecnología, Spain).

References

1. Ábrahám IM, Han S-K, Todman MG, Korach KS, Herbison AE (2003) Estrogen receptor β mediates rapid estrogen actions on gonadotropin-releasing hormone neurons in vivo. J Neurosci 23:5771–5777
2. Adashi EY (1984) Clomiphene citrate: mechanism(s) and site(s) of action – a hypothesis revisited. Fertil Steril 42:331–344
3. Adashi EY, Hsueh AJ, Bambino TH, Yen SS (1981) Disparate effect of clomiphene and tamoxifen on pituitary gonadotropin release in vitro. Am J Physiol Endocrinol Metab 240:E125–130
4. Azuma K, Horie K, Inoue S, Ouchi Y, Sakai R (2004) Analysis of estrogen receptor α signalling complex at the plasma membrane. FEBS Lett 577:339–344
5. Baker VL, Draper M, Paul S, Allerheiligen S, Glant M, Shifren J, Jaffe RB (1998) Reproductive endocrine and endometrial effects of raloxifene hydrochloride, a selective estrogen receptor modulator, in women with regular menstrual cycles. J Clin Endocrinol Metab 83:6–13
6. Bellido C, Martín de las Mulas J, Tena-Sempere M, Aguilar R, Alonso R, Sánchez-Criado JE (2003) Tamoxifen induces gonadotropin-releasing hormone self-priming through an estroge-dependent progesterone receptor expressión in the gonadotrope of the rat. Neuroendocrinology 77:425–435
7. Blaustein JD (2004) Minireview: neuronal steroid hormona receptors: they're not just for hormones anymore. Endocrinology 145:1075–1081

8. Blum A, Hathaway L, Mincemoyer R, Schenke WH, Casco G, Waclawiw MA, Panza MA, Cannon III RO (2000) Hormonal, lipoprotein, and vascular effects of the selective estrogen receptor modulator raloxifene in hypercholesteronomic men. Am J Cardiol 85:1491–1494
9. Bowe J, Li XF, Sugden D, Katzellenenbogen JA, Katzellenenbogen BS, O'Byrne KT (2003) The effects of the phytoestrogen, coumestrol, on gonadotropin-releasing hormone (GnRH) mRNA expression in GT1-7 GnRH neurones. J Neuroendocrinol 15:105–108
10. Buelke-Sam J, Bryant HU, Francis PC (1998) The selective estrogen receptor modulator, raloxifene: an overview of nonclinical pharmacology and reproductive and developmental testing. Reprod Toxicol 12:217–221
11. Butler JA, Sjöberg M, Coen CW (1999) Evidence for oestrogen receptor α-immunoreactivity in gonadotrophin-releasing hormone-expressing neurones. J Neuroendocrinol 11:331–335
12. Byers M, Kuiper GGJM, Gustaffsson J-A, Park-Sarge O-K (1997) Estrogen receptor-β mRNA expression in rat ovary: down regulation by gonadotropins. Mol Endocrinol 11:172–182
13. Byrne B, Fowler PL, Templeton A (1996) Role of progesterone and nonsteroidal ovarian factors in regulating gonadotropin-releasing hormone self-priming in vitro. J Clin Endocrinol Metab 81:1454–1459
14. Chappell PE, Levine JE (2000) Stimulation of gonadotropin-releasing homone surges by estrogen. I. Role of hypothalamic progesterone receptors. Endocrinology 141:1477–1485
15. Chen Z, Zheng H, Dong KW (2001) Identification of negative and positive estrogen response elements in human GnRH upstream promoter in the placental JEG-3 cells. Mol Cell Endocrinol 184:125–134
16. Cheng WC, Yen ML, Hsdu SHJ, Chen KH, Tsai KS (2004) Effects of raloxifene, one of the selective estrogen receptor modulators, on pituitary-ovary axis and prolactin in postmenopausal women. Endocrine 23:215–218
17. Childs GV, Unabia G, Komak S (2001) Differential expression of estradiol receptors alpha and beta by gonadotrophs during the estrous cycle. J Histochem Cytochem 49:665–666
18. Chongthammakun S, Teresawa E (1993) Negative feedback effects of estrogen on luteinizing hormone-releasing hormone release occur in pubertal, but not prepubertal, ovariectomized female rhesus monkeys. Endocrinology 132:735–743
19. Christian HC, Morris JF (2002) Rapid actions of 17β-oestradiol on a subset of lactotrophs in the rat pituitary. J Physiol 539.2:557–566
20. Condon TP, Dykshoon-Bosch MA, Kelly MJ (1988) Episodic luteinizing-hormone release in the ovariectomized female guinea pig: rapid inhibition by estrogen. Biol Reprod 38:121–126
21. Conneely OM (2001) Perspective: female steroid hormone action. Endocrinology 142:2194–2199
22. Coombes RC, Haynes BP, Dowsett M, Quigley M, English J, Judson IR, Griggs LJ, Potter GA, McCague R, Jarman M (1995) Idoxifene: report of a phase I study in patients with metastatic breast cancer. Cancer Res 55:1070–1074
23. Couse JF, Korach KS (1999) Estrogen receptor null mice: what have we learned and where will they lead us? Endocr Rev 20:358–417
24. Demay F, De Monti M, Tiffoche C, Vaillant C, Thieulant ML (2001) Steroid-independent activation of ER by GnRH in gonadotrope pituitary cells. Endocrinology 142:3340–3347

25. de Koning J, Lambalk CB, Helmerhorst FM, Helder MN (2001) Is GnRH self-priming an obligatory feature of the reproductive cycle? Hum Reprod 16:209–214
26. Docke F, Ledwon P, Sturzebecher B, Rohde W, Dorner G (1989) Oestrogen priming for the positive oestrogen feedback: site of action. Exp Clin Endocrinol 94:55–60
27. Docke F, Rohde W, Sturzebecher B, Ledwon P, Dorner G (1990) Evidence that desensitization of the negative feedback of oestrogen and priming for the positive feedback of oestrogen depend upon a common mechanism of oestrogen action in rats. J Endocrinol 126:395–402
28. Donath J, Nishino Y (1998) Effect of partial versus pure antiestrogens on ovulation and the pituitary-ovarian axis in the rat. J Steroid Biochem Mol Biol 66:247–254
29. Dong KW, Chen ZG, Cheng KW, Yu KL (1996) Evidence for estrogen receptor-mediated regulation of human gonadotropin-releasing hormone promoter activity in human placental cells. Mol Cell Endocrinol 117:241–246
30. Doran PM, Riggs BL, Atkinson EJ, Khosla S (2001) Effects of raloxifene, a selective estrogen receptor modulator, on bone turnover markers and serum sex steroid and lipid levels in elderly men. J Bone Miner Res 16:2118–2125
31. Dorling AA, Todman MG, Korach KS, Herbison AE (2003) Critical role for estrogen receptor alpha in negative feedback regulation of gonadotropin-releasing hormone mRNA expression in the female mouse. Neuroendocrinology 78:204–209
32. Drouin J, Labrie F (1981) Interactions between 17 beta-estradiol and progesterone in the control of luteinizing hormone and follicle-stimulating hormone release in rat anterior pituitary cells in culture. Endocrinology 108:52–57
33. Drouva SV, Laplante E, Gautron JP, Kordon C (1984) Effects of 17 beta-estradiol on LH-RH release from rat mediobasal hypothalamic slices. Neuroendocrinology 38: 152–157
34. Dupont S, Krust A, Gansmuller A, Dierich A, Chambon P, Mark M (2000) Effect of single and compound knockouts of estrogen receptors alpha (ERα) and β (ERβ) on muse reproductive phenotypes. Development 127:4277–4291
35. El Majdoubi M, Sahu A, Plant TM (1998) Effect of estrogen on hypothalamic transforming growth factor alpha and gonadotropin-releasing hormone gene expression in the female rhesus monkey (*Macaca mulatta*). Neuroendocrinology 67: 228–235
36. Ellmen J, Hakulinen P, Partanen A, Hayes DF (2003) Estrogenic effects of toremifen and tamoxifen in postmenopausal breast cancer patients. Breast Cancer Res Treat 82:103–111
37. Engel JB, Felberbaum RE, Eilers W, Polack S, Ortmann O, Diedrich K (2002) Clomiphene-induced LH surges and cetrorelix. Reprod Biomed Online 5:109–111
38. Evans NP, Dahl GE, Glover BH, Karsch FJ (1994) Central regulation of pulsatile gonadotropin-releasing hormone (GnRH) secretion by estradiol during the period leading up to the preovulatory GnRH surge in the ewe. Endocrinology 134:1806–1811
39. Eyigor O, Jennes L (1997) Expression of glutamate receptor subunit mRNAs in gonadotropin-releasing hormone neurons during the sexual maturation of the female rat. Neuroendocrinology 66:122–129
40. Fabian CJ, Kimler BF, Anderson J,Tawfik OW, Mayo MS, Burak Jr WE, O'Shaugnessy JA, Albain KS, Hyams DM, Budd GT, Ganz PA, Sauter ER, Beenken SW, Grizzle WE, Fruehauf JP, Arneson DW, Bacus JW, Lagios MD, Johnson KA, Browne D (2004) Breast cancer chemoprevention phase I evaluation of biomarker modulation by ar-

zoxifene, a third generation selective estrogen receptor modulator. Clin Cancer Res 10:5403–5417

41. Fink G (1988) Gonadotropin secretion and its control. In: Knobil E, Neill J (eds) The physiology of reproduction. Raven, New York, pp 1349–1377
42. Fink G (1995) The self-priming effect of LHRH: a unique servomechanism and possible cellular model of memory. Front Neuroendocrinol 16:18–190
43. Fink G (2000) Neuroendocrine regulation of pituitary function: general principles. In: Conn PM, Freeman ME (eds) Neuroendocrinology in physiology and medicine. Humana, Totowa, NJ, pp 107–134
44. Florio P, Quirici B, Casarosa E, Lombardi I, Luisi M, Genazzani AD, Petraglia F, Genazzani AR (2001) Neuroendocrine effects of raloxifene hydrochloride in postmenopausal women. Gynecol Endocrinol 15:359–366
45. Flugge G, Oertel WH, Wuttke W (1986) Evidence for estrogen-receptive GABAergic neurons in the preoptic/anterior hypothalamus area of the rat brain. Neuroendocrinology 43:1–5
46. Fowler PA, Templeton A (1996) The nature and function of putative gonadotropin surge-attenuating/inhibiting factor (GnSAF/IF). Endocr Rev 17:103–120
47. Fowler PA, Spears N (2004) The cultured rodent follicle as a model for investigations on gonadotropin surge-attenuating factor (GnSAF) production. Reproduction 127:679–688
48. Fowler PA, Sorsa-Leslie T, Cash P, Dunbar B, Melvin W, Wilson Y, Mason HD, Harris W (2002) A 60–66 Kda protein with gonadotropin surge attenuating factor bioactivity is produced by human ovarian granulose cells. Mol Hum Reprod 8:823–832
49. Fowler PA, Sorsa-Leslie T, Harris W, Mason HD (2003) Ovarian gonadotropin surge-attenuating factor (GnSAF): where are we after 20 years of research? Reproduction 126:689–699
50. Freeman ME (1994) The neuroendocrine control of the varian cycle of the rat. In: Knobil E, Neill JD (eds) The physiology of reproduction, 2nd edn. Raven, New York, vol 2, pp 613–658
51. Gao X, Petroff BK, Oluola O, Georg G, Terranova PF, Rozman KK (2002) Endocrine disruption by indole-3-carbinol and tamoxifen: blockage of ovulation. Toxicol Appl Pharmacol 183:179–188
52. Garas A, Trypsianis G, Kallitsaris A, Milingos S, Messinis IE (2004) Effects of clomiphene and reloxifene on gonadatrophin secretion in postmenopausal women: evidence of nongenomic action. Clin Endocrinol 61:256–262
53. Geisler J, Ekse D, Hosch S, Lønning PE (1995a) Influence of droloxifene (3-hydroxytamoxifen), 40 mg daily, on plasma gonadotrophins, sex hormone binding globulin and estrogen levels in postmenopausal breast cancer patients. J Steroid Biochem Mol Biol 55:193–195
54. Geisler J, Haarstad H, Gündersen S, Raabe N, Kvinnsland S, Lønning PE (1995b) Influence of treatment with the anti-oestrogen 3-hydroxytamoxifen (droloxifene) on plasma sex hormone levels in postmenopausal breast cancer patients. J Endocrinol 146:359–363
55. Genazzani AR, Lombardi I, Borgioli G, di Bono I, Casarosa E, Gambacciani M, Palumbo M, Genazzani AD, Luisi M (2003) Adrenal function under long-term raloxifene administration. Gynecol Endocrinol 17:159–168
56. Glass CK, Rosenfeld MG (2000) The coregulator exchange in transcriptional functions of nuclear receptors. Genes Dev 14:121–141
57. González D, Bellido C, Aguilar R, Garrido-Gracia JC, Hernández G, Alonso R, Sánchez-Criado JE (2000) Luteinizing hormone secretion elicited in a ligand-independent

activation of progesterone receptor manner at pituitary level in the rat: differential effect of two selective estrogen receptor modulators. Neurosci Lett 289:111–114
58. Guelmes P, Abreu P, Sánchez-Criado JE, Prieto L, Alonso R, Hernández G (2003) Differential effects of selective estrogen receptor modulators on luteinizing hormone-releasing hormone-induced luteinizing hormone secretion and inositol phosphate accumulation in female rat pituitary glands. J Physiol 548.P:5P.P147
59. Guerra B, Díaz M, Alonso R, Marín M (2004) Plasma membrane oestrogen receptor mediates neuroprotection against β-amyloid toxicity through activation of Raf-1/MEK/ERK cascade. J Neurochem 91:99–109
60. Henderson SR, Baker C, Fink G (1977) Oestradiol-17beta and pituitary responsiveness to luteinizing hormone releasing factor in the rat: a study using rectangular pulses of oestradiol-17 beta monitored by non-chromatographic radioimmunoassay. J Endocrinol 73:441–453
61. Herbison AE (1998) Multimodal influence of estrogen upon gonadotropin-releasing hormone neurons. Endocr Rev 19:302–330
62. Herbison AE, Pape J-R (2001) New evidence for estrogen receptors in gonadotropin-releasing hormone neurons. Front Neuroendocrinol 22:292–308
63. Herbison AE, Skynner MJ, Sim JA (2001) Lack of detection of estrogen receptor-α transcripts in mouse gonadotropin-relesing hormone neurons. Endocrinology 142:493
64. Hernández G, Hernández-Jiménez JG, Guelmes P, Sánchez-Criado JE, Bellido C, Martínez-Morales JR, Prieto L, Marín F, Glidewell-Kenney C, López FJ, Alonso R (2003) Reduction of pituitary sensitivity to gonadotropin-releasing hormone (GnRH) and subsequent ovulation blockade after treatment with the selective estrogen receptor modulator LY117018-HCl. Reproduction 125:597–606
65. Hiroi H, Inoue S, Watanabe T, Goto W, Orimo A, Momoeda M, Tsutsumi O, Taketani Y, Muramatsu M (1999) Differential immunolocalization of estrogen receptor α and β in rat ovary and uterus. J Mol Endocrinol 22:34–44
66. Hotchkiss J, Konbill E (1994) The menstrual cycle and its neuroendocrine control. In: Knobil E, Neill JD (eds) The physiology of reproduction, 2nd edn. Raven, New York, vol 2, pp 711–749
67. Hrabovszky E, Shughrue PJ, Merchenthaler I, Hajszán T, Carpenter CD, Liposits Z, Petersen SL (2000) Detection of estrogen receptor-β messenger ribonucleic acid and ^{125}I-estrogen binding sites in luteinizing hormone-releasing hormone neurons of the rat brain. Endocrinology 141:3506–3509
68. Hrabovszky E, Steinhauser AM, Barabás K, Shughrue PJ, Petersen SL, Merchenthaler I, Liposits Z (2001) Estrogen receptor-β immunoreactivity in luteinizing hormone-releasing hormone neurons of the rat brain. Endocrinology 142:3261–3264
69. Jarry H, Leonhardt S, Wuttke W (1991) Gamma-aminobutyric acid neurons in the preoptic/anterior hypothalamic area synchronize the phasic activity of the gonadotropin-releasing hormone pulse generator in ovariectomized rats. Neuroendocrinology 53:261–267
70. Jarry H, Leonhardt S, Schwarze T, Wuttke W (1995) Preoptic rather than mediobasal hypothalamic amino acid neurotransmitter release regulates GnRH secretion during the estrogen-induced LH surge in the ovariectomized rat. Neuroendocrinology 62:479–486
71. Jordan VC, Morrow M (1999) Tamoxifen, raloxifen and the prevention of breast cancer. Endocr Rev 20:253–278

72. Jordan VC, Fritz NF, Tormey DC (1987a) Long-term adjuvant therapy with tamoxifen: effects on sex hormone binding globulin and antithrombin III. Cancer Res 47:4517–4519
73. Jordan VC, Fritz NF, Tormey DC (1987b) Endocrine effects of adjuvant chemotherapy and long-term tamoxifen administration on node-positive patients with breast cancer. Cancer Res 47:624–630
74. Jordan VC, Fritz NF, Langan-Fahey S, Thompson M, Tormey DC (1991) Alterations of endocrine parameters in premenopausal women with breast cancer during long-term adjuvant therapy with tamoxifen as the single agent. J Natl Cancer Inst 83:1488–1491
75. Jordan VC, Morrow M (1999) Tamoxifen, raloxifene and the prevention of breast cancer. Endocr Rev 20:253–278
76. Kallo I, Butler JA, Barkovics-Kallo M, Goubillon ML, Coen CW (2001) Oestrogen receptor beta-immunoreactivity in gonadotropin releasing hormone-expressing neurones: regulation by oestrogen. J Neuroendocrinol 13:741–748
77. Kelly MJ, Rønnekleiv OK, Ibrahim N, Lagrange AH, Wagner EJ (2002) Estrogen modulation of K^+ channel activity in the hypothalamic neurons involved in the control of the reproductive axis. Steroids 67:447–456
78. Kilic-Okman T, Kucuk M, Altaner S (2003) Comparison of the effects of letrozole and clomiphene citrate on ovarian follicles, endometrium, and hormone levels in the rat. Fertil Steril 80:1330–1332
79. Kimura F, Funabashi T (1998) Two subgroups of gonadotropin-releasing hormone neurons control gonadotropin secretion in rats. News Physiol Sci 13:225–231
80. Kostoglou-Athanassiou I, Ntalles K, Gogas J, Markopoulos C, Alevizou-Terzaki V, Athanassiou P, Georgiou E, Proukakis C (1997) Sex hormones in postmenopausal women with breast cancer on tamoxifen. Horm Res 47:116–120
81. Krege JH, Hodgin JB, Couse JF, Enmark E, Warner M, Mahler JF, Sar M, Korach KS, Gustafsson JA, Smithies O (1998) Generation and reproductive phenotypes of mice lacking estrogen receptor β. Proc Natl Acad Sci USA 95:15677–15682
82. Kuiper GGJM, Enmark E, Pelto-Huikko M, Nilsson S, Gustafsson J-A (1996) Cloning of a novel estrogen receptor expressed in rat prostate and ovary. Proc Natl Acad Sci USA 93:5925–5930
83. Kuiper GGJM, Carlsson B, Grandient K, Enmark E, Haggblad J, Nilsson S, Gustaffsson JA (1997) Comparison of the ligand binding specificity and transcript tissue distribution of estrogen receptors α and β. Endocrinology 138:863–870
84. Lagrange AH, Rønnekleiv, Kelly MJ (1995) Estradiol-17β and μ-Opioid peptides rapidly hyperpolarize GnRH neurons: a cellular mechanism of negative feedback? Endocrinology 136:2341–2344
85. Lasco A, Cannavo S, Gaudio A, Morabito N, Basile G, Nicita-Mauro V, Frisina N (2002) Effects of long-lasting raloxifene treatment on serum prolactin and gonadotropin levels in postmenopausal women. Eur J Endocrinol 147:461–465
86. Le WW, Bergohrn KA, Rassnick S, Hoffman GE (1999) Periventricular preoptic ara neurons coactivated with luteinizing hormone (LH)-releasing hormone (LHRH) neurons at the time of of the LH surge are LHRH afferents. Endocrinology 140:510–519
87. Legan SJ, Tsai HW (2003) Oestrogen receptor-alpha and beta immunoreactivity in gonadotropin-releasing hormone neurons after ovariectomy and chronic exposure to oestradiol. J Neuroendocrinol 15:1164–1170
88. Lehman MH, Karsch FJ (1993) Do gonadotropin-releasing hormone, tyrosine hydroxylase-, and β-endorphin-immunoreactive neurons contain estrogen recep-

tors? A double-label immunocytochemical study in the Suffolk ewe. Endocrinology 133:887–895

89. Leipheimer RE, Gallo RV (1983) Acute and long-term changes in central and pituitary mechanisms regulating pulsatile luteinizing hormone secretion after ovariectomy in the rat. Neuroendocrinology 37:421–426
90. Levine NE (1997) New concepts of neuroendocrine regulation of gonadotropin surges in rats. Biol Reprod 56:293–302
91. Levine JE, Norman RL, Gliessman PM, Oyama TT, Bangsberg DR, Spies HG (1985) In vivo gonadotropin-releasing hormone release and serum luteinizing hormone measurements in ovariectomized, estrogen-treated rhesus macaques. Endocrinology 117:711–721
92. Levine JE, Bauer-Dantoin AC, Besecke LM, Conaghan LA, Legan SJ, Meredith JM, Strobl FJ, Urban JH, Vogelsong KM, Wolfe AM (1991) Neuroendocrine regulation of luteinizing hormone pulse generator in the rat. Recent Prog Horm Res 47:97–153
93. Levine JE, Chappel P, Besecke LM, Bauer-Dantoin AC, Wolfe AM, Porkka-Heiskanen T, Urban JH (1995) Amplitude and frequency modulation of pulsatile luteinizing hormone-releasing hormone release. Cell Mol Neurobiol 15:117–139
94. Long GG, Cohen IR, Gries CL, Young JK, Francis PC, Capen CC (2001) Proliferative lesions of ovarian granulosa cells and reversible hormonal changes induced in rats by a selective estrogen receptor modulator. Toxicol Pathol 29:719–726
95. Lønning PE, Johannessen DC, Lien EA, Ekse D, Fotsis T, Adlercreutz H (1995) Influence of tamoxifen on sex hormones, gonadotrophins and sex hormone binding globulin in postmenopausal breast cancer patients. J Steroid Biochem Mol Biol 52:491–496
96. López F, Donoso A, Negro-Vilar A (1990) Endogenous excitatory aminoacids regulate the estradiol-induced LH surge in ovariectomized rats. Endocrinology 126:1771–1773
97. Lubahn DB, Moyer JS, Golding TS, Couse JF, Korach KS, Smithies O (1993) Alteration of reproductive function but not prenatal sexual development after insertional disruption of the mouse estrogen receptor gene. Proc Natl Acad Sci USA 90:11162–11166
98. Lustig RH, Pfaff DW, Fishman J (1988) Opioidergic modulation of the oestradiol-induced LH surge in the rat: roles of ovarian steroids. J Endocrinol 116:55–69
99. Mallory DS, Gallo RV (1990) Medial preoptic-anterior hypothalamic area involvement in the suppression of pulsatile LH release by a mu-opiod agonist in the ovariectomized rat. Brain Res Bull 25:251–257
100. Marín R, Guerra B, Morales A, Díaz M, Alonso R (2003) An estrogen membrane receptor participates in the neuroprotective action of estradiol against amyloid β-peptide$_{1-40}$-induced toxicity in SN56 neurons. J Neurochem 85:1180–1189
101. Marín R, Guerra B, Alonso R, Ramírez CM, Díaz M (2005) Estrogen activates classical and alternative mechanisms to orchestrate neuroprotection. Curr Neurovas Res 2:287–301
102. Martínez-Morales JR, Morales A, Marín R, Hernández-Jiménez JG, Acevedo A, Guerra B, Hernández G, López-Coviella I, Prieto L, Alonso R (2001) Estrogen modulates norepinephrine-induced accumulation of adenosine cyclic monophosphate in a subpopulation of immortalized luteinizing hormone-releasing hormone secreting neurons from the mouse hypothalamus. Neurosci Lett 298:61–64
103. McDonnell DP (1999) The molecular pharmacology of SERMs. Trends Endocrinol Metab 10:301–311
104. McDonnell DP (2003) Mining the complexities of the estrogen signalling pathways for novel therapeutics. Endocrinology 144:4237–4240

105. McDonnell DP, Connors CE, Wijayaratne A, Chang C-Y, Norris JD (2002) Definition of the molecular and cellular activities of selective estrogen receptor modulators. Recent Prog Hor Res 57:295–316
106. McKenna NJ, Xu J, Nawasz Z, Tsai SY, O'Malley BW (1999) Nuclear receptor coactivators: multiple enzymes, multiple complexes, multiple functions. J Steroid Biochem Mol Biol 69:3–12
107. Mellon PL, Windle JJ, Goldsmith PC, Padula CA, Roberts JL, Weiner RI (1990) Immortalization of hypothalamic GnRH neurons by genetically targeted tumorigenesis. Neuron 5:1–10
108. Messinis IE, Nillius SJ (1982) Comparison between tamoxifen and clomiphene for induction of ovulation. Acta Obstet Gynecol Scand 61:377–379
109. Messinis IE, Templeton A (1990) Anti-oestrogen effect of clomiphene citrate in oestrogen-treated, hypogonadal women. Hum Reprod 5:150–152
110. Meyers MJ, Sun J, Carlson KE, Marriner A, Katznellenbogen BS, Katzenellenbogen JA (2001) Estrogen receptor-β potency-selective ligands: structure-activity relationship studies of diarylpropionitriles and their acetylene and polar analogues. J Med Chem 44:4230–4251
111. Mitchner NA, Garlick C, Ben-Jonathan N (1998) Cellular distribution and gene regulation of estrogen receptors α and β in the rat pituitary gland. Endocrinology 139:976–3983
112. Mitsushima D, Jinnai K, Kimura F (1997) Possible role of $GABA_A$ receptor system in the timing of proestrous LH surge in rats. Endocrinology 138:1944–1948
113. Miyake A, Tasaka K, Sakumoto T, Kawamura Y, Nagahara Y, Aono T (1983) Clomiphene citrate induces luteinizing hormone release through hypothalamic hormone-releasing hormone in vitro. Acta Endocrinol 103:289–292
114. Moenter SM, Caraty A, Karsch FJ (1990) The estradiol-induced surge of gonadotropin-releasing homone in the ewe. Endocrinology 127:1375–1384
115. Moenter SM, Caraty A, Locatelli A, Karsch FJ (1991) Pattern of gonadotropin-releasing hormone (GnRH) secretion leading up to ovulation in the ewe: existence of a preovulatory GnRH surge. Endocrinology 129:1175–1182
116. Morales A, Díaz M, Ropero AB, Nadal A, Alonso R (2003) Estradiol modulates acetylcholine-induced Ca^{2+} signals in LHRH-releasing GT1–7 cells through a membrane binding site. Eur J Neurosci 18:2505–2514
117. Nadal A, Díaz M, Valverde M A (2001) The estrogen trinity: membrane, cytosolic, and nuclear effects. News Physiol Sci 16:251–255
118. Navarro CE, Abdul Saeed S, Murdock C, Martínez-Fuentes AJ, Arora KK, Krsmanovic LZ, Catt KJ (2003) Regulation of cyclic adenosine 3′,5′-monophosphate signaling and pulsatile neurosecretion by G_i-coupled plasma membrane estrogen receptors in immortalized gonadotropin-releasing hormone neurons. Mol Endocrinol 17:1792–1804
119. Nishihara E, Nagayama Y, Inoue S, Hiroi H, Muramatsu M, Yamashita S, Koji T (2000) Ontogenic changes in the expression of estrogen receptor α and β in rat pituitary gland detected by immunohistochemistry. Endocrinology 141:615–620
120. Norfleet AM, Thomas ML, Gametchu B, Watson CS (1999) Estrogn receptor-α detected on the plasma membrane of aldehyde-fixed GH_3/B6F10 rat pituitary tumor cells by enzyme-linked immunocytochemistry. Endocrinology 140:3805–3814
121. Nunemaker CS, De Fazio RA, Moenter SM (2002) Estradiol-sensitive afferents modulate long-term episodic firing patterns of GnRH neurons. Endocrinology 143:2284–2292

122. Ondo J, Mansky T, Wuttke W (1982) In vivo GABA release from the medial preoptic area of diestrous and ovariectomized rats. Exp Brain Res 4669–4672
123. Pappas TC, Gametchu B, Yannariello-Brown J, Collins TJ, Watson CS (1994) Membrane oestrogen receptor in GH3B6 cells are associated with rapid oestrogen-induced release of prolactin. Endocrine 2:813–822
124. Pasqualini C, Guivarch D, Boxberg YV, Nothias F, Vincent J-D, Vernier P (1999) Stage- and region-specific expression of estrogen receptor α isoforms during ontogeny of the pituitary gland. Endocrinology 140:2781–2789
125. Patisaul HB, Aultman EA, Bielsky IF, Young LJ, Wilson ME (2003) Immediate and residual effects of tamoxifen and ethynylestradiol in the female rat hypothalamus. Brain Res 978:185–193
126. Pelletier G, Labrie C, Labrie F (2000) Localization of oestrogen receptor α, oestrogen receptor β and androgen receptors in the rat reproductive organs. J Endocrinol 165:359–370
127. Pelletier G, Labrie C, Martel C, Li S, Labrie F (2001) Role of extra-ovarian oestrogens in the regulation of gonadotropin releasing hormone mRNA expression in the rat brain. J Neuroendocrinol 13:678–682
128. Petersen SL, McCrone S, Keller M, Shores S (1995) Effects of estrogen and progesterone on luteinizing hormone-releasing hormone messenger ribonucleic acid levels: consideration of temporal and neuroanatomical variables. Endocrinology 136:3604–3610
129. Petersen SL, Ottem EN, Carpenter CD (2003) Direct and indirect regulation of gonadotropin-releasing hormone neurons by estradiol. Biol Reprod 69:1771–1778
130. Ping L, Mahesh VB, Wiedmeier VT, Brann DW (1994) Release of glutamate and aspartate from the preoptic area during the progesterone-induced LH surge: In vivo microdialysis studies. Neuroendocrinology 59:318–324
131. Pinilla L, González LC, Tena-Sempere M, Aguilar E (2001) Evidence for an estrogen-like action of raloxifene upon the hypothalamic-pituitary unit: raloxifene inhibits luteinizing hormone secretion and stimulates prolactin secretion in ovariectomized female rats. Neurosci Lett 311:149–152
132. Prevot V, Croix D, Rialas CM, Poulain P, Fricchione GL, Stefano GB, Beauvillain JC (1999) Estradiol coupling to endothelial nitric oxide stimulates gonadotropin-releasing hormone release from rat median eminence via a membrane receptor. Endocrinology 140:652–659
133. Prevot V, Bouret S, Croix D, Takumi T, Jennes L, Mitchell V, Beauvillain JC (2000) Evidence that members of the TGFβ superfamily play a role in regulation of the GnRH neuroendocrine axis: Expression of a type I serine-threonine kinase receptor for TGRβ and activin in GnRH neurones and hypothalamic areas of the female rat. J Neuroendocrinol 12:677–670
134. Qiu J, Bosch MA, Tobias SC, Grandy DK, Scanlan TS, Ronnekleiv OK, Kelly MJ (2003) Rapid signaling of estrogen in hypothalamic neurons involves a novel G-protein-coupled estrogen receptor that activates protein kinase C. J Neurosci 23:9529–9540
135. Rance NE, Uswandi SV (1996) Gonadotropin-releasing hormone gene expression is increased in the medio basal hypothalamus in postmenopausal women. J Clin Endocrinol Metab 81:3540–3546
136. Ravdin PM, Fritz NF, Tormey DC, Jordan VC (1988) Endocrine status of postmenopausal node-positive breast cancer patients following adjuvant chemotherapy and long-term tamoxifen. Cancer Res 48:1026–1029
137. Razandi M, Pedram A, Merchenthaler I, Greene GL, Levin ER (2004) Plasma membrane estrogen receptors exist and function as dimers. Mol Endocrinol 18:2854–2865

138. Reindollar R, Koltun W, Parsons A, Rosen A, Siddhanti S, Plouffe Jr L (2002) Effects of oral raloxifene on serum estradiol levels and other markers of estrogenicity. Fertil Steril 78:469–472
139. Rosie R, Thomson E, Fink G (1990) Oestrogen positive feedback stimulates the synthesis of LHRH mRNA in neurones of the rostral diencephalons of the rat. J Endocrinol 124:285–289
140. Roy D, Angelini NL, Belsham DD (1999) Estrogen directly represses gondotropin-releasing hormone (GnRH) gene expression in estrogen receptor-α (ERα)- and ERβ-expressing GT1-7 GnRH neurons. Endocrinology 140:5045–5053
141. Sánchez-Criado JE, Guelmes P, Bellido C, González M, Hernández G, Aguilar R, Garrido-Gracia JC, Bello AR, Alonso R (2002) Tamoxifen but not other selective estrogen receptor modulators antagonizes estrogen actions on luteinizing hormone secretion while inducing gonadotropin-releasing hormone self-priming in the rat. Neuroendocrinology 76:203–213
142. Sánchez-Criado JE, Martín de las Mulas J, Bellido C, Tena-Sempere M, Aguilar R, Garrido-Gracia JC (2004) Biological role of pituitary estrogen ERalpha and ERbeta on progesterone receptor expressión and action ando on gonadotropin and prolactin secretion in the rat. Neuroendocrinology 79:247–258
143. Sánchez-Criado JE, Martín de las Mulas J, Bellido C, Aguilar R, Garrido-Gracia JC (2005) Gonadotrope oestrogen receptor-α and -β and progestrone receptor immunoreactivity alter ovariectomy and exposure to oestradiol benzoote, tamoxifen or raloxifen in the rat: correlation with LH secretion. J Endocrinol 184:59–68
144. Sánchez-Criado JE, Bellido C, Aguilar R, Garrido-Gracia JC (2005) A paradoxical inhibitory effect of oestradio-17beta on GnRH self-priming in pituitaries from tamoxifen treated rats. J Endocrinol 186:43–49
145. Sarkar DK, Fink G (1980) Luteinizing hormone releasing factor in pituitary stalk plasma from long-term ovariectomized rats: effects of steroids. J Endocrinol 86:511–524
146. Sarkar DK, Chiappa SA, Fink G, Sherwood NM (1976) Gonadotropin-releasing hormone surge in pro-oestrous rats. Nature 264:461–463
147. Saunders PTK, Maguire SM, Gaughan J, Millar MR (1997) Expression of oestrogen receptor beta (ERbeta) in multiple rat tissues visualised by immunohistochemistry. J Endocrinol 154:R13–R16
148. Schreihofer DA, Resnick EM, Soh AY, Shupnik MA (1999) Transcriptional regulation by a naturally occurring truncated rat estrogen receptor (ER), truncated ER product-1 (TERP-1). Mol Endocrinol 13:320–329
149. Schreihofer DA, Stoler MH, Shupnik MA (2000) Differential expression and regulation of estrogen receptors (ERs) in rat pituitary cell lines: estrogen decreases ERα protein and estrogen responsiveness. Endocrinology 141:2174–2184
150. Schreihofer DA, Resnick EM, Lin VY, Shupnik MA (2001) Ligand-independent activation of pituitary ER: dependence on PKA-stimulated pathways. Endocrinology 142:3361–3368
151. Schreihofer DA, Rowe DF, Rissman EF, Scordalakes EM, Gustaffsson JA, Shupnik MA (2002) Estrogen receptor-α (ERα), but not ERβ, modulates estrogen stimulation of the ERα-truncated variant, TERP-1. Endocrinology 143:4196–4202
152. Schuiling GA, Pols-Valkhof N, Koiter TR (1985) Clomiphene citrate can mimic the augmentative (positive) but not the depressing (negative) effect of estradiol on the LHRH-stimulated release of LH and FSH by the pituitary gland of the long-term ovariectomized rat. Experientia 41:1060–1063

153. Scott RE, Wu-Peng XS, Pfaff DW (2002) Regulation and expression of progesterone receptor mRNA isoforms A and B in the male and female hypothalamus and pituitary following oestrogen treatment. J Neuroendocrinol 14:175–183
154. Scully KM, Gleiberman AS, Lindzey J, Lubhan DB, Korach KS, Rosenfeld MG (1997) Role of estrogen receptor-α in the anterior pituitary gland. Mol Endocrinol 11:674–681
155. Sharifi N, Reuss AE, Wray S (2002) Prenatal LHRH neurons in nasal explant cultures express estrogen receptor beta transcript. Endocrinology 143: 2503–2507
156. Shen ES, Meade EH, Pérez MC, Deecher DC, Negro-Vilar A, López FJ (1998) Expression of functional estrogen receptors and galanin messenger ribonucleic acid in immortalized luteinizing hormone-releasing hormone neurons: estrogenic control of galanin gene expression. Endocrinology 139:939–948
157. Shimizu I, Terakawa N, Aono T, Tanizawa O, Matsumoto K (1986) Clomiphene citrate induces pituitary GnRH receptors in ovariectomized rats: possible role in induction of ovulation. Acta Endocrinol 111:179–184
158. Shivers BD, Harlan RE, Morrell JI, Pfaff DW (1983) Absence of oestradiol concentration in cell nuclei of LHRH-immunoreactive neurones. Nature 304:345–347
159. Shughrue PJ, Lane MV, Merchenthaler I (1997) Regulation of progesterone receptor messenguer ribonucleic acid in the rat medial preoptic nucleus by estrogenic and antiestrogenic compounds: an in situ hybridization study. Endocrinology 138:5476–5484
160. Shupnik MA (1996) Gonadotropin gene modulation by steroids and gonadotropin-releasing hormone. Biol Reprod 54:279–286
161. Shupnik MA (2002) Oestrogen receptor, receptor variants and oestrogen actions in the hypothalamic-pituitary axis. J Neuroendocrinol 14:85–94
162. Skynner MJ, Sim JA, Herbison AE (1999) Detection of estrogen receptor α and β messenger ribonucleic acid in adult gonadotropin-releasing hormone neurons. Endocrinology 140:5195–5201
163. Smith CL, O'Malley BW (2004) Coregulator function: a key to understanding tissue specificity of selective receptor modulators. Endocr Rev 25:45–71
164. Speight A, Popkin R, Watts AG, Fink G (1981) Oestradiol-17β increases pituitary responsiveness by a mechanism that involves the release and the priming effect of luteinizing hormone releasing factor. J Endocrinol 88:301–308
165. Spergel DJ, Kruth U, Hanley DF, Sprengel R, Seeburg PH (1999) GABA- and glutamate-activated channels in green fluorescent protein-tagged gonadotropin-releasing hormone neurons in transgenic mice. J Neurosci 19:2037–2050
166. Stauffer SR, Coletta CJ, Tedesco R, Nishiguchi G, Carlson K, Sun J, Katzenellenbogen BS, Katzenellenbogen JA (2000) Pyrazole ligands: structure-affinity/activity relationships and receptor-alpha-selective agonists. J Med Chem 43:4934–4947
167. Sullivan KA, Witkin JW, Ferin M, Silverman AJ (1995) GnRH neurons in the rhesus macaque are not immunoreactive for the estrogen receptor. Brain Res 685:198–200
168. Sun J, Meyers MJ, Fink BE, Rajendran R, Katzenellenbogen JA, Katzenellenebogen BS (1999) Novel ligands that function as selective estrogens or antiestrogens for estrogen receptor-α or estrogen receptor-β. Endocrinology 140:800–804
169. Suter KJ, Wuarin J-P, Smith BN, Dudek FE, Moenter SM (2000) Whole-cell recordings from preoptic/hypothalamic slices reveal burst firing in gondotropin-releasing hormone neurons identified with green fluorescent protein in transgenic mice. Endocrinology 141:3731–3736

170. Szabo M, Kilen SM, Nho SJ, Schwartz NB (2000) Progesterone receptor A and B messenger ribonucleic acid levels in the anterior pituitary of rats are regulated by estrogen. Biol Reprod 62:95–102
171. Számel I, Hindy I, Vincze B, Eckhardt S, Kangas L, Hajba A (1994) Influence of toremifene on the endocrine regulation in breast cancer patients. Eur J Cancer 30:154–158
172. Számel I, Hindy I, Vincze B, Budai B, Kangas L, Hajba A, Lammintausta R (1995) Endocrine mechanism of action of toremifene at the level of the central nervous system in advanced breast cancer patients. Cancer Chemother Pharmacol 42:241–246
173. Tébar M, Bellido C, Aguilar R, Sánchez-Criado JE (1994) Inappropriate ovarian feedback in basal gonadotropin secretion in 4-day cyclic rat treated with mifepristone: role of endogenous estradiol. J Endocrinol Invest 17:425–430
174. Tébar M, Ruiz A, Sánchez-Criado JE (1998) Involvement of estrogen and follicle-stimulating hormone on basal and luteinizing hormone (LH)-releasing hormone-stimulated LH secretion in RU486-induced 3-day estrous cycle in the rat. Biol Reprod 58:615–619
175. Temple JL, Laing E, Sunder A, Wray S (2004) Direct action of estradiol on gonadotropin-reelasing hormone-1 neuronal activity via a transcription-dependent mechanism. J Neurosci 24:6326–6333
176. Tena-Sempere M, Navarro VM, Mayen A, Bellido C, Sánchez-Criado JE (2004) Regulation of estrogen receptor (ER) isoform messenger RNA expressión by different ligands in female rat pituitary. Biol Reprod 70:671–678
177. Terakawa N, Shimizu I, Tsutsumi H, Aono T, Matsumoto K (1985) A possible role of clomiphene citrate in the control of pre-ovulatory LH surge during induction of ovulation. Acta Endocrinol 109:58–63
178. Terakawa N, Shimizu I, Aono T, Tanizawa O, Matsumoto K (1986) Dexamethasone inhibits the effects of oestrogen on the pituitary gland in rats. Acta Endocrinol 112:64–70
179. Terasawa E (2001) Luteinizing hormone-releasing hormone (LHRH) neurons: mechanism of pulsatile LHRH release. Vitam Horm 63:91–129
180. Toney TW, Katznellenbogen BS (1986) Antiestrogen action in the medial basal hypothalamus and pituitary on immature female rats: insights concerning relationships among estrogen, dopamine, and prolactin. Endocrinology 119:2661–2669
181. Tsai MJ, O'Malley BW (1994) Molecular mechanisms of action of steroid/thyroid receptor superfamiliy members. Annu Rev Biochem 63:451–486
182. Turgeon JL, McDonnell DP, Martin KA, Wise PM (2004) Hormone therapy: physiological complexity belies therapeutic simplicity. Science 304:1269–1273
183. Uebelhart B, Herrmann F, Pavo I, Draper MW, Rizzoli R (2004) Raloxifene treatment is associated with increased serum estradiol and decreased bone remodeling in healthy middle-aged men with low sex hormone levels. J Bone Miner Res 19:1518–1524
184. Vaillant C, Chesnel F, Schausi D, Tiffoche C, Thieulant M-L (2002) Expression of estrogen receptor subtypes in rat pituitary gland during pregnancy and lactation. Endocrinology 143:4249–4258
185. Valverde MA, Parker MG (2002) Classical and novel steroid actions: a unified but complex view. Trends Biochem Sci 27:172–173
186. Van den Pol AN, Wuarin J, Dudek FE (1990) Glutamate, the dominant excitatory transmitter in neuroendocrine regulation. Science 250:1276–1278
187. Waring DW, Turgeon JL (1992) A pathway for luteinizing hormone-releasing hormone self-potentiation: cross-talk with the progesterone receptor. Endocrinology 130:3275–3282

188. Watson RE, Langrub MC, Landis JW (1992) Further evidence that most luteinizing hormone-releasing hormone neurons are not directly estrogen-responsive: simultaneous localization of luteinizing hormone-releasing hormone and estrogen-receptor immunoreactivity in the guinea pig brain. J Neuroendocrinol 4:311–318
189. Weisner JB, Koeng JI, Krulich L, Moss RL (1984) Site of action for β-endorphin-induced changes in plasma luteinizing hormone and prolactin in the ovariectomized rat. Life Sci 34:1463–1473
190. Wersinger SR, Haisenleder DJ, Lubahn DB, Rissman EF (1999) Steroid feedback on gonadotropin release and pituitary gonadotropin subunit mRNA in mice lacking a functional estrogen receptor α. Endocrine 11:137–143
191. Wiegand SJ, Terasawa E (1982) Discrete lesions reveal functional heterogeneity of suprachiasmatic structures in regulation of gonadotropin secretion in the female rat. Neuroendocrinology 34:395–44
192. Wierman ME, Kepa JK, Sun W, Gordon DF, Wood WM (1992) Estrogen negatively regulates rat gonadotropin releasing hormone (rGnRH) promoter activity in transfected placental cells. Mol Cell Endocrinol 86:1–10
193. Wilson ME, Price RH, Handa RJ (1998) Estrogen receptor-β messenger ribonucleic acid expression in the pituitary gland. Endocrinology 139:5151–5156
194. Xia L, Van Vugt D, Alston EJ, Luckhaus J, Ferin M (1992) A surge of gonadotropin-releasing hormone accompanies the estradiol-induced gonadotropin surge in the rhesus monkey. Endocrinology 131:2812–2820
195. Yin P, Kawashima K, Arita J (2002) Direct actions of estradiol on the anterior pituitary gland are required for hypothalamus-dependent lactotrope proliferation and secretory surges of luteinizing hormone but not of prolactin in female rats. Neuroendocrinology 75:392–401
196. Zhou W, Koldzic-Zivanovic N, Clarke CH, de Beun R, Wassermann K, Bury PS, Cunningham KA, Thomas ML (2002) Selective estrogen receptor modulator effects in the rat brain. Neuroendocrinology 75:24–33

Chapter 6

Pure Antiestrogens

Carlos Hermenegildo

6.1 Introduction

An antiestrogen is a compound that blocks the action of estrogens. According to McGregor and Jordan (1998), antiestrogens can be classified into two major groups:

6.1.1 Type I

This group is made up of compounds exhibiting mixed estrogenic/antiestrogenic actions in the laboratory. These compounds are also known as SERMs (selective estrogen receptor modulators) and include both triphenylethylene derivatives (such as tamoxifen, toremifene, idoxifene, or droloxifene) and benzothiophenes (raloxifene) (Bryant and Dere 1998). The agonist–antagonist profile for a given compound is tissue and species specific. Tamoxifen, for instance, inhibits estrogen-stimulated growth of breast cancer cells (antagonistic activity) but stimulates endometrial proliferation (agonistic activity). Tamoxifen is a pure estrogen antagonist in the chick but partial estrogen agonist in the mouse, rat, and human (Baker and Jaffe 1996).

6.1.2 Type II

Type II antiestrogens, pure antiestrogens, or selective estrogen receptor downregulators (SERDs) (Howell et al. 2004b) have no estrogen-like properties in laboratory assays.

To illustrate the different actions of both groups of antiestrogens, Table 6.1 presents the tissue-specific effects obtained with the administration of type I (tamoxifen and raloxifene) and type II (ICI 164384 and fulvestrant) antiestrogens in preclinical studies.

The pure antiestrogens were discovered about 20 years ago by Wakeling and collaborators (Wakeling and Bowler 1987). To date, a few distinct compounds

Table 6.1. Tissue-associated estrogen activities of various estrogen receptor ligands based on preclinical studies. We present the effects of two estrogen receptor agonists (17β-estradiol and 17α-ethynyl estradiol), two selective estrogen receptor modulators (SERMs, tamoxifen, and raloxifene), and two pure antiestrogens (fulvestrant and ICI 164384) (from Bryant and Dere 1998)

Compound	Mammary tissue	Uterus metabolism	Bone	Cholesterol
17β-estradiol 17α-ethynyl estradiol	Agonist	Agonist	Agonist	Agonist
Tamoxifen	Antagonist	Partial agonist	Agonist	Agonist
Raloxifene	Antagonist	Antagonist	Agonist	Agonist
ICI 164384 Fulvestrant	Antagonist	Antagonist	Antagonist	Antagonist

of this group have been discovered. All of them are able to bind to the estrogen receptor (ER) without any estrogenic activity, either in vitro or in vivo, in any studied species or tissues, including all estrogen target tissues such as uterus, mammary gland, ovary, or bone.

The main potential utility of antiestrogens would be the treatment of advanced breast cancer after failure of long-term tamoxifen therapy. Nevertheless, pure antiestrogens could also find application in gynecology and in other non-malignant conditions (Gradishar and Jordan 1997). In April 2002, fulvestrant was the first pure antiestrogen approved by the Food and Drug Administration for clinical practice (Bross et al. 2003).

The aim of the present review is to update the recent discoveries on the mechanisms of action, biological effects, clinical trials, and potential clinical utility of pure antiestrogens.

6.2 Chemical Structure and Classification

The main compounds that have demonstrated a pure antiestrogenic activity in the laboratory are the following (Fig. 6.1):

1. **ICI 164384.** This is the first pure antiestrogen discovered (Wakeling and Bowler 1987). This compound is a 7α-alkylamine derivative of 17β-estradiol, with a 16-atom carbon chain in the 7α position.
2. **Fulvestrant.** Also called ICI 182780 and Faslodex, this compound is also a 7α-alkylamine derivative of 17β-estradiol, developed from ICI 164384

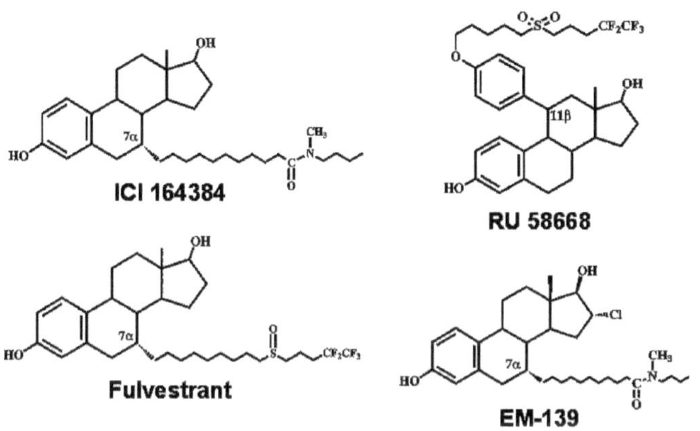

Fig. 6.1. Chemical structures of pure antiestrogens. Chemical structures of ICI 164384, fulvestrant, RU 58668, and EM-139 are presented (MacGregor and Jordan 1998)

to improve the bioavailability and the biological profile of its activity: the amide moiety was replaced by other polar groups and the terminal alkyl function was fluorinated. Those molecular changes made fulvestrant more potent, and its affinity for ERs approximately is 4–5 times higher than that of ICI 164384 (Wakeling et al. 1991). Since both compounds are poorly soluble and have low oral activity, they are being used as depot injections in clinical studies. Fulvestrant is the only pure antiestrogen approved for the treatment of hormone-sensitive breast cancer in postmenopausal women with disease progression following antiestrogen therapy (Bross et al. 2002, 2003).

3. **RU 58668.** This is a 17β-estradiol derivative compound, substituted in the 11β-position with a long hydrophobic side chain, producing a spatial arrangement similar to the 7α-substituted compounds in relation to the plane of steroid nucleus (Van de Velde et al. 1994, 1996).
4. **EM-139.** This compound is also a 7α derivative of 17β-estradiol, with a structure similar to that of ICI 164384 (Doualla-Bell et al. 1995).

Other compounds, such as ZK-703 and ZK-253, are currently under preclinical testing, and preliminary data show a pure antiestrogen activity in xenograft breast cancer models (Hoffmann et al. 2004).

6.3 Mechanism of Action

Pure antiestrogens are distinguishable form other SERMs in terms of their mechanism of action, although both classes of agent mediate their effects through the two types of estrogen receptors (ERα and ERβ).

Type I antiestrogens are competitive inhibitors of the binding of estrogens to ER. As demonstrated for raloxifene, these compounds seem to form a complex with the ER that retains partial transcription activity as a result of imperfect changes in the tertiary structure of the complex (Brzozowski et al. 1997). Due to this partial agonistic activity, type I antiestrogens show a wide range of biological functions, from complete antagonism to partial agonism, depending upon the species, tissue, or target genes studied (Bryant and Dere 1998).

Pure antiestrogens also act as competitive inhibitors of the estradiol–ER complex. For instance, ICI 164384 is a competitive antagonist of both ERα and ERβ (Barkhem et al. 1998). In MCF-7 cells, similar amounts of estradiol and RU58668 are bound to ER (Jensen and Khan 2004).

Distinct mechanisms of action have been ascribed to pure antiestrogens (Fig. 6.2). According to one proposal, pure antiestrogens impede the dimerization of two ER–ligand complexes, preventing binding to DNA and, as a consequence, gene activation (Fawell et al. 1990). However, it was later reported that the pure antiestrogen–ER complex is able to bind to EREs, as has been demonstrated for ICI 164384 and RU 58668 (Barsalou et al. 1998), though the transcription unit formed is inactive (Pink and Jordan 1996).

Pure antiestrogens also exert a unique mechanism of action: they decrease intracellular levels of ER (Wakeling 2000). Fulvestrant is able to bind to newly

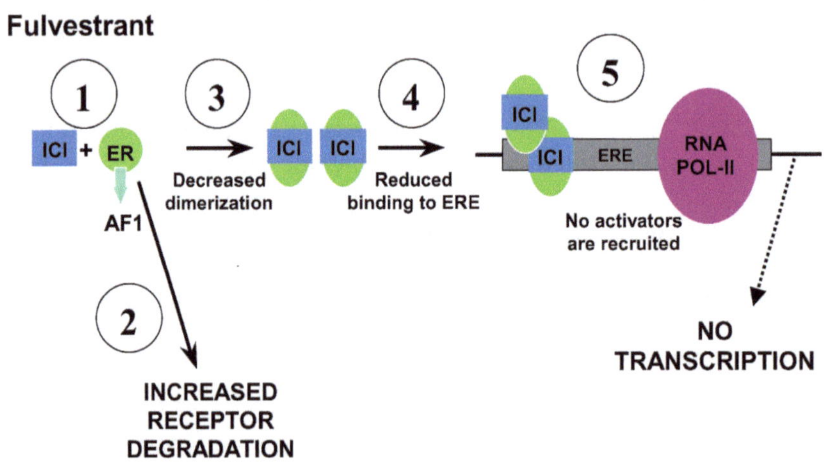

Fig. 6.2. Proposed mechanisms of action of pure antiestrogens (fulvestrant). **1** Fulvestrant (ICI) binds to estrogen receptor (ER). **2** Fulvestrant binding to ER accelerates receptor degradation ("ER down-regulator"). **3** Rate of dimerization and nuclear localization of fulvestrant–ER complex is reduced. **4** Reduced binding of fulvestrant–ER to ERE. **5** No transcription of estrogen-responsive genes; since AF-1 and AF-2 are inactive, no coactivators are recruited and the activity of RNA polymerase II is not activated (or inhibited) (Wakeling 2000)

synthesized ER in cell cytoplasm, modifying the cytoplasm–nucleus net flux of the ER by diminishing its transport into the nucleus. The paralyzed receptors are then rapidly destroyed (Dauvois et al. 1993) in a process implying an increased turnover of ER by the ubiquitin–proteasome pathway, since the complex formed between ER and fulvestrant causes a high ubiquitination and rapid destruction of the receptor (Wijayaratne and McDonnell 2001).

Also, RU 58668 modifies the subcellular distribution of ER, appearing as clusters in the perinuclear region of cytoplasm, without association to specific cellular structures. This means that after RU 58668 treatment, ER is sequestered in the cytoplasm associated to short half-life proteins (probably induced by RU 58668 treatment) that impede its entry into the nucleus (Devin-Leclerc et al. 1998).

As a consequence of the above-cited studies, it has been suggested that the title of pure antiestrogen should be given to those compounds that are capable of blocking the entry of the ER into the nucleus. This mechanism of action would be the essential difference between pure antiestrogens and SERMs (type I antiestrogens). In this sense, type I antiestrogens induce an increase in the amount of ER in the cell nucleus, while pure antiestrogens diminish it (and therefore they can also be named SERDs) (Devin-Leclerc et al. 1998; Howell et al. 2004b).

In explaining these observed differences between both classes of antiestrogens, it has been proposed that the large side chains in the pure antiestrogen molecules are responsible for the mechanism of differences observed in the action. The binding of estradiol, raloxifene, and ICI 164384 to ER has been studied by crystallography. Raloxifene and ICI 164384 bind to the same aminoacids as estradiol, but the side chain of both compounds interacts differently with several amino acids of the binding domain. Such interaction modifies the tertiary structure of the complex, which may explain the differences in their actions (Brzozowski et al. 1997; Schafer et al. 1999; Pike et al. 2001; Lonard and Smith 2002).

In addition to their interference with ER physiology, alternative mechanisms of action have been reported that help to explain the antiestrogenic potential of pure antiestrogens. Among other things, pure antiestrogens seem to inhibit some enzymatic activities involved in estrogen synthesis. EM-139 was the first pure antiestrogen reported to inhibit an enzyme, 17β-hydroxysteroid dehydrogenase, thus reducing the peripheral conversion of estrone into estradiol (Li et al. 1995). Additionally, fulvestrant has been reported to inhibit aromatase activity in vitro. This inhibition is not due to down-regulation of the aromatase transcript; on the contrary, its activity remains inhibited even after the pure antiestrogen is removed from the cells, suggesting that fulvestrant remains bound to the enzyme (Long et al. 1998).

Finally, it has been suggested that fulvestrant, in addition to its antiestrogenic activity, has also significant antiprogestin activity, comparable to the activity of the antiprogestin RU-486 (Nawaz et al. 1999).

6.4 Effects of Pure Antiestrogens

The majority of the actions of pure antiestrogens have been described in studies designed in cell cultures (effects in vitro) or in experiments performed in animals. During the last few years, only a few clinical studies have been completed. The main objective of the majority of the studies has been to demonstrate the pure antiestrogenic action of these compounds.

6.4.1 In Vitro Studies

These studies have been focused on the effects of pure antiestrogens on gene expression, on cell growth and proliferation, and on the effects on different growth factors.

6.4.1.1 *Effects on Gene Expression*

In a study of global gene expression in MCF-7 cells, fulvestrant antagonized estradiol action on > 95% of estradiol-regulated genes. Moreover, the antagonism of fulvestrant was not accompanied by partial agonism, in comparison with the other tested compounds (raloxifene and hydroxytamoxifen), supporting the full pure antiestrogen activity of this compound. There were also genes specifically down-regulated by fulvestrant, and the majority of these genes appear to be regulators of the cell cycle, cell proliferation, and DNA synthesis. Therefore, by down-regulating the expression of these genes, fulvestrant has an additional beneficial effect against the proliferation of breast cancer cells (Frasor et al. 2004).

6.4.1.2 *Effects on Cell Growth and Proliferation*

In the initial studies with pure antiestrogens, both ICI 164384 and fulvestrant inhibited cell growth and arrested the cell cycle in the G_1 phase. These effects were two orders of magnitude more potent than those achieved with tamoxifen in the same experimental conditions (Wakeling and Bowler 1987).

When used in tumor cells, fulvestrant was initially described as a potent, competitive growth inhibitor of ER-positive, human breast cancer MCF-7 cells, whose growth is stimulated by estradiol. The compound was ineffective in tumor cell lines without ER, such as MDA-MB-231. The inhibitory effects were more pronounced with fulvestrant than with tamoxifen in the same cell line (Wakeling et al. 1991).

6.4.1.3 *Effects on Growth Factors*

Pure antiestrogens have been demonstrated to block some of the effects of estrogens on growth factors. Estrogens increase the transforming growth factor α (TGFα) production, which in turn stimulates cell growth and, in a process that implies the epidermal growth factor (EGF), increases cell replication. ICI 164384 and fulvestrant block estradiol-stimulated TGFα production (Wakeling et al. 1989; MacGregor and Jordan 1998; Tong et al. 2002).

Fulvestrant has been reported to decrease both insulin-like growth factor I (IGF-I) stimulated cell growth and IGF-I receptor mRNA (Huynh et al. 1996). Moreover, in the human fetal osteoblast cell line (hFOB/ER9 cells), both ICI 164384 and fulvestrant blocked the estradiol-induced increase in IGF-I mRNA levels (Kassem et al. 1998).

6.4.2 Experiments in Animals

To date, all the experiments done in animals with pure antiestrogens have disregarded any estrogenic actions of these compounds. Some of the described effects are presented here, arranged by the tissue or organ where they have been described (Table 6.2).

6.4.2.1 *Breast*

The main potential utility of the pure antiestrogens is in the treatment of breast cancer. Several studies on their effects on the breast demonstrate both the pure antiestrogenic action of the tested compounds and their beneficial effects on breast cancer treatment. In experiments conducted in nude mice xenotransplanted with two different human estradiol-dependent breast tumors, a single injection of fulvestrant provided an antitumor efficacy equivalent to that of daily tamoxifen treatment for at least 4 weeks (Wakeling et al. 1991). Additionally, RU 58668 was able to induce up to 30% disappearance of MCF-7 breast

Table 6.2. Effects of pure antiestrogens on experimental animals

Organ	Effect	Animal	Antiestrogen	Reference
Breast	Mammary atrophy	Rat	Fulvestrant	(Lim et al. 2001)
	Antitumor	Nude mice	Fulvestrant	(Wakeling et al. 1991)
Uterus	Development block	Immature rat	Fulvestrant	(Wakeling et al. 1991)
	Involution	Mature rat	Fulvestrant	(Wakeling et al. 1991)
	Involution	Monkey	Fulvestrant	(Dukes et al. 1992, 1993)
	Block of endometrial tumor progression	Athymic mice	ICI 164384	(Gottardis et al. 1990)
Skeleton	Decreased trabecular bone density	Rat	ICI 164384	(van Bezooijen et al. 1998)
	Reduced bone volume	Rat	Fulvestrant	(Gallagher et al. 1993)
Cardiovascular effects	Block of cholesterol-lowering activity of estradiol	Rat	Fulvestrant	(Lundeen et al. 1997)
	Block of vascular smooth muscle cell proliferation	Rat	ICI 164384	(Cathapermal et al. 1998)
	Block of estradiol-induced increase in blood flow in aorta	Rabbit	Fulvestrant	(Hegele-Hartung et al. 1997)

cancer tumors implanted in nude mice (Van de Velde et al. 1995). Moreover, a 3-week treatment with fulvestrant in control rats induced a great mammary atrophy, as a consequence of an increased epithelial cell apoptosis (Lim et al. 2001).

6.4.2.2 *Uterus*

The effects of pure antiestrogens in the uterus have also been extensively studied, since it is an estrogen-dependent organ and the target of the main side effects of tamoxifen therapy, such as endometrial hyperplasia, hypertrophy of glandular epithelium, or even focal cellular atypia (Sourla et al. 1997).

Fulvestrant has demonstrated high antiuterotrophic potency in several animal models. This compound has been reported to block the uterus development in immature rats (Wakeling et al. 1991) and to promote the involution of uterus in adult normal (Dukes et al. 1993) and ovariectomized monkeys (Dukes et al. 1992). In vivo, RU 58668 displayed a total antiuterotrophic activity in mice and rats without exhibiting any agonistic effect (Van de Velde et al. 1994).

When studied in a model of human endometrial carcinoma, such as EnCa101 tumors in athymic mice, ICI 164384 not only showed no stimulatory activity on tumor progression but also blocked the tamoxifen-stimulated growth of the tumor (Gottardis et al. 1990).

The overall uterine effects obtained in animals treated with the different compounds make it possible to assume that pure antiestrogens could be used in the treatment of endometrial disorders and endometrial carcinoma (Gradishar and Jordan 1997).

6.4.2.3 *Skeleton*

The effects of the pure antiestrogens on the skeleton are controversial, although it seems ICI 164384 and fulvestrant decrease bone density. It has been demonstrated that treatment of rats with the pure antiestrogen ICI 164384 induced a significant decrease in trabecular bone mineral density, comparable to that observed after ovariectomy (van Bezooijen et al. 1998). Administration of fulvestrant to adult female rats reduced bone volume at the proximal tibial metaphysis and increased the osteoclast surface. When administered to ovariectomized rats, fulvestrant inhibited the estradiol-stimulated cancellous bone formation, while affecting neither longitudinal nor periosteal tibial growth (Gallagher et al. 1993).

6.4.2.4 *Cardiovascular Effects*

Estrogens are thought to exert their cardiovascular effects by acting on blood lipoproteins or by direct effects on blood vessels. In studies performed in rats, fulvestrant had no effect on plasma cholesterol levels. When administered along with estradiol, however, it blocked the cholesterol-lowering activity of estradiol (Lundeen et al. 1997).

By acting on the vessel wall, estradiol significantly inhibited superoxide anion-induced vascular smooth muscle cell proliferation, whereas the pure antiestrogen ICI 164384 reversed the inhibitory effect of estradiol (Cathapermal et al. 1998). Fulvestrant also reversed the estradiol-induced increase in blood flow in rabbit aorta (Hegele-Hartung et al. 1997).

6.4.3 Clinical Studies

There is very little information concerning the performance of pure antiestrogens in clinical conditions, and all studies have been done with fulvestrant.

6.4.3.1 *Pharmacokinetics*

Pure antiestrogenic activity must be sustained over time to achieve its effects, mainly an effective inhibition of estrogen-controlled proliferation. Therefore, exposure to fulvestrant via chronic administration is required. Since oral delivery is not an appropriate route of administration, fulvestrant is administered by a long-acting, intramuscular formulation (Robertson and Harrison 2004). It is given as a 250 mg dose in a prolonged-release intramuscular formulation. Plasma concentrations of fulvestrant are measurable up to 28 d after dosing, with peak plasma concentrations occurring 1 – 11 d after dosing, reaching C_{max} values of about 6 ng/ml (Robertson and Harrison 2003).

6.4.3.2 *Tolerability.*

In general, fulvestrant is well tolerated in studies conducted in healthy volunteers (Addo et al. 2002) and in clinical trials (Howell et al. 2002, 2004a; Osborne et al. 2002). The most common adverse effects are nausea, asthenia, pain, vasodilatation, and headache (Robertson et al. 2003; Howell et al. 2004a). In trials in which fulvestrant was compared to anastrazole (an aromatase inhibitor), the incidence of adverse events relevant to endocrine therapy (gastrointestinal disturbances, hot flushes, vaginitis, weight gain, thromboembolic disease, urinary tract infection, and joint disorders) were similar for both groups, with the exception of joint disorder incidence, which was lower with fulvestrant (Robertson et al. 2003). In the trial comparing fulvestrant with tamoxifen, the incidence of hot flushes was lower in patients treated with fulvestrant, without any difference in the other above-mentioned adverse events relevant to endocrine therapy (Howell et al. 2004a).

6.4.3.3 *Clinical Efficacy Studies*

The first clinical trial of fulvestrant was conducted to assess its tolerance, pharmacokinetics, and short-term biological effects in women with primary breast cancer. Control group patients received no treatment. The treated patients received daily intramuscular injections of fulvestrant at doses of 6 or 18 mg for 7 d prior to primary breast surgery. There were no effects on serum gonadotropin or sex hormone binding globulin levels, suggesting a lack of agonist activity of the compound at the pituitary or hepatic level. Fulvestrant significantly reduced the tumor expression of ER, progesterone receptor, and Ki67, a nuclear antigen whose expression is closely related to cell proliferation (DeFriend et al. 1994). Similar, comparative studies performed with tamoxifen and fulvestrant showed no effect of tamoxifen on tumor expression of ER (McClelland et al. 1996).

In tumor samples derived from the study of DeFriend (DeFriend et al. 1994), ER protein content was suppressed by fulvestrant, whereas the levels of EGF receptor (EGFR) and its ligand TGFα were unaltered by treatment. Since a loss of endocrine sensitivity has been attributed to tumors with elevated levels of EGFR and TGFα, treatment with fulvestrant preserves the hormone response of tumor cells (McClelland et al. 1996).

Fulvestrant has also been administered to premenopausal women. The administration of 12 mg/d for 7 d in the follicular phase prior to hysterectomy produced no changes in luteinizing hormone (LH) and follicle-stimulating hormone (FSH) levels or in ovarian function. As expected, fulvestrant caused a potent antiestrogenic action in the endometrium, blocking the physiological increase of the endometrial thickness (Thomas et al. 1994). In another study of similar design, fulvestrant administration prior to hysterectomy reduced endometrial ER and Ki67 expression (Dowsett et al. 1995).

The effect of long-term treatment (up to 33 months) with fulvestrant in patients with advanced tamoxifen-resistant breast cancer was first studied in a small group of patients ($n = 19$) in phase I/II clinical trials (Howell et al. 1995, 1996). A clinical benefit (complete response + partial response + stable disease $\geq$ 24 weeks) rate of 69% was obtained in patients treated with fulvestrant, without serious side effects from the treatment. Moreover, the high level of response suggested that fulvestrant was not cross-resistant with tamoxifen. The LH and FSH levels rose after suspension of tamoxifen and then remained stable thereafter, suggesting no effect of fulvestrant on the pituitary-hypothalamic axis. There were no significant changes in serum levels of prolactin, the sex-hormone-binding globulin (SHBG). Compared to the effects of tamoxifen, which reduces serum levels of LH and FSH (Willis et al. 1977) and reduces LDL and cholesterol levels and increases SHBG, HDL, and triglycerides levels (Sakai et al. 1978; Love et al. 1990), those of long-term treatment with fulvestrant did not modify levels of total cholesterol, LDL-cholesterol, HDL-cholesterol, or tryglycerides (Howell et al. 1996).

Three randomized phase III trials have evaluated the efficacy of fulvestrant. The first two trials were designed to compare the efficacy of fulvestrant

(250 mg) with anastrazole (1 mg), an inhibitor of aromatase, for the treatment of postmenopausal women with advanced disease previously treated with antiestrogenic therapy (mainly tamoxifen) (Howell et al. 2002; Osborne et al. 2002). Trial 0021, conducted in North America, and trial 0020, conducted in Europe, Australia, and South Africa, were designed to allow the combination of their results (Morris and Wakeling 2002). In both trials, fulvestrant (total $n = 851$ patients) was at least as effective as anastrazole, with time to disease progression of disease slightly higher (Howell et al. 2002; Osborne et al. 2002). The combined analysis of both trials revealed that time to disease progression of disease was significantly higher (30%) in the fulvestrant-treated group (Morris and Wakeling 2002).

In the third phase III trial, fulvestrant was compared with tamoxifen in 587 postmenopausal patients with metastatic/locally advanced breast cancer previously untreated for advanced disease. At a median followup of 14.5 months, there was no significant difference between fulvestrant and tamoxifen for time to progression. Nevertheless, fulvestrant showed only noninferiority to tamoxifen in the receptor-positive group, and the time to treatment failure was significantly worse for fulvestrant when all patients were considered (Howell et al. 2004a). Data analysis reflects a higher rate of early progressions in the fulvestrant group. Moreover, pharmacokinetic studies demonstrate that fulvestrant takes 3–6 months to reach steady-state plasma levels, suggesting that either a loading dose or doses of fulvestrant may be required (Howell et al. 2004b).

6.5 Clinical Utility

The main potential clinical utility of the pure antiestrogens is their use as a second-line treatment in patients with tamoxifen-resistant breast cancer. Tamoxifen is, for the moment, the first option in breast cancer expressing ER, but in a number of patients, tumors develop resistance to tamoxifen (Jordan 1993). Different hypotheses have been proposed to explain this resistance: alterations in tamoxifen metabolism (Osborne et al. 1991), specific mutations on the genes encoding RE protein (which could explain the fact that an antiestrogen transmits an estrogenic signal) (Jiang et al. 1992), alterations induced by tamoxifen in the gene regulation mechanisms (Johnston et al. 1997), and others, such as alterations in ER phosphorylation and direct effects on genes (MacGregor and Jordan 1998).

Pure antiestrogens, which act by different mechanisms of action, probably are not affected by the mechanisms of tamoxifen resistance. As a result, those compounds might be a good choice as second-line hormonotherapy of breast cancer after failure of tamoxifen treatment, as has been reported in clinical trials (DeFriend et al. 1994; Howell et al. 1995, 1996, 2004a; Morris and Wakeling 2002).

It seems reasonable that pure antiestrogens might be used as a good alternative to tamoxifen in the treatment of breast cancer, due to their beneficial effects, without increasing the risk of endometrium cancer (Simard et al. 1997).

Nevertheless, their potential use in large treatments will depend on systemic actions, since the beneficial effects may be counterbalanced by deleterious consequences on the cardiovascular (Hegele-Hartung et al. 1997) and skeletal systems (Gallagher et al. 1993). Moreover, most pure antiestrogens have a poor oral bioavailability. Therefore, the use of other routes of administration, such as intravenously, is mandatory. In some cases, to circumvent such problems, the production of nanospheres loaded with the pure antiestrogen RU 58668 has been tested (Ameller et al. 2004).

Finally, therapeutic sequencing of different hormonal agents is fast becoming a common clinical practice, and fulvestrant is a good treatment choice to extend the opportunity for using endocrine therapies before reliance upon cytotoxic chemotherapy is necessary. Further research is required in order to evaluate the optimal sequence, both in clinical practice as well as in the laboratory, to choose the correct treatment of breast cancer in each person after the appearance of tamoxifen-induced drug resistance (Robertson 2004; Osipo et al. 2004; Johnston 2004; Robertson et al. 2005).

Acknowledgements

The preparation of this review was supported by Grant 03/0831 from Fondo de Investigación Sanitaria, Madrid, Spain.

References

1. Addo S, Yates RA, Laight A (2002) A phase I trial to assess the pharmacology of the new oestrogen receptor antagonist fulvestrant on the endometrium in healthy postmenopausal volunteers. Br J Cancer 87:1354–1359
2. Ameller T, Marsaud V, Legrand P, Gref R, Renoir JM (2004) Pure antiestrogen RU 58668-loaded nanospheres: morphology, cell activity and toxicity studies. Eur J Pharm Sci 21:361–370
3. Baker VL, Jaffe RB (1996) Clinical uses of antiestrogens. Obstet Gynecol Surv 51:45–59
4. Barkhem T, Carlsson B, Nilsson Y, Enmark E, Gustafsson J, Nilsson S (1998) Differential response of estrogen receptor alpha and estrogen receptor beta to partial estrogen agonists/antagonists. Mol Pharmacol 54:105–112
5. Barsalou A, Gao W, Anghel SI, Carriere J, Mader S (1998) Estrogen response elements can mediate agonist activity of anti-estrogens in human endometrial Ishikawa cells. J Biol Chem 273:17138–17146
6. Bross PF, Baird A, Chen G, Jee JM, Lostritto RT, Morse DE, Rosario LA, Williams GM, Yang P, Rahman A, et al. (2003) Fulvestrant in postmenopausal women with advanced breast cancer. Clin Cancer Res 9:4309–4317

7. Bross PF, Cohen MH, Williams GA, Pazdur R (2002) FDA drug approval summaries: fulvestrant. Oncologist 7:477–480
8. Bryant HU, Dere WH (1998) Selective estrogen receptor modulators: an alternative to hormone replacement therapy. Proc Soc Exp Biol Med 217:45–52
9. Brzozowski AM, Pike AC, Dauter Z, Hubbard RE, Bonn T, Engstrom O, Ohman L, Greene GL, Gustafsson JA, Carlquist M (1997) Molecular basis of agonism and antagonism in the oestrogen receptor. Nature 389:753–758
10. Cathapermal S, Lavigne MC, Leong-Son M, Alibadi T, Ramwell PW (1998) Stereoisomer-specific inhibition of superoxide anion-induced rat aortic smooth-muscle cell proliferation by 17beta-estradiol is estrogen receptor dependent. J Cardiovasc Pharmacol 31:499–505
11. Dauvois S, White R, Parker MG (1993) The antiestrogen ICI 182780 disrupts estrogen receptor nucleocytoplasmic shuttling. J Cell Sci 106:1377–1388
12. DeFriend DJ, Howell A, Nicholson RI, Anderson E, Dowsett M, Mansel RE, Blamey RW, Bundred NJ, Robertson JF, Saunders C, et al. (1994) Investigation of a new pure antiestrogen (ICI 182780) in women with primary breast cancer. Cancer Res 54:408–414
13. Devin-Leclerc J, Meng X, Delahaye F, Leclerc P, Baulieu EE, Catelli MG (1998) Interaction and dissociation by ligands of estrogen receptor and Hsp90: the antiestrogen RU 58668 induces a protein synthesis-dependent clustering of the receptor in the cytoplasm. Mol Endocrinol 12:842–854
14. Doualla-Bell F, Bonneau MJ, Labrie F, Fortier MA (1995) Differential effects of a steroidal antiestrogen, EM-139, on prostaglandin and cyclic adenosine 3′,5′-monophosphate production in the circular and longitudinal layers of bovine myometrium. Biol Reprod 52:1358–1363
15. Dowsett M, Howell R, Salter J, Thomas NM, Thomas EJ (1995) Effects of the pure antioestrogen ICI 182780 on oestrogen receptors, progesterone receptors and Ki67 antigen in human endometrium in vivo. Hum Reprod 10:262–267
16. Dukes M, Miller D, Wakeling AE, Waterton JC (1992) Antiuterotrophic effects of a pure antioestrogen, ICI 182,780: magnetic resonance imaging of the uterus in ovariectomized monkeys. J Endocrinol 135:239–247
17. Dukes M, Waterton JC, Wakeling AE (1993) Antiuterotrophic effects of the pure antioestrogen ICI 182,780 in adult female monkeys (Macaca nemestrina): quantitative magnetic resonance imaging. J Endocrinol 138:203–210
18. Fawell SE, White R, Hoare S, Sydenham M, Page M, Parker MG (1990) Inhibition of estrogen receptor-DNA binding by the "pure" antiestrogen ICI 164,384 appears to be mediated by impaired receptor dimerization. Proc Natl Acad Sci USA 87:6883–6887
19. Frasor J, Stossi F, Danes JM, Komm B, Lyttle CR, Katzenellenbogen BS (2004) Selective estrogen receptor modulators: discrimination of agonistic versus antagonistic activities by gene expression profiling in breast cancer cells. Cancer Res 64:1522–1533
20. Gallagher A, Chambers TJ, Tobias JH (1993) The estrogen antagonist ICI 182,780 reduces cancellous bone volume in female rats. Endocrinology 133:2787–2791
21. Gottardis MM, Ricchio ME, Satyaswaroop PG, Jordan VC (1990) Effect of steroidal and nonsteroidal antiestrogens on the growth of a tamoxifen-stimulated human endometrial carcinoma (EnCa101) in athymic mice. Cancer Res 50:3189–3192
22. Gradishar WJ, Jordan VC (1997) Clinical potential of new antiestrogens. J Clin Oncol 15:840–852
23. Hegele-Hartung C, Fritzemeier KH, Diel P (1997) Effects of a pure antiestrogen and progesterone on estrogen-mediated alterations of blood flow and progesterone receptor expression in the aorta of ovariectomized rabbits. J Steroid BioChem Mol Biol 63:237–249

24. Hoffmann J, Bohlmann R, Heinrich N, Hofmeister H, Kroll J, Kunzer H, Lichtner RB, Nishino Y, Parczyk K, Sauer G, et al. (2004) Characterization of new estrogen receptor destabilizing compounds: effects on estrogen-sensitive and tamoxifen-resistant breast cancer. J Natl Cancer Inst 96:210–218
25. Howell A, DeFriend D, Robertson J, Blamey R, Walton P (1995) Response to a specific antioestrogen (ICI 182780) in tamoxifen-resistant breast cancer. Lancet 345:29–30
26. Howell A, DeFriend DJ, Robertson JF, Blamey RW, Anderson L, Anderson E, Sutcliffe FA, Walton P (1996) Pharmacokinetics, pharmacological and anti-tumour effects of the specific anti-oestrogen ICI 182780 in women with advanced breast cancer. Br J Cancer 74:300–308
27. Howell A, Robertson JF, Quaresma AJ, Aschermannova A, Mauriac L, Kleeberg UR, Vergote I, Erikstein B, Webster A, Morris C (2002) Fulvestrant, formerly ICI 182,780, is as effective as anastrozole in postmenopausal women with advanced breast cancer progressing after prior endocrine treatment. J Clin Oncol 20:3396–3403
28. Howell A, Robertson JFR, Abram P, Lichinitser MR, Elledge R, Bajetta E, Watanabe T, Morris C, Webster A, Dimery I, et al. (2004a) Comparison of fulvestrant versus tamoxifen for the treatment of advanced breast cancer in postmenopausal women previously untreated with endocrine therapy: a multinational, double-blind, randomized trial. J Clin Oncol 22:1605–1613
29. Howell SJ, Johnston SRD, Howell A (2004b) The use of selective estrogen receptor modulators and selective estrogen receptor down-regulators in breast cancer. Best Pract Res Clin Endocrinol Metab 18:47–66
30. Huynh H, Nickerson T, Pollak M, Yang X (1996) Regulation of insulin-like growth factor I receptor expression by the pure antiestrogen ICI 182780. Clin Cancer Res 2:2037–2042
31. Jensen EV, Khan SA (2004) A two-site model for antiestrogen action. Mech Age Develop 125:679–682
32. Jiang SY, Langan-Fahey SM, Stella AL, McCague R, Jordan VC (1992) Point mutation of estrogen receptor (ER) in the ligand-binding domain changes the pharmacology of antiestrogens in ER-negative breast cancer cells stably expressing complementary DNAs for ER. Mol Endocrinol 6:2167–2174
33. Johnston S (2004) Fulvestrant and the sequential endocrine cascade for advanced breast cancer. Br J Cancer 90(Suppl 1):S15–S18
34. Johnston SR, Lu B, Dowsett M, Liang X, Kaufmann M, Scott GK, Osborne CK, Benz CC (1997) Comparison of estrogen receptor DNA binding in untreated and acquired antiestrogen-resistant human breast tumors. Cancer Res 57:3723–3727
35. Jordan VC (1993) A current view of tamoxifen for the treatment and prevention of breast cancer. Br J Pharmacol 110:507–517
36. Kassem M, Okazaki R, Harris SA, Spelsberg TC, Conover CA, Riggs BL (1998) Estrogen effects on insulin-like growth factor gene expression in a human osteoblastic cell line with high levels of estrogen receptor. Calcif Tissue Int 62:60–66
37. Li S, Levesque C, Geng CS, Yan X, Labrie F (1995) Inhibitory effects of medroxyprogesterone acetate (MPA) and the pure antiestrogen EM-219 on estrone (E1)-stimulated growth of dimethylbenz(a)anthracene (DMBA)-induced mammary carcinoma in the rat. Breast Cancer Res Treat 34:147–159
38. Lim KB, Ng CY, Ong CK, Ong CS, Tran E, Nguyen TT, Chan GM, Huynh H (2001) Induction of apoptosis in mammary gland by a pure anti-estrogen ICI 182780. Breast Cancer Res Treat 68:127–138
39. Lonard DM, Smith CL (2002) Molecular perspectives on selective estrogen receptor modulators (SERMs): progress in understanding their tissue-specific agonist and antagonist actions. Steroids 67:15–24

40. Long BJ, Tilghman SL, Yue W, Thiantanawat A, Grigoryev DN, Brodie AM (1998) The steroidal antiestrogen ICI 182,780 is an inhibitor of cellular aromatase activity. J Steroid BioChem Mol Biol 67:293–304
41. Love RR, Newcomb PA, Wiebe DA, Surawicz TS, Jordan VC, Carbone PP, DeMets DL (1990) Effects of tamoxifen therapy on lipid and lipoprotein levels in postmenopausal patients with node-negative breast cancer. J Natl Cancer Inst 82:1327–1332
42. Lundeen SG, Carver JM, McKean ML, Winneker RC (1997) Characterization of the ovariectomized rat model for the evaluation of estrogen effects on plasma cholesterol levels. Endocrinology 138:1552–1558
43. MacGregor JI, Jordan VC (1998) Basic guide to the mechanisms of antiestrogen action. Pharmacol Rev 50:151–196
44. McClelland RA, Gee JM, Francis AB, Robertson JF, Blamey RW, Wakeling AE, Nicholson RI (1996) Short-term effects of pure anti-oestrogen ICI 182780 treatment on oestrogen receptor, epidermal growth factor receptor and transforming growth factor-alpha protein expression in human breast cancer. Eur J Cancer 32A: 413–416
45. Morris C, Wakeling A (2002) Fulvestrant ('Faslodex')-a new treatment option for patients progressing on prior endocrine therapy. Endocr Relat Cancer 9:267–276
46. Nawaz Z, Stancel GM, Hyder SM (1999) The pure antiestrogen ICI 182,780 inhibits progestin-induced transcription. Cancer Res 59:372–376
47. Osborne CK, Coronado E, Allred DC, Wiebe V, DeGregorio M (1991) Acquired tamoxifen resistance: correlation with reduced breast tumor levels of tamoxifen and isomerization of trans-4-hydroxytamoxifen. J Natl Cancer Inst 83:1477–1482
48. Osborne CK, Pippen J, Jones SE, Parker LM, Ellis M, Come S, Gertler SZ, May JT, Burton G, Dimery I, et al. (2002) Double-blind, randomized trial comparing the efficacy and tolerability of fulvestrant versus anastrozole in postmenopausal women with advanced breast cancer progressing on prior endocrine therapy: results of a North American trial. J Clin Oncol 20:3386–3395
49. Osipo C, Liu H, Meeke K, Jordan VC (2004) The consequences of exhaustive antiestrogen therapy in breast cancer: estrogen-induced tumor cell death. Exp Biol Med 229: 722–731
50. Pike AC, Brzozowski AM, Walton J, Hubbard RE, Thorsell AG, Li YL, Gustafsson JA, Carlquist M (2001) Structural insights into the mode of action of a pure antiestrogen. Structure 9:145–153
51. Pink JJ, Jordan VC (1996) Models of estrogen receptor regulation by estrogens and antiestrogens in breast cancer cell lines. Cancer Res 56:2321–2330
52. Robertson JF, Harrison M (2004) Fulvestrant: pharmacokinetics and pharmacology. Br J Cancer 90(Suppl 1):S7–10
53. Robertson JF, Harrison MP (2003) Equivalent single-dose pharmacokinetics of two different dosing methods of prolonged-release fulvestrant ('Faslodex') in postmenopausal women with advanced breast cancer. Cancer Chemother Pharmacol 52:346–348
54. Robertson JF, Osborne CK, Howell A, Jones SE, Mauriac L, Ellis M, Kleeberg UR, Come SE, Vergote I, Gertler S, et al. (2003) Fulvestrant versus anastrozole for the treatment of advanced breast carcinoma in postmenopausal women: a prospective combined analysis of two multicenter trials. Cancer 98:229–238
55. Robertson JFR (2004) Selective oestrogen receptor modulators/new antioestrogens: a clinical perspective. Cancer Treat Rev 30:695–706
56. Robertson JFR, Come SE, Jones SE, Beex L , Kaufmann M, Makris A, Nortier JWR, Possinger K, Rutqvist LE (2005) Endocrine treatment options for advanced breast cancer – the role of fulvestrant. Eur J Cancer 41:346–356

57. Sakai F, Cheix F, Clavel M, Colon J, Mayer M, Pommatau E, Saez S (1978) Increases in steroid binding globulins induced by tamoxifen in patients with carcinoma of the breast. J Endocrinol 76:219–226
58. Schafer JI, Liu H, Tonetti DA, Jordan VC (1999) The interaction of raloxifene and the active metabolite of the antiestrogen EM-800 (SC 5705) with the human estrogen receptor. Cancer Res 59:4308–4313
59. Simard J, Labrie C, Belanger A, Gauthier S, Singh SM, Merand Y, Labrie F (1997) Characterization of the effects of the novel non-steroidal antiestrogen EM-800 on basal and estrogen-induced proliferation of T-47D, ZR-75-1 and MCF-7 human breast cancer cells in vitro. Int J Cancer 73:104–112
60. Sourla A, Luo S, Labrie C, Belanger A, Labrie F (1997) Morphological changes induced by 6-month treatment of intact and ovariectomized mice with tamoxifen and the pure antiestrogen EM-800. Endocrinology 138:5605–5617
61. Thomas EJ, Walton PL, Thomas NM, Dowsett M (1994) The effects of ICI 182,780, a pure anti-oestrogen, on the hypothalamic- pituitary-gonadal axis and on endometrial proliferation in pre- menopausal women. Hum Reprod 9:1991–1996
62. Tong GM, Rajah TT, Zang XP, Pento JT (2002) The effect of antiestrogens on TGF-beta-mediated chemotaxis of human breast cancer cells. Anticancer Res 22:103–106
63. van Bezooijen RL, Que I, Ederveen AG, Kloosterboer HJ, Papapoulos SE, Lowik CW (1998) Plasma nitrate + nitrite levels are regulated by ovarian steroids but do not correlate with trabecular bone mineral density in rats. J Endocrinol 159:27–34
64. Van de Velde P, Nique F, Bouchoux F, Bremaud J, Hameau MC, Lucas D, Moratille C, Viet S, Philibert D, Teutsch G (1994) RU 58668, a new pure antiestrogen inducing a regression of human mammary carcinoma implanted in nude mice. J Steroid Bio Chem Mol Biol 48:187–196
65. Van de Velde P, Nique F, Bremaud J, Hameau MC, Philibert D, Teutsch G (1995) Exploration of the therapeutic potential of the antiestrogen RU 58668 in breast cancer treatment. Ann NY Acad Sci 761:164–175
66. Van de Velde P, Nique F, Planchon P, Prevost G, Bremaud J, Hameau MC, Magnien V, Philibert D, Teutsch G (1996) RU 58668: further in vitro and in vivo pharmacological data related to its antitumoral activity. J Steroid BioChem Mol Biol 59:449–457
67. Wakeling AE (2000) Similarities and distinctions in the mode of action of different classes of antioestrogens. Endocr Relat Cancer 7:17–28
68. Wakeling AE, Bowler J (1987) Steroidal pure antioestrogens. J Endocrinol 112:R7–10
69. Wakeling AE, Dukes M, Bowler J (1991) A potent specific pure antiestrogen with clinical potential. Cancer Res 51:3867–3873
70. Wakeling AE, Newboult E, Peters SW (1989) Effects of antioestrogens on the proliferation of MCF-7 human breast cancer cells. J Mol Endocrinol 2:225–234
71. Wijayaratne AL, McDonnell DP (2001) The human estrogen receptor-alpha is a ubiquitinated protein whose stability is affected differentially by agonists, antagonists, and selective estrogen receptor modulators. J Biol Chem 276:35684–35692
72. Willis KJ, London DR, Ward HW, Butt WR, Lynch SS, Rudd BT (1977) Recurrent breast cancer treated with the antioestrogen tamoxifen: correlation between hormonal changes and clinical course. Br Med J 1:425–428

Part II

Clinical Area

Chapter 7

Physiological Regulation of Bone Metabolism and Estrogen Agonism

Miguel Angel García-Pérez

The adult skeleton is periodically remodeled by transitory anatomic structures that contain juxtaposed osteoclast and osteoblast teams and that replace old bone with new bone. The purpose of this remodeling is both to prevent bone aging and repair the damage that occurs as well as to guarantee a contribution of minerals, especially calcium, to body cells for their correct function. In the last few years, due mainly to the research in molecular biology and cellular differentiation and to studies of genetically manipulated mice, it has been possible to discover many aspects both of the cellular and molecular bases of this bone remodeling as well as of the differentiation and function of the two main implied cell types: osteoblasts and osteoclasts.

This chapter will focus mainly on the effects that the modulation of the estrogen receptor (ER) determines on bone metabolism. This information will contribute to a better understanding of the data presented in the next chapter, which is dedicated to demonstrated SERM actions on bone. Much of our knowledge on the role of ER agonism in the field derives from the observation of the action of estrogens. Particular attention will be paid in this chapter to the role that estrogens have in normal bone remodeling and the one that is established when the protection of sex steroids ceases during menopause. Certainly, estrogens and androgens slow the rate of bone remodeling and protect against bone loss. Conversely, loss of estrogen leads to an increased rate of remodeling and inclines the balance between bone resorption and formation in favor of the former.

The regulation of this process is very complex because there are many cytokines and growth factors implicated and because systemic hormones control production of numerous local mediators in the bone microenvironment. Nevertheless, it has recently been possible to expand our knowledge of the factors that govern this bone remodeling with the discovery of decisive molecules for the differentiation and function of osteoclasts. These molecules are proteins belonging to the tumor necrosis factor (TNF) superfamily: osteoprotegerin (OPG), the receptor activator of nuclear factor-κB ligand (RANKL), and their receptor RANK. Nevertheless, other molecules such as TNF-α, IL-1, and IL-6 are important mediators during bone remodeling, in particular after estrogen deficiency.

7.1 Normal Bone Remodeling

The skeleton is a specialized and dynamic organ subjected to continuous regeneration. In adult skeleton, this process, known as bone remodeling, consists of the renovation of old bone by new bone in the same anatomical place (Frost 1973). In adult vertebrates, 10% of the skeletal bone mass is replaced every year, amounting to a complete structural overhaul every decade. Bone resorption and formation are closely linked within spatiotemporal anatomic structures called the basic multicellular unit (BMU) (Parfitt 1994). A working and mature BMU consists of an osteoclast team in the front degrading bone followed by an osteoblast team forming new bone (Fig. 7.1). Although the role of this bone remodeling in the mature skeleton is not completely clarified, it is believed that it serves not only to repair damage, to prevent bone aging and the underlying consequences, but also to assure appropriate blood levels of calcium, which is needed for cell function (Manolagas 2000).

The two main arguments in favor of bone remodeling being principally an autocrine–paracrine function are that bone remodeling occurs simultaneously in multiple locations and that cells of osteoblast lineage participate in osteoclast differentation (Rodan et al. 1981; Lacey et al. 1998; Simonet et al. 1997; Yasuda et al. 1998). Early progenitors of hematopoietic lineage differentiate into osteoclasts when they receive appropriate signals from stromal/osteoblastic (stromal/OB) support cells. These support cells express M-CSF and RANKL to promote differentiation of osteoclast progenitors. In addition, the process is subject to both negative and positive control by a complex network of transcriptional regulators, of circulating hormones, and of locally produced cytokines acting on RANKL and OPG synthesis such as parathyroid hormone (PTH), 1,25-vitamin D3 (vitamin D3), TNF-α, IL-1, and IL-6 (Manolagas et al. 1995).

The factors responsible for the initiation of a BMU are unknowns, although there is evidence to suggest that osteocytes are implicated (Verborgt et al. 2000). The osteocytes are the most abundant cells in bone, and they derive from osteoblasts that have been absorbed into the bone matrix as a consequence of the bone-forming function of osteoblasts. Osteocytes communicate with each other and with the cells that line the bone surface via an extensive canalicular network (Jilka 2003), so that they can detect areas of bone that should be repaired and transmit the appropriate signals to osteoprogenitors in BM to begin a new BMU (Jilka 2003). The mechanism by which bone cells reach BMUs await full clarification, especially in those parts of the skeleton where hematopoietic marrow is sparse or absent. In these parts, the circulatory route

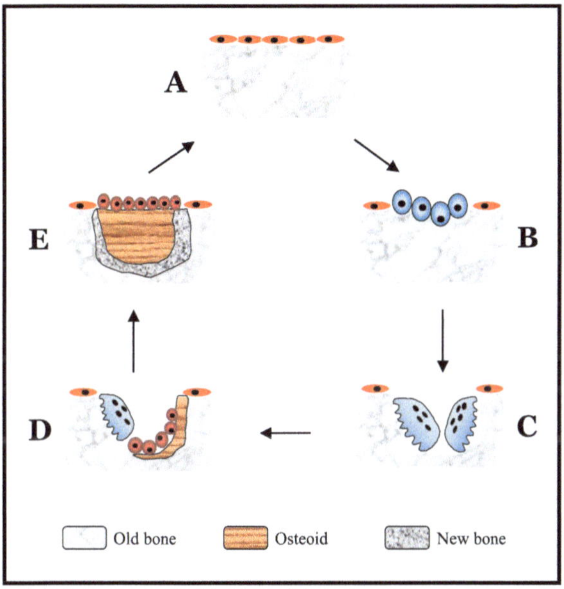

Fig. 7.1. Bone remodeling cycle in basic multicellular unit (BMU). After microdamage to bone, or following mechanical stress or chemical or cellular signaling, a BMU will originate. The preosteoclasts, which are related to macrophages, appear and, by means of different stages, in which the activation of several genes intervenes, and after the action of soluble cytokines, they transform into multinucleated osteoclasts. The mature osteoclasts resorb bone (**A–C**). While advancing the BMU, new osteoclasts are continuously activated and start resorption. After resorption, osteoclasts disappear (probably by apoptosis), and this or other poorly known signals, such as bone-derived growth factors that are released by resorption, probably attract osteoblasts (**D**). Osteoblasts start the formation of new bone by secreting osteoid that later mineralizes (**E**). The final osteoblasts turn into lining, while some of the osteoblasts turn into osteocytes that remain in the bone, connected by long cell processes that can sense mechanical stresses to the bones called canaliculi

is the only route by which osteoclasts can reach bone, although this is not valid for osteoblasts since preosteoblasts are not known to circulate (Parfitt 2000). Recruitment of osteoblasts can be due to the release of growth factors from the bone matrix during bone resorption, to derived signals from endothelial cells that participate in the BMU, to differentiation of the near stromal cells, or even to differentiation of cells that initially displayed a vascular phenotype (Parfitt 2000, 2001).

7.2 Executive Cells: Osteoblasts and Osteoclasts

The most important cells implied in bone remodeling are the osteoclasts and osteoblast, although in this process different cellular types such as endothelial cells, stromal cells, lining cells, osteocytes, and T-cells participate. Bone formation is a complex process involving the commitment of osteoprogenitor cells, the proliferation of preosteoblasts, and their differentiation into mature and functional osteoblasts. Osteoblasts come from multipotential undifferentiated mesenchymal stem cells that are able to form cartilage, bone, muscle cells, or adipocytes after induction by hormonal or local factors. Several experiments have demonstrated that adipocytes and osteoblasts share a common precursor cell (Pittenger et al. 1999; Triffitt 1996). This cell differentiates into one or the other cell depending on the expression of specific transcription factors. Thus, the expression of peroxisome proliferator activated receptor $\gamma 2$ (PPAR$\gamma 2$) is requested for commitment to the adipocyte lineage, whereas mesenchymal cells expressing Cbfa1/Runx2 are committed to osteoblast lineage (Rodan et al. 1997).

Many transcription factors and proteins are involved not only in the formation and differentiation of osteoblasts but also in their inhibition. Among them, bone morphogenetic proteins (BMPs) and core binding factor a1 (Cbfa1) are crucial molecules in bone biology because they induce differentiation of mesenchymal cells toward cells of osteoblastic lineage (Canalis et al. 2003). The BMPs are members of the TGF-β superfamily of proteins that includes TGF-β, activins, and inhibins. BMPs are the only factors able to initiate osteoblastogenesis from noncommitted progenitors (Abe et al. 2000). An essential function of BMPs is to induce the differentiation of mesenchymal cells toward cells of osteoblastic lineage and promote osteoblast maturation and function, which requires interactions between BMPs and other factors like Smad and Cbfa1 (Yamaguchi et al. 1996). BMPs are modulated by numerous secreted factors such as Noggin, Chordin, SOST, and Gremlin, which inhibit BMP action by binding BMPs (Lee et al. 2000; Balemans et al. 2002). Cbfa1 is a specific transcription factor of osteoblasts whose deficiency causes an arrest of osteoblast development, absence of osteoblasts, and lack of bone formation (Ducy et al. 1997). Several studies have demonstrated that Cbfa1 is crucial also for postnatal differentiation and maintenance of osteoblasts and for the function of mature osteoblasts (Ducy et al. 1998, 1999). Regulation of osteoblastogenesis is much more complex and involves a large number of genes, but it is not the topic of this chapter (Canalis et al. 2003; Balemans et al. 2002; Harada et al, 2003; Ducy et al. 2000).

Once stem cells are committed to the osteoblast lineage, proliferating osteoprogenitors become preosteoblasts, cell growth declines, and there is a progressive expression of differentiation markers by osteoblasts (Stein et al. 1996). Osteoblastic differentiation is characterized by the sequential expression of alkaline phosphatase (ALP), an early marker of osteoblastic phenotype, followed by the synthesis and deposition of collagen type I, bone matrix proteins, and glycosaminoglycans and an increased expression of osteocalcin and bone sialoprotein at the onset of mineralization. When bone matrix has been deposited and calcified, most of the osteoblasts reduce their activity of matrix synthesis and become flattened lining cells. Around 10% of the osteoblasts are absorbed into the matrix synthesized by themselves and thus becoming osteocytes, which remain connected to each other by cytoplasmic extensions located in canaliculi. This allows for the transfer of molecules and nutrients from the older bone to the bone surface. Due to the proximity of the bone matrix, the osteocytes and lining cells sense external mechanical signals and transfer this information to other cells by changes in integrins and the cytoskeletal network. More than half of the osteoblasts undergo apoptosis when bone formation concludes (Jilka et al. 1998).

Osteoclasts are large, highly specialized, and polarized multinucleated cells with a characteristic trait. Their cell membrane has folds and invaginations at the interface with the bone surface called "*ruffled border*". Resorption occurs under this membrane in a microcompartment localized between the ruffled border and the bone matrix. Osteoclasts resorb bone by means of producing hydrogen ions to solubilize the mineral phase and to secrete proteolitic enzymes to degrade the organic matrix. To function, osteoclasts should be attached to the bone surface and secrete several enzymes such as tartrate-resistant acid phosphatase (TRAP; a phenotypic marker of these cells), cathepsins, and matrix metalloproteases (Blair 1998; Boyle et al. 2003). The acidification of the mineralized matrix depends on proton production by carbonic anhydrase II, whose deficiency induces osteopetrosis due to a lack of bone resorption (Sly et al. 1983). In addition, indicating the importance of cathepsin K, knockout mice of this protein exhibit an inhibition of bone resorption and display an osteopetrotic phenotype (Gowen et al. 1999). The most important integrin responsible for osteoclast attachment to bone is the vitronectin receptor ($\alpha V\beta 3$). If this integrin is inhibited, bone resorption is impaired, thus showing the importance of attachment to the bone for osteoclast function (Helfrich et al. 1992).

Osteoclasts are derived from hematopoietic stem cells of the monocyte-macrophage lineage, which also produces monocytes and macrophages (Kurihara et al. 1989; Roodman 1996). The point at which the committed osteoclast progenitor separates from the macrophage lineage is not clear, but when it receives the appropriate signal, this progenitor abandons the BM and goes to bone either by means of circulation or by direct migration. Deletion of gene encoding for molecules that regulate osteoclastogenesis (OCS) results in osteopetrosis due to a failure in osteoclast formation, and, in occasions, an absence of macrophages also occurs. The transcription factor PU.1 is critical for both the initial commitment of both cellular types, since its deficiency results in osteopetrosis with neither osteoclasts nor macrophages (Tondravi et al.

1997). Macrophage-colony stimulating factor (M-CSF) is needed for both early as well as for committed progenitors, promoting proliferation and survival (Kodama et al. 1991). The absence of c-Fos, however, results in osteopetrosis in the absence of osteoclasts, but with normal macrophage numbers, showing a step that allows for the differentiation of osteoclast and macrophage lineages (Grigoriadis et al. 1994). Other crucial proteins for the formation and differentiation of osteoclasts, whose discovery has been one of the most remarkable contributions to osteoclast biology in recent years and to which an entire section of this chapter is dedicated, are RANKL, RANK, and OPG (Lacey et al. 1998; Simonet et al. 1997; Anderson et al. 1997).

7.3
Role of Proinflammatory Cytokines in Bone Resorption

Early stages of hematopoiesis and OCS progress along similar pathways; therefore it is normal that cytokines and growth factors implied in hematopoiesis also affect the development of osteoclasts. The first evidence of this implication came from the discovery that supernatants of activated human monocytes stimulated bone resorption (Horton et al. 1972). This activity was called *osteoclast-activating factor* (OAF) and later identified as interleukin 1 (IL-1) (Dewhirst et al. 1985). Afterwards, IL-6 and TNF-α were identified, which, like IL-1, are essential mediators in inflammatory responses. Many other cytokines that stimulate bone resorption like IL-3, IL-11, IL-15, IL-17, and GM-CSF and others that inhibit it such as IL-4, IL-10, IL-18, and IFN-γ were also identified (Manolagas 2000; Manolagas et al. 1995; Jilka 1998). All these agents directly affect OCS or indirectly act as local regulators of the action of systemic hormones like PTH, vitamin D3, and estrogens. This chapter will focus on the involvement of the cytokines most implicated in bone resorption such as IL-1, TNF-α, and IL-6.

Interleukin 1 (IL-1) is produced mainly by activated monocytes-macrophages, and its principal action is to stimulate thymocytes. A pleiotropic cytokine, IL-1 induces the expression of a large diversity of cytokines such as IL-6, leukaemia inhibitory factor (LIF), and other proinflammatory molecules (Dimarello 1994). IL-1 and TNF-α carry out as part of their function increasing the expression of NF-κB and JNK (c-Jun N-terminal kinase). The importance of IL-1 in OCS is demonstrated because the IL-1-receptor-deficient mouse is resistant to ovariectomy (OVX)-induced bone loss (Lorenzo et al. 1998). The importance in pathological bone loss is also illustrated by the fact that treatment with IL-1 receptor antagonist slows down bone erosion for patients affected with rheumatoid arthritis (Kwan et al. 2004). IL-1 increases osteoclast differentiation rather than mature osteoclast activity, and infusion of IL-1 into mice induces hypercalcemia and bone resorption. Finally, IL-1 and TNF-α

stimulate OCS by inducing the expression of RANKL, and it has been demonstrated that IL-1 mediates the osteoclastogenic effect of TNF-α by enhancing stromal cell expression of RANKL (Wei et al. 2005).

Tumor necrosis factor α (TNF-α) is a multifunctional cytokine produced by activated monocytes-macrophages. TNF-α is one of the most potent osteoclastogenic cytokines produced in inflammation, and, in addition, TNF-α induces IL-1 synthesis. Like the other known stimulators of bone resorption, it acts through osteoblastic cells; however, it has been demonstrated that TNF-α is able to induce osteoclast formation from stromal-depleted macrophages, with potency similar to that of RANKL (Kobayashi et al. 2000). TNF-α is able to induce bone resorption in vitro (Thomson et al. 1987) as well as in vivo (Köning et al. 1988). Osteoclasts induced by TNF-α have the capacity to form resorption pits on dentine slices only in the presence of IL-1α. TNF-α, together with IL-1, plays an important role in bone resorption in inflammatory diseases (Kobayashi et al. 2000). Inhibition of TNF by TNF binding protein (TNFbp) completely prevents bone loss and osteoclast formation (Kimble et al. 1997).

Interleukin-6 (IL-6) is a member of the gp130 cytokine family and is constitutively produced by several cells of bone microenvironment, particularly by osteoblasts and their precursors (Heymann et al. 2000). The main function in bone is on OCS and bone resorption, and its effects are connected to those of IL-1, TNF-α, and PTHrP. IL-6 induces osteoclastlike formation by inducing IL-1 synthesis, and the addition of anti-IL-1 inhibits osteoclast formation by IL-6 (Kurihara et al. 1990). Moreover, IL-6 mediates the effects of TNF-α and enhances PTHrP-induced hypercalcemia and bone resorption by increasing the osteoclast progenitor pool and differentiation into mature osteoclasts (Devlin et al. 1998).

Independently, if these cytokines can exert their bone resorption functions without RANKL, they all stimulate the production of RANKL for stromal/OB cells, and conversely RANKL is able to increase IL-1 and TNF-α synthesis in vitro. To complicate this scenario, these systems of cytokines connect with the network of systemic hormones, such as PTH, PTH-related protein (PTHrP), vitamin D3, estrogens, androgens, glucocorticoids, and T4, since the hormones regulate the production of many of these cytokines by stromal/OB cells (Manolagas et al. 1995; Bellido et al. 1995; Lakatos et al. 1997).

7.4 The RANKL/RANK/OPG System

During the 1970s data on the expression of receptors for known stimulators of bone resorption, like PTH and vitamin D3, demonstrated that these receptors were not present on osteoclasts or their precursor cells, but were on osteoblasts (Rodan et al. 1981). Moreover, cellular interactions between stromal/OB cells and hematopoietic cells of BM are critical for osteoclast development, and this requirement of interaction became a common denominator for all known OCS stimulators (Kelly et al. 1998). These precedents served to formulate the hypothesis that in the surface of these cells exists an "*osteoclast differentiating factor*" (ODF) (Suda et al. 1992). The molecular mechanism of dependence that OCS has with stromal/OB cells has been explained recently with the discovery of a new bone system of cytokines belonging to the TNF superfamily of receptors and ligands. These crucial proteins for the differentiation and function of osteoclasts are RANKL, its receptor RANK, and OPG.

RANKL, also known as TRANCE, OPGL, or ODF, was cloned almost simultaneously by 4 groups (Lacey et al. 1998; Yasuda et al. 1998; Anderson et al. 1997; Wong et al. 1997). RANKL is expressed in stromal/OB cells, and its expression is increased for factors that induce bone resorption as glucocorticoids, IL-1, IL-6, IL-11, IL-17, TNF-α, PGE2, PTH, or vitamin D3 (Lacey et al. 1998; Yasuda et al. 1998). RANKL stimulates the differentiation and survival of osteoclast precursors, activates to mature osteoclast, and prolongs its lifespan by inhibiting its apoptosis (Lacey et al. 1998; Yasuda et al. 1998). RANKL, together with M-CSF, is necessary and sufficient to carry out all the steps of OCS, even in the absence of stromal cells. The administration of RANKL to the mouse induces a severe osteoporosis, hypercalcemia, and rapid bone loss (Lacey et al. 1998). Conversely, RANKL-deficient mice have a severe osteopetrosis phenotype with the absence of mature osteoclasts, defects in the dental eruption, and several defects in the maturation of T- and B-cells and in the formation of the lymphatic node (Kong et al. 1999a; Kong et al. 1999b). Several agents regulate RANKL expression (Table 7.1). Thus, IL-1, IL-6, TNF-α, vitamin D3, and PTH are compounds that stimulate the production of RANKL, whereas TGF-β is the main factor that inhibits RANKL expression (Khosla 2001; Hofbauer et al. 2000; Suda et al. 1999). Estrogens do not seem to modulate the in vitro expression of RANKL, although the OVX accompanies an increase in the expression of RANKL (Suda et al. 1999) and OPG (Hofbauer et al. 1999).

The receptor for RANKL is RANK, also known as ODAR (Anderson et al. 1997; Hsu et al. 1999). RANK is expressed in osteoclast precursors, mature osteoclasts, condrocytes, fibroblasts, and immune system cells (Anderson et al. 1997; Hsu et al. 1999). The binding of RANKL with RANK on preosteoclasts initiates the OCS and the activation of osteoclasts (Anderson et al. 1997; Hsu et al. 1999; Nakagawa et al. 1998). RANK-deficient mice display a phenotype characterized by osteopetrosis and several defects in the immune system similar to that observed in RANKL-deficient mice (Dougall et al. 1999). Consistent with this hypothesis, RANK-deficient mice are resistant to bone resorption induced by TNF-α, IL-1β, or vitamin D3 (Li et al. 2000). In agreement with this, mice deficient in molecules implied in the transduction pathway from RANK like TRAF-6 or NF-κB1/NK-κB2 also show an osteopetrotic phenotype,

Table 7.1. Regulators of RANKL, RANK, and OPG expression

	RANKL	RANK	OPG	Reference
PTH	$\Uparrow$		$\Downarrow$	(Yasuda et al. 1998; Lee et al. 1991)
Vitamin D3	$\Uparrow$		$\Uparrow$	(Yasuda et al. 1998; Hofbauer et al. 1998)
Estrogen	#		$\Uparrow$	(Hofbauer et al. 1999)
Calcium	$\Uparrow$		$\Uparrow$	(Ahlen et al. 2002; Takami et al. 2000)
Glucocorticoids	$\Uparrow$		$\Downarrow$	(Gao et al. 1998)
BMP-2			$\Uparrow$	(Hofbauer et al. 1998)
IL-1	$\Uparrow$		$\Uparrow$	(Hofbauer et al. 1999)
TNF-α	$\Uparrow$		$\Uparrow$	(Hofbauer et al. 1999)
IL-6	$\Uparrow$	$\Downarrow$	$\Uparrow$	(Palmqvist et al. 2002)
IL-11	$\Uparrow$		$\Uparrow$	(Yasuda et al. 1998; Ahlen et al. 2002)
IL-17	$\Uparrow$			(Nakashima et al. 2000)
TGF-β	$\Downarrow$		$\Uparrow$	(Murikami et al. 1998)
IL-4 + α-CD3 (T-cells)	$\Uparrow$	$\Uparrow$		(Anderson et al. 1997)
TGF-β+α-CD3 (T-cells)	$\Uparrow$	$\Uparrow$		(Anderson et al. 1997; Quinn et al. 2001)
CD40L (dendritic cells)		$\Uparrow$	$\Uparrow$	(Anderson et al. 1997; Yun et al. 1998)
Cyclosporine A	$\Uparrow$		$\Downarrow$	(Hofbauer et al. 2001)
Rapamycin	$\Uparrow$		$\Downarrow$	(Hofbauer et al. 2001)

$\Uparrow$ increase expression; $\Downarrow$ decrease expression; # unchanged

demonstrating that signals through RANK are necessary for the differentiation and activation of osteoclasts (Lomaga et al. 1999; Iotsova et al. 1997). Unlike RANKL and OPG, the expression of RANK on osteoclastic cells is stable, with few variations for osteopetrotic agents (Hofbauer et al. 2000). In the immune system, however, the expression of RANKL in T-cells is activated for IL-4 and TGF-β, while the expression of RANK on dendritic cells is upregulated by CD40-L (Table 7.1) (Anderson et al. 1997).

The osteoprotegerin (OPG), also known as OCIF, TR1, or FDCR-1, is the first soluble protein that belongs to the TNF superfamily (Simonet et al. 1997; Kwon et al. 1998; Yun et al. 1998). Unlike RANK and RANKL, OPG is expressed in high concentrations in a variety of tissues and cellular types such as skin, bones, large arteries, and the gastrointestinal tract (Simonet et al. 1997). In bone, OPG is produced by stromal/OB cells (Hofbauer et al. 1999) and works as a "decoy receptor" for RANKL, competing with RANK for binding RANKL. Therefore, OPG is a potent inhibitor of the OCS. In vitro, OPG inhibits the differentiation and survival of osteoclast precursors, blocks their activation, and induces their apoptosis (Lacey et al. 1998; Yasuda et al. 1998; Hofbauer et al.

1999). OPG in vivo overexpression induces severe osteopetrosis similar to that in RANKL- and RANK-deficient mice, although without showing the effects on the immune system of these (Simonet et al. 1997). OPG-deficient mice show a severe osteoporosis, an arterial calcification that suggests a role in the vascular system, and an altered B-cell maturation and antibody response (Yun et al. 2001). OPG is also produced by osteoblasts in response to anabolic agents such as estrogens and BMPs, and administration of recombinant OPG to the mouse results in an increase of bone mass and prevents the bone loss induced by OVX (Simonet et al. 1997; Yasuda et al. 1998; Udagawa et al. 2000). The production of OPG is stimulated by IL-1, TNF-α, TGF-β, BMP-2, BMP-7, vitamin D3, 17β-estradiol, and calcium, while it is diminished by PGE2, glucocorticoids, PTH, and cyclosporine A (Hofbauer et al. 2000; Suda et al. 1999).

The proposed model to explain OCS is schematized in Fig. 7.2. Several agents, induced or not for estrogen deficiency, stimulate the expression of RANKL on stromal/OB cells. The binding of RANKL with its receptor RANK on osteoclastic precursors, together with M-CSF, is a necessary and sufficient condition to carry out all the steps in the formation and differentiation of the osteoclasts. Undoubtedly all this is much more complex than what is described here since at least 24 genes that positively and negatively regulate OCS have been described (Boyle et al. 2003).

Inflammation and autoimmunity often are associated with the destruction of bone, but the molecular link between these two processes had long been unclear. The role of bone in the generation of immune system cells is evident since they are formed in the marrow housed within the bone; however, the role of these cells on bone is not so clear. RANKL and RANK were described initially in activated T-cells and in dendritic cells, respectively, where they have functions in the regulation of cellular lifespan and immunomodulation (Anderson et al. 1997; Wong et al. 1997). Recently the term *osteoimmunology* has been coined to describe the link between the immune system and bone (Arron et a. 2000). Several data support this idea:

1. T-cell-deficient mice do not lose bone after OVX (Cenci et al. 2000).
2. Activated monocytes or T-cells can induce OCS through the secretion of proresorptive cytokines IL-1, TNF-α, and IL-11, which upregulate RANKL in osteoblasts (Hofbauer et al. 1999).
3. Activated T-cells also express RANKL (Anderson et al. 1997).
4. The systemic activation of T-cells leads to a RANKL-dependent increase of OCS (Kong et al. 1999b).
5. Mice lacking CTLA4, in which T-cells are systemically activated, exhibit osteoporosis (Kong et al. 1999b).

Nevertheless, T-cells also secrete cytokines, including IFN-γ, IL-12, IL-18, TGF-β, and IFN-β, which inhibit the pro-osteoclastogenic effects of RANKL.

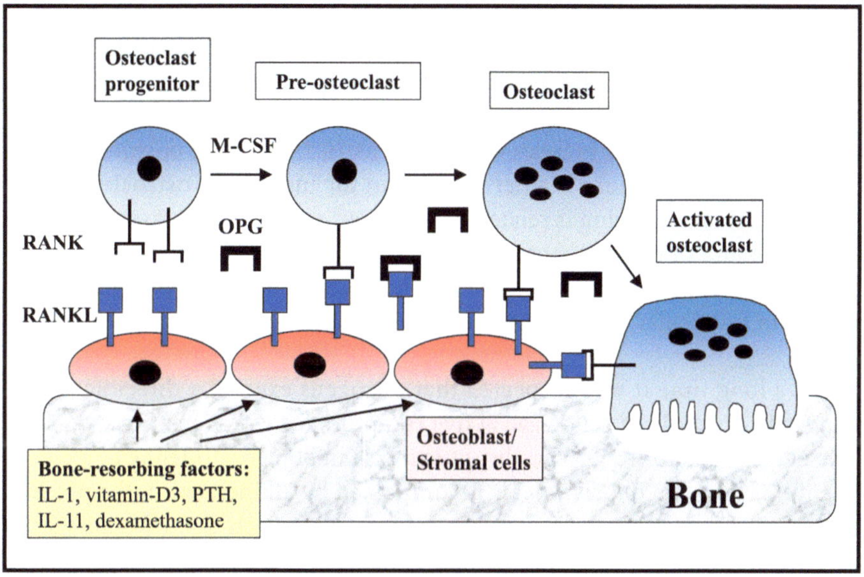

Fig. 7.2. Osteoclastogenesis. Several bone resorbing factors such as IL-1, TNF-α, vitamin D3, and dexamethasone stimulate the expression of RANKL on the membranes of stromal/OB cells, although it can be secreted into circulation. The binding of RANKL with RANK on osteoclast precursors, together with M-CSF, is the signal required to initiate and maintain all steps of the OCS. The OPG is another member of the TNF superfamily and acts as a decoy receptor for RANKL. OPG is secreted by stromal/OB cells and inhibits osteoclast formation by blocking the RANKL/RANK signal pathway

Therefore, T-cells participate in bone loss during inflammation or when T-cells are chronically activated (rheumatoid arthritis, periodontitis, infections, bone prothesis) and recently have been implicated in postmenopausal bone loss (Cenci et al. 2000, 2003; Roggia et al. 2001).

7.5 Bone Remodeling After Estrogen Deficiency

Osteoporosis is a consequence of the reduction of skeletal mass caused by an imbalance between bone resorption and bone formation. The loss of gonadal function and aging are the two main factors that contribute to the development of osteoporosis. Around the fourth or fifth decade of life, men and women lose bone at a rate of 0.3–0.5% per year. After menopause, the rate of bone loss increases to 10% a year (Nordin et al. 1990; Riggs et al. 1986, 1998). The bone loss due to estrogen withdrawal is associated with increments in both bone resorption as well as in bone formation, with the former exceeding the latter. This indicates the birth of new BMUs or an increase in the lifespan of current BMUs (Manolagas 2000). Estrogen deficiency increases the activation frequency (*birth rate*) of BMUs, which leads to higher bone turnover and induces a remodeling imbalance by prolonging the resorption phase (osteoclast apoptosis is reduced (Hughes et al. 1996)) and a shortening of the formation phase (osteoblast apoptosis is increased (Manolagas 2000)). Unlike postmenopausal bone loss, in which there is a net increase in the number of osteoclasts, bone loss associated with aging is related to a reduced offer of osteoblasts in relation to the demand of the newly created BMUs (Erikson et al. 1990). Both types of bone loss affect different bone types; while postmenopausal bone loss occurs mainly in trabecular bone, the age-associated one occurs primarily in cortical bone.

For a long time it was suspected that estrogens exerted a direct action on bone cells since these cells have active receptors for estrogens (Eriksen et al. 1988; Oursler et al. 1991). The abrupt increase in bone remodeling as a consequence of estrogen deprivation is accompanied by an increase in the production of several cytokines and growth factors (Manolagas 2000; Manolagas et al. 1995; Jilka 1998; Pacifici et al. 1998). Many studies on bone estrogen action have focused on the role of cytokines and molecules such as IL-1, IL-6, TNF-α, GM-CSF, M-CSF, and PGE2 (Fig. 7.3). These factors induce bone resorption, and their expression increases with estrogen deficiency and decreases with estrogen administration (Manolagas 2000; Manolagas et al. 1995; Hofbauer et al. 2000; Riggs et al. 1998; Pacifici et al. 1998). In 1987 it was demonstrated that cultures of monocytes from osteoporotic women have higher levels of IL-1 than those in women with normal bone turnover (Pacifici et al. 1987). These authors also demonstrated an increase in the production of IL-1 and TNF for cultures of monocytes from women subjected to OVX but not if these women took estrogens (Pacifici et al. 1991). In mice, treatment with inhibitors of IL-1 and TNF prevents bone loss induced by OVX (Yamamoto et al. 1996), and OVX is not followed by bone loss in IL-1 type I receptor (IL-1RI)-deficient mice or in mice that overexpress a soluble form of the TNF receptor, that which makes them unable to respond to TNF-α (Ammann et al. 1997). Moreover, treatment of ovariectomized mice with an inhibitor of TNF, such as TNF-binding protein (TNFbp), prevents bone loss induced by OVX (Kimble et al. 1997).

While studies have repeatedly demonstrated that IL-1 and TNF-α are potent inductors of bone loss after OVX, the role of IL-6 is more uncertain. The IL-6-deficient mouse does not lose bone mass after OVX, although it has increased bone turnover (Poli et al. 1994), while the mouse overexpressing IL-6 does not present osteoporosis, which seems to be a contradiction (Kitamura et al. 1995). Moreover, neutralizing antibodies against IL-6 prevents an increase in osteoclast number after OVX (Kimble et al. 1997; Jilka et al. 1992), although it does not prevent bone loss after OVX, nor does it diminish in vivo bone resorption (Kimble et al. 1997). All this suggests that IL-6 contributes to the expansion

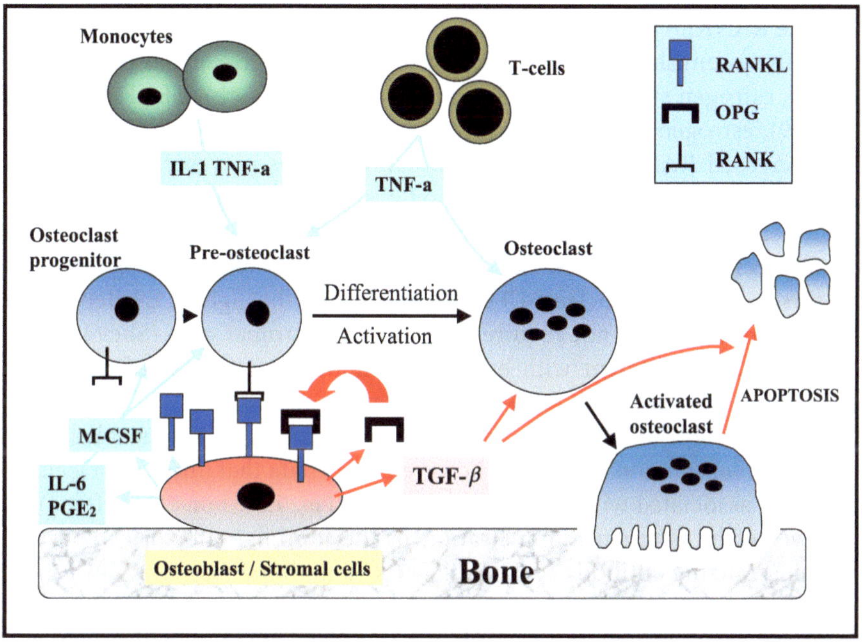

Fig. 7.3. Osteoclastogenesis after estrogen deficiency. Estrogen deprivation leads to an increase in the synthesis of RANKL for stromal/OB cells of the BM. This increase in the expression of RANKL leads to an increase in OCS. Estrogen deficiency also induces the synthesis and secretion of cytokines, such as IL-6 and M-CSF, that increase the number of preosteoclasts in the BM, and thus increases OCS. Nonetheless, certain cells of the immune system, such as monocytes and T-cells, intervene in the process when the supply of estrogens fails. These cells secrete IL-1 and TNF-α that are powerful inductors of OCS. When estrogens or agonists of estrogen receptors like raloxifene are administered, the synthesis and secretion of many of the mentioned cytokines diminish and the synthesis and liberation of OPG and TGF-β are stimulated. These molecules inhibit OCS by inhibiting the RANKL/RANK signal pathway and by promoting osteoclast apoptosis

of osteoclasts from hematopoietic precursors, although it does not seem to be a dominant factor in estrogen-deficiency-induced bone loss (Manolagas 2000; Hofbauer et al. 2000).

In summary, IL-1 and TNF-α activate mature osteoclasts indirectly via a primary effect on osteoblasts and by inhibiting osteoclast apoptosis. In addition, they increase osteoclast formation either by directly stimulating the proliferation of osteoclast precursors or by increasing the pro-osteoclastogenic capacity of bone stromal cells. Although in vitro TNF-α and IL-1 can apparently induce the development of TRAP+ osteoclasts in the absence of RANKL/RANK, all data seem to indicate that TNF-α and IL-1 potentiate osteoclast development via the activation of common second messenger systems, such as NF-κB activation, and that the effects on OCS require the RANKL/RANK system (Jones et al. 2002).

If the RANKL/OPG system is a final effector on the biology of osteoclasts, then this system should be the basis for the antiresorptive effects of estrogen. Indeed, estrogen stimulates OPG synthesis for osteoblastic cells (Hofbauer et al. 1999), estrogen deficiency induced by OVX results in a decrease in OPG and increased RANKL production, an action that is prevented by estradiol administration, and OPG administration prevents bone loss induced by OVX (Simonet et al. 1997; Hofbauer et al. 2000; Hofbauer 1999). In addition, estrogen can suppress RANKL and M-CSF-induced differentiation of myelomonocytic precursors into multinucleated TRAP+ osteoclasts through an ER-dependent mechanism that does not require mediation by stromal cells (Shevde et al. 2000). Finally, treatment with estradiol inhibits the response of osteoclast precursors to the action of RANKL (Srivastava et al. 2001).

As previously stated, T-cells intervene in bone loss that is established in states of inflammation. There are, however, more data that implicate T-cells in bone loss associated with estrogen deficiency (Fig. 7.3). Bone loss after OVX is prevented by estrogen administration, by the administration of TNFbp, and by a neutralizing antibody to TNF-α. There is no bone loss after OVX in T-cell-deficient mice (Cenci et al. 2000). In addition, it has been shown that enhanced T-cell production of TNF is a key mechanism by which estrogen deficiency induces bone loss in vivo (Roggia et al. 2001). Activated T-cells also produce IFN-γ, which strongly suppresses OCS by interfering with the RANKL/RANK signaling pathway via the induction of TRAF6 degradation that results in an inhibition of the RANKL-induced activation of NF-κB and JNK (Takayanagi et al. 2000). OVX increases TNF levels in BM by increasing the production of TNF by T-cells, which is induced by a complex mechanism driven by IFN-γ (Cenci et al. 2003; Gao et al. 2004). This cytokine augments antigen presentation by enhancing MHCII expression on BM macrophages through induction of class II transactivator (CIITA) expression (Cenci et al. 2003). Upregulation of antigen presentation results, in turn, in increased T-cell activation, proliferation, and lifespan. Therefore, TNF produced by T-cells plays a pivotal role in the mechanism of estrogen-deficiency-induced bone loss. The mechanism by which OVX upregulates the production of IFN-γ remains undetermined, but TFG-β could be involved since it has been reported that TFG-β represses the production of IFN-γ by directly targeting T-cells and inhibiting their proliferation and differentiation (Kehrl et al. 1986; Gorelik et al. 2002).

7.6 Effects of Estrogen and Agonist of Estrogen Receptor on Bone Cells

Bone cells contain estrogen receptors (Eriksen et al. 1988; Oursler et al. 1991; Vidal et al. 1999). Estrogens act directly on osteoblasts and affect cell proliferation and the expression of many genes coding for enzymes, bone matrix proteins, transcription factors, and hormone receptors, as well as growth factors and cytokines (Spelsberg et al. 1999). It has been shown that estrogen inhibits the synthesis of IL-1, IL-6, TNF-α, and IL-11, as well as IL-6 synthesis in response to IL-1 (Manolagas 2000; Jilka 1998; Jilka et al. 1992; Kimble et al. 1996). Estrogen has also been shown to induce the synthesis of BMP-6, OPG, TGF-β, NF-κB, and c-Fos (Stein et al. 1995; Tau et al. 1998; Rickard et al. 1998). The main in vivo action of estrogens on the skeleton is to inhibit bone resorption. This action is indirect since it implies the regulation of cytokines and growth factor production by osteoblasts. Estrogens should have a direct action on osteoclasts, however, since active ERs have been described on osteoclasts. The most important action is probably that estrogens induce osteoclast apoptosis (Hughes et al. 1996; Kameda et al. 1997). This estrogen-mediated induction of apoptosis may be enhanced in vivo by TGF-β since this molecule produces osteoclast apoptosis and its production is increased by estrogens (Hughes et al. 1996). Estrogens have also shown the capacity to inhibit the expression of TRAP, to increase the induction in the expression of an IL-1 decoy receptor gene (Sunyer et al. 1999), and to inhibit certain steps in the RANK-JNK signal transduction pathway by suppressing activation of MKK4 and JNK, and c-Jun expression and its subsequent AP-1 transactivation of transcription (Srivastava et al. 2001, 1999). Some evidence suggests that estrogens increase osteoblast formation, differentiation, proliferation, and function, although results vary among the different model systems (Manolagas 2000; Chow et al. 1992; Gohel et al. 1999).

It has been proposed that estrogen's effects may be mediated by different cell signaling pathways. It has been described that the antiapoptotic effect of estradiol on osteoblasts and osteocytes can be mediated for rapid, nongenomic, and sex-nonspecific signaling through the ligand binding domain of the ER that is localized exclusively in the cell membrane (Kousteni et al. 2001). In addition, investigators have identified a synthetic ligand called estren that reverses bone loss in ovariectomized females (Kousteni et al. 2002), which activates only a subset of these pathways, suggesting that bypassing the traditional estrogen pathways can prevent bone loss without the associated side effects on reproductive organs. This compound exhibits no classical sex steroid hormone activity, and it is a potent activator of the rapid cell-membrane-mediated Src-MAPK pathways in cell culture models that induce a rapid activation of MAPK (Kousteni et al. 2003). This extranuclear mode of action of estren has led to the definition of a new class of pharmacotherapeutic agents called ANGELS (Activators of Nongenotropic Estrogen-like Signaling) (Manolagas et al. 2002).

The beneficial role of estrogen replacement therapy (ERT) to prevent bone loss has been largely demonstrated (Nelson et al. 2002; Wells et al. 2002). Recently, however, the results of the great clinical study WHI (Women's Health Initiative) was published in which several side effects, such as an increase in breast cancer incidence and several vascular problems of ERT, were reported (Kobayashi et al. 2000; Rossouw et al. 2002). All of this has led to the large present effort to find new alternatives to ERT. Some of these alternatives are phytoestrogens and SERMs (Selective Estrogen Receptor Modulators).

The ideal SERM would have the beneficial effects of estrogen in bone without the undesirable effects in the breast and uterus, the current gold standard being raloxifene. SERMs are compounds that bind to estrogen receptors and exhibit estrogen agonistic effects on bone and lipid metabolism and estrogen antagonistic effects on uterine endometrium and breast tissue. Because of its tissue selectivity, raloxifene may have fewer side effects than is typically observed with ERT. The beneficial role of raloxifene in bone loss, in the decrease in bone fractures (Delmas et al. 1997; Ettinger et al. 1999), in the decrease in the incidence of breast cancer (Cummings et al. 1999), and in cardiovascular problems (Barrett-Connor et al. 2002) is well established. It has been demonstrated in osteoporotic postmenopausal women that raloxifene decreases levels of the cytokines involved in bone resorption such as IL-6 and TNF-α. This suggests that modulation of soluble factors could play a pivotal role in the mechanisms of the osteoprotective effect of raloxifene (Gianni et al. 2004).

Raloxifene, like 17β-estradiol, significantly reduces the number of osteoclasts in culture, inhibits bone resorption in a pit assay, increases osteoblast proliferation, increases Cbfa1 transcription factor mRNA, prevents the TNF-α-induced IL-1β increase, and stimulates TGF-β expression in rat bone (Taranta et al. 2002; Tou et al. 2001; Yang et al. 1996). Moreover, it has been shown that raloxifene can suppress RANKL and M-CSF-induced differentiation of myelomonocytic precursors into multinucleated TRAP+ osteoclasts through an ER-dependent mechanism that does not require mediation by stromal cells (Shevde et al. 2000). Raloxifene decreases levels of RANKL (Cheung et al. 2003) and stimulates OPG production and inhibits IL-6 production by human osteoblasts, and therefore, since OPG production increases with osteoblastic maturation, enhancement of OPG production by raloxifene could be related to the stimulatory effects on osteoblastic differentiation (Viereck et al. 2003). It seems, however, that the stimulation of bone formation by raloxifene differs from that of estradiol (Qu et al. 1999). Finally, raloxifene, like estradiol, directly decreases the expression of beta3-integrin mRNA and protein, which suggests that the inhibitory action of raloxifene and estradiol on bone resorption may affect adhesion and, like estradiol, prevent the increase in B-cells induced by OVX (Saintier et al. 2004; Onoe et al. 2000).

7.7 Conclusions

Bone metabolism has quickly become a topic of fascinating research. The bone, far from being a metabolically inactive tissue, is a tissue where different cell types and different molecules carry out numerous and varied functions. This has been due largely to the discovery of the RANKL/RANK/OPG system of cytokines. These new molecules are decisive in OCS, bone metabolism, and bone loss, but they are also important for other tissues and cells. Indeed, these proteins are critical in several systems: the immune system, where they have functions that affect cell survival and the immunomodulation of T-, B-, and dendritic cells; the vascular system; and the endocrine system.

This chapter has focused on normal bone remodeling and that which is established after estrogen deficiency. Bone remodeling is regulated not only by this new system of cytokines, but also by other molecules, especially when gonadal function ceases. This constitutes a complex scenario in which transcription factors, systemic hormones, growth factors, and cytokines, together with a variety of cells like osteoclasts, osteoblasts, osteocytes, endothelial cells, lining cells, T-cells, B-cells, and dendritic cells, cohabit and interrelate.

All these discoveries have generated new therapeutic possibilities based on the use of OPG and on inhibitors of the RANKL/RANK signaling pathway, not only for the treatment of postmenopausal bone loss, but also for other pathologies. Special mention should be made of the new therapeutic possibilities constituted by ANGELS, since everything seems to indicate that research is at the threshold of a new way of inhibiting bone loss without the side effects of classic ERT.

References

1. Frost HM (1973) Bone remodeling and its relationships to metabolic bone disease. Charles C. Thomas, Springfield, MA
2. Parfitt AM (1994) Osteonal and hemi-osteonal remodeling: the spatial and temporal framework for signal traffic in adult human bone. J Cell Biochem 55:273–286
3. Manolagas SC (2000) Birth and death of bone cells: basic regulatory mechanisms and implications for the pathogenesis and treatment of osteoporosis. Endocr Rev 21:115–137
4. Rodan GA, Martin TJ (1981) Role of osteoblast in hormonal control of bone resorption – a hypothesis. Calcif Tissue Int 33:349–351
5. Lacey DL, Timms E, Tan HL, Kelley MJ, Dunstan CR, Burgess T, Elliott R, Colombero A, Elliott G, Scully S, Hsu H, Sullivan J, Hawkins N, Davy E, Capparelli C, Eli A, Qian YX, Kaufman S, Sarosi I, Shalhoub V, Senaldi G, Guo J, Delaney J, Boyle WJ (1998) Osteoprotegerin ligand is a cytokine that regulates osteoclast differentiation and activation. Cell 93:165–176
6. Simonet WS, Lacey DL, Dunstan CR, Kelley M, Chang MS, Luthy R, Nguyen HQ, Wooden S, Bennett L, Boone T, Shimamoto G, DeRose M, Elliott R, Colombero A,

Tan HL, Trail G, Sullivan J, Davy E, Bucay N, Renshaw-Gegg L, Hughes TM, Hill D, Pattison W, Campbell P, Boyle WJ (1997) Osteoprotegerin: a novel secreted protein involved in the regulation of bone density. Cell 89:309–319

7. Yasuda H, Shima N, Nakagawa N, Mochizuki SI, Yano K, Fujise N, Sato Y, Goto M, Yamaguchi K, Kuriyama M, Kanno T, Murakami A, Tsuda E, Morinaga T, Higashio K (1998) Identity of osteoclastogenesis inhibitory factor (OCIF) and osteoprotegerin (OPG): a mechanism by which OPG/OCIF inhibits osteoclastogenesis in vitro. Endocrinology 139:1329–1337
8. Manolagas SC, Jilka RL (1995) Bone marrow, cytokines, and bone remodeling. Emerging insights into the pathophysiology of osteoporosis. N Engl J Med 332:305–311
9. Verborgt O, Gibson GJ, Schaffer MB (2000) Loss of osteocyte integrity in association with microdamage and bone remodeling after fatigue in vivo. J Bone Miner Res 15:60–67
10. Jilka RL (2003) Biology of the basic multicellular unit and the pathophysiology of osteoporosis. Med Pediatr Oncol 41:182–185
11. Parfitt AM (2000) The mechanism of coupling: a role for the vasculature. Bone 26:319–323
12. Parfitt AM (2001) The bone remodeling compartment: a circulatory function for bone lining cells. J Bone Miner Res 16:1583–1585
13. Pittenger MF, Mackay AM, Beck SC, Jaiswal RK, Douglas R, Mosca JD (1999) Multilineage potential of adult human mesenchymal stem cells. Science 284:143–147
14. Triffitt JT (1996) The stem cell of the osteoblast. In: Bilezikian JP, Raisz LG, Rodan GA (eds) Principles of bone biology. Academic, San Diego, pp 39–50
15. Rodan GA, Harada SI (1997) The missing bone. Cell 89:677–680
16. Canalis E, Economides AN, Gazzerro E (2003) Bone morphogenetic proteins, their antagonist, and the skeleton. Endocr Rev 24:218–235
17. Abe E, Yamamoto M, Taguchi Y, Lecka-Czernik B, O'Brien CA, Economides AN, Stahl N, Jilka RL, Manolagas SC (2000) Essential requirement of BMPs-2/4 for both osteoblast and osteoclast formation in murine bone marrow cultures from adult mice: antagonism by noggin. J Bone Miner Res 15:663–673
18. Yamaguchi A, Ishizuya T, Kintou N, Wada Y, Katagiri T, Wozney JM, Rosen V, Yoshiki S (1996) Effects of BMP-2, BMP-4, and BMP-6 on osteoblastic differentiation of bone marrow-derived stromal cell lines, ST2 and MC3T3-G2/PA6. Biochem Biophys Res Commun 220:366–371
19. Lee KS, Kim HJ, Li QL, Chi XZ, Ueta C, Komori T, Wozney JM, Kim EG, Choi JY, Ryoo HM, Bae SC (2000) Runx2 is a common target of transforming growth factor beta1 and bone morphogenetic protein 2, and cooperation between Runx2 and Smad5 induces osteoblast-specific gene expression in the pluripotent mesenchymal precursor cell line C2C12. Mol Cell Biol 20:8783–8792
20. Balemans W, Van Hul W (2002) Extracellular regulation of BMP signaling in vertebrates: a cocktail of modulators. Dev Biol 250:231–250
21. Ducy P, Zhang R, Geoffroy V, Ridall AL, Karsenty G (1997) Osf2/Cbfa1: a transcriptional activator of osteoblast differentiation. Cell 89:747–754
22. Ducy P, Karsenty G (1998) Genetic control of cell differentiation in the skeleton. Curr Opin Cell Biol 10:614–619
23. Ducy P, Starbuck M, Priemel M, Shen J, Pinero G, Geoffroy V, Amling M, Karsenty G (1999) A Cbfa1-dependent genetic pathway controls bone formation beyond embryonic development. Genes Dev 13:1025–1036
24. Harada S, Rodan GA (2003) Control of osteoblast function and regulation of bone mass. Nature 423:349–355

25. Ducy P, Schinke T, Karsenty G (2000) The osteoblast: a sophisticated fibroblast under central surveillance. Science 289:1501–1504
26. Stein GS, Lian JB, Stein JL, van Wijnen AJ, Frenkel B, Montecino M (1996) Mechanism regulating osteoblast and proliferation. In: Bilezikian JP, Raisz LG, Rodan GA (eds) Principles of bone biology. Academic, New York, pp 69–86
27. Jilka RL, Weinstein RS, Bellido T, Parfitt AM, Manolagas SC (1998) Osteoblast programmed cell death (apoptosis): modulation by growth factors and cytokines. J Bone Miner Res 13:793–802
28. Blair HC (1998) How the osteoclast degrades bone. Bioessays 20:837–846
29. Boyle WJ, Simonet WS, Lacey DL (2003) Osteoclast differentiation and activation. Nature 423:337–342
30. Sly WS, Hewett-Emmett D, Whyte MP, Yu YS, Tashian RE (1983) Carbonic anhydrase II deficiency identified as the primary defect in the autosomal recessive syndrome of osteopetrosis with renal tubular acidosis and cerebral calcification. Proc Natl Acad Sci USA 80:2752–2756
31. Gowen M, Lazner F, Dodds R, Kapadia R, Feild J, Tavaria M, Bertoncello I, Drake F, Zavarselk S, Tellis I, Hertzog P, Debouck C, Kola I (1999) Cathepsin K knockout mice develop osteopetrosis due to a deficit in matrix degradation but not demineralization. J Bone Miner Res 14:1654–1663
32. Helfrich MH, Nesbitt SA, Dorey EL, Horton MA (1992) Rat osteoclasts adhere to a wide range of RGD (Arg-Gly-Asp) peptide-containing proteins, including the bone sialoproteins and fibronectin, via a beta 3 integrin. J Bone Miner Res 7:335–343
33. Kurihara N, Suda T, Miura Y, Nakauchi H, Kodama H, Hiura K, Hakeda Y, Kumegawa M (1989) Generation of osteoclasts from isolated hematopoietic progenitor cells. Blood 74:1295–1302
34. Roodman GD (1996) Advances in bone biology: the osteoclast. Endocr Rev 17:308–332
35. Tondravi MM, McKercher SR, Anderson K, Erdmann JM, Quiroz M, Maki R, Teitelbaum SL (1997) Osteopetrosis in mice lacking haematopoietic transcription factor PU.1. Nature 386:81–84
36. Kodama H, Yamasaki A, Nose M, Niida S, Ohgame Y, Abe M, Kumegawa M, Suda T (1991) Congenital osteoclast deficiency in osteopetrotic (op/op) mice is cured by injections of macrophage colony-stimulating factor. J Exp Med 173:269–272
37. Grigoriadis AE, Wang ZQ, Cecchini MG, Hofstetter W, Felix R, Fleisch HA, Wagner EF (1994) c-Fos: a key regulator of osteoclast-macrophage lineage determination and bone remodeling. Science 266:443–448
38. Anderson DM, Maraskovsky E, Billingsley WL, Dougall WC, Tometsko ME, Roux ER, Teepe MC, DuBose RF, Cosman D, Galibert L (1997) A homologue of the TNF receptor and its ligand enhance T-cell growth and dendritic-cell function. Nature 390:175–179
39. Horton JE, Raisz LG, Simmons HA, Oppenheim JJ, Mergenhagen SE (1972) Bone resorbing activity in supernatant fluid from cultured human peripheral blood leukocytes. Science 177:793–795
40. Dewhirst FE, Stashenko PP, Mole JE, Tsurumachi T (1985) Purification and partial sequence of human osteoclast-activating factor: identity with interleukin 1 beta. J Immunol 135:2562–2568
41. Jilka RL (1998) Cytokines, bone remodeling, and estrogen deficiency: a 1998 update. Bone 23:75–81
42. Dimarello CA (1994) The interleukin-1 family: 10 years of discovery. FASEB J 8:1314–1325

43. Lorenzo JA, Naprta A, Rao Y, Alander C, Glaccum M, Widmer M, Gronowicz G, Kalinowski J, Pilbeam CC (1998) Mice lacking the type I interleukin-1 receptor do not lose bone mass after ovariectomy. Endocrinology 139:3022–3025
44. Kwan TS, Padrines M, Theoleyre S, Heymann D, Fortun Y (2004) IL-6, RANKL, TNF-alpha/IL-1: interrelations in bone resorption pathophysiology. Cytokine Growth Factor Rev 15:49–60
45. Wei S, Kitaura H, Zhou P, Ross FP, Teitelbaum SL (2005) IL-1 mediates TNF-induced osteoclastogenesis. J Clin Invest 115:282–290
46. Kobayashi K, Takahashi N, Jimi E, Udagawa N, Takami M, Kotake S, Nakagawa N, Kinosaki M, Yamaguchi K, Shima N, Yasuda H, Morinaga T, Higashio K, Martin TJ, Suda T (2000) Tumor necrosis factor alpha stimulates osteoclast differentiation by a mechanism independent of the ODF/RANKL-RANK interaction. J Exp Med 191:275–286
47. Thomson BM, Mundy GR, Chambers TJ (1987) Tumor necrosis factors alpha and beta induce osteoblastic cells to stimulate osteoclastic bone resorption. J Immunol 138:775–779
48. Köning A, Muhlbauer RC, Fleisch H (1988) Tumor necrosis factor alpha and interleukin-1 stimulate bone resorption in vivo as measured by urinary [^{3}H]tetracycline excretion from prelabeled mice. J Bone Miner Res 3:621–627
49. Kimble RB, Bain S, Pacifici R (1997) The functional block of TNF but not of IL-6 prevents bone loss in ovariectomized mice. J Bone Miner Res 12:935–941
50. Heymann D, Rousselle AV (2000) gp130 Cytokine family and bone cells. Cytokine 12:1455–1468
51. Kurihara N, Bertolini D, Suda T, Akiyama Y, Roodman GD (1990) IL-6 stimulates osteoclast-like multinucleated cell formation in long term human marrow cultures by inducing IL-1 release. J Immunol 144:4226–4230
52. Devlin RD, Reddy SV, Savino R, Ciliberto G, Roodman GD (1998) IL-6 mediates the effects of IL-1 or TNF, but not PTHrP or 1,25(OH)2D3, on osteoclast-like cell formation in normal human bone marrow cultures. J Bone Miner Res 13:393–399
53. Bellido T, Jilka RL, Boyce BF, Girasole G, Broxmeyer H, Dalrymple SA, Murray R, Manolagas SC (1995) Regulation of interleukin-6, osteoclastogenesis, and bone mass by androgens. The role of the androgen receptor. J Clin Invest 95:2886–2895
54. Lakatos P, Foldes J, Horvath C, Kiss L, Tatrai A, Takacs I, Tarjan G, Stern PH (1997) Serum interleukin-6 and bone metabolism in patients with thyroid function disorders. J Clin Endocrinol Metab 82:78–81
55. Kelly KA, Tanaka S, Baron R, Gimble JM (1998) Murine bone marrow stromally derived BMS2 adipocytes support differentiation and function of osteoclast-like cells in vitro. Endocrinology 139:2092–2101
56. Suda T, Takahashi N, Martin TJ (1992) Modulation of osteoclast differentiation. Endocr Rev 13:66–80
57. Wong BR, Rho J, Arron J, Robinson E, Orlinick J, Chao M, Kalachikov S, Cayani E, Bartlett FS, III, Frankel WN, Lee SY, Choi Y (1997) TRANCE is a novel ligand of the tumor necrosis factor receptor family that activates c-Jun N-terminal kinase in T cells. J Biol Chem 272:25190–25194
58. Kong YY, Yoshida H, Sarosi I, Tan HL, Timms E, Capparelli C, Morony S, Oliveira-dos-Santos AJ, Van G, Itie A, Khoo W, Wakeham A, Dunstan CR, Lacey DL, Mak TW, Boyle WJ, Penninger JM (1999a) OPGL is a key regulator of osteoclastogenesis, lymphocyte development and lymph-node organogenesis. Nature 397:315–323
59. Kong YY, Feige U, Sarosi I, Bolon B, Tafuri A, Morony S, Capparelli C, Li J, Elliott R, McCabe S, Wong T, Campagnuolo G, Moran E, Bogoch ER, Van G, Nguyen LT,

Ohashi PS, Lacey DL, Fish E, Boyle WJ, Penninger JM (1999b) Activated T cells regulate bone loss and joint destruction in adjuvant arthritis through osteoprotegerin ligand. Nature 402:304–309
60. Khosla S (2001) Minireview: the OPG/RANKL/RANK system. Endocrinology 142: 5050–5055
61. Hofbauer LC, Heufelder AE (2000) Clinical review 114: hot topic. The role of receptor activator of nuclear factor-kappaB ligand and osteoprotegerin in the pathogenesis and treatment of metabolic bone diseases. J Clin Endocrinol Metab 85:2355–2363
62. Suda T, Takahashi N, Udagawa N, Jimi E, Gillespie MT, Martin TJ (1999) Modulation of osteoclast differentiation and function by the new members of the tumor necrosis factor receptor and ligand families. Endocr Rev 20:345–357
63. Hofbauer LC, Khosla S, Dunstan CR, Lacey DL, Spelsberg TC, Riggs BL (1999) Estrogen stimulates gene expression and protein production of osteoprotegerin in human osteoblastic cells. Endocrinology 140:4367–4370
64. Hsu H, Lacey DL, Dunstan CR, Solovyev I, Colombero A, Timms E, Tan HL, Elliott G, Kelley MJ, Sarosi I, Wang L, Xia XZ, Elliott R, Chiu L, Black T, Scully S, Capparelli C, Morony S, Shimamoto G, Bass MB, Boyle WJ (1999) Tumor necrosis factor receptor family member RANK mediates osteoclast differentiation and activation induced by osteoprotegerin ligand. Proc Natl Acad Sci USA 96:3540–3545
65. Nakagawa N, Kinosaki M, Yamaguchi K, Shima N, Yasuda H, Yano K, Morinaga T, Higashio K (1998) RANK is the essential signaling receptor for osteoclast differentiation factor in osteoclastogenesis. BioChem Biophys Res Commun 253:395–400
66. Dougall WC, Glaccum M, Charrier K, Rohrbach K, Brasel K, De Smedt T, Daro E, Smith J, Tometsko ME, Maliszewski CR, Armstrong A, Shen V, Bain S, Cosman D, Anderson D, Morrissey PJ, Peschon JJ, Schuh J (1999) RANK is essential for osteoclast and lymph node development. Genes Dev 13:2412–2424
67. Li J, Sarosi I, Yan XQ, Morony S, Capparelli C, Tan HL, McCabe S, Elliott R, Scully S, Van G, Kaufman S, Juan SC, Sun Y, Tarpley J, Martin L, Christensen K, McCabe J, Kostenuik P, Hsu H, Fletcher F, Dunstan CR, Lacey DL, Boyle WJ (2000) RANK is the intrinsic hematopoietic cell surface receptor that controls osteoclastogenesis and regulation of bone mass and calcium metabolism. Proc Natl Acad Sci USA 97:1566–1571
68. Lomaga MA, Yeh WC, Sarosi I, Duncan GS, Furlonger C, Ho A, Morony S, Capparelli C, Van G, Kaufman S, van der HA, Itie A, Wakeham A, Khoo W, Sasaki T, Cao Z, Penninger JM, Paige CJ, Lacey DL, Dunstan CR, Boyle WJ, Goeddel DV, Mak TW (1999) TRAF6 deficiency results in osteopetrosis and defective interleukin-1, CD40, and LPS signaling. Genes Dev 13:1015–1024
69. Iotsova V, Caamano J, Loy J, Yang Y, Lewin A, Bravo R (1997) Osteopetrosis in mice lacking NF-kappaB1 and NF-kappaB2. Nat Med 3:1285–1289
70. Kwon BS, Wang S, Udagawa N, Haridas V, Lee ZH, Kim KK, Oh KO, Greene J, Li Y, Su J, Gentz R, Aggarwal BB, Ni J (1998) TR1, a new member of the tumor necrosis factor receptor superfamily, induces fibroblast proliferation and inhibits osteoclastogenesis and bone resorption. FASEB J 12:845–854
71. Yun TJ, Chaudhary PM, Shu GL, Frazer JK, Ewings MK, Schwartz SM, Pascual V, Hood LE, Clark EA (1998) OPG/FDCR-1, a TNF receptor family member, is expressed in lymphoid cells and is up-regulated by ligating CD40. J Immunol 161:6113–6121
72. Hofbauer LC, Gori F, Riggs BL, Lacey DL, Dunstan CR, Spelsberg TC, Khosla S (1999) Stimulation of osteoprotegerin ligand and inhibition of osteoprotegerin production by glucocorticoids in human osteoblastic lineage cells: potential paracrine mechanisms of glucocorticoid-induced osteoporosis. Endocrinology 140:4382–4389

73. Yun TJ, Tallquist MD, Aicher A, Rafferty KL, Marshall AJ, Moon JJ, Ewings ME, Mohaupt M, Herring SW, Clark EA (2001) Osteoprotegerin, a crucial regulator of bone metabolism, also regulates B cell development and function. J Immunol 166:1482–1491
74. Udagawa N, Takahashi N, Yasuda H, Mizuno A, Itoh K, Ueno Y, Shinki T, Gillespie MT, Martin TJ, Higashio K, Suda T (2000) Osteoprotegerin produced by osteoblasts is an important regulator in osteoclast development and function. Endocrinology 141:3478–3484
75. Arron JR, Choi Y (2000) Bone versus immune system. Nature 408:535–536
76. Cenci S, Weitzmann MN, Roggia C, Namba N, Novack D, Woodring J, Pacifici R (2000) Estrogen deficiency induces bone loss by enhancing T-cell production of TNF-alpha. J Clin Invest 106:1229–1237
77. Hofbauer LC, Lacey DL, Dunstan CR, Spelsberg TC, Riggs BL, Khosla S (1999) Interleukin-1beta and tumor necrosis factor-alpha, but not interleukin-6, stimulate osteoprotegerin ligand gene expression in human osteoblastic cells. Bone 25:255–259
78. Cenci S, Toraldo G, Weitzmann MN, Roggia C, Gao Y, Qian WP, Sierra O, Pacifici R (2003) Estrogen deficiency induces bone loss by increasing T cell proliferation and lifespan through IFN-gamma-induced class II transactivator. Proc Natl Acad Sci USA 100:10405–10410
79. Roggia C, Gao Y, Cenci S, Weitzmann MN, Toraldo G, Isaia G, Pacifici R (2001) Up-regulation of TNF-producing T cells in the bone marrow: a key mechanism by which estrogen deficiency induces bone loss in vivo. Proc Natl Acad Sci USA 98:13960–13965
80. Nordin BE, Need AG, Chatterton BE, Horowitz M, Morris HA (1990) The relative contributions of age and years since menopause to postmenopausal bone loss. J Clin Endocrinol Metab 70:83–88
81. Riggs BL, Melton LJ III (1986) Involutional osteoporosis. N Engl J Med 314: 1676–1686
82. Riggs BL, Khosla S, Melton LJ III (1998) A unitary model for involutional osteoporosis: estrogen deficiency causes both type I and type II osteoporosis in postmenopausal women and contributes to bone loss in aging men. J Bone Miner Res 13:763–773
83. Hughes DE, Dai A, Tiffee JC, Li HH, Mundy GR, Boyce BF (1996) Estrogen promotes apoptosis of murine osteoclasts mediated by TGF-beta. Nat Med 2:1132–1136
84. Eriksen EF, Hodgson SF, Eastell R, Cedel SL, O'Fallon WM, Riggs BL (1990) Cancellous bone remodeling in type I (postmenopausal) osteoporosis: quantitative assessment of rates of formation, resorption, and bone loss at tissue and cellular levels. J Bone Miner Res 5:311–319
85. Eriksen EF, Colvard DS, Berg NJ, Graham ML, Mann KG, Spelsberg TC, Riggs BL (1988) Evidence of estrogen receptors in normal human osteoblast-like cells. Science 241:84–86
86. Oursler MJ, Osdoby P, Pyfferoen J, Riggs BL, Spelsberg TC (1991) Avian osteoclasts as estrogen target cells. Proc Natl Acad Sci USA 88:6613–6617
87. Pacifici R (1998) Cytokines, estrogen, and postmenopausal osteoporosis – the second decade. Endocrinology 139:2659–2661
88. Pacifici R, Rifas L, Teitelbaum S, Slatopolsky E, McCracken R, Bergfeld M, Lee W, Avioli LV, Peck WA (1987) Spontaneous release of interleukin 1 from human blood monocytes reflects bone formation in idiopathic osteoporosis. Proc Natl Acad Sci USA 84:4616–4620
89. Pacifici R, Brown C, Puscheck E, Friedrich E, Slatopolsky E, Maggio D, McCracken R, Avioli LV (1991) Effect of surgical menopause and estrogen replacement on cytokine release from human blood mononuclear cells. Proc Natl Acad Sci USA 88: 5134–5138

90. Yamamoto T, Ozono K, Kasayama S, Yoh K, Hiroshima K, Takagi M, Matsumoto S, Michigami T, Yamaoka K, Kishimoto T, Okada S (1996) Increased IL-6-production by cells isolated from the fibrous bone dysplasia tissues in patients with McCune-Albright syndrome. J Clin Invest 98:30–35
91. Ammann P, Rizzoli R, Bonjour JP, Bourrin S, Meyer JM, Vassalli P, Garcia I (1997) Transgenic mice expressing soluble tumor necrosis factor-receptor are protected against bone loss caused by estrogen deficiency. J Clin Invest 99:1699–1703
92. Poli V, Balena R, Fattori E, Markatos A, Yamamoto M, Tanaka H, Ciliberto G, Rodan GA, Costantini F (1994) Interleukin-6 deficient mice are protected from bone loss caused by estrogen depletion. EMBO J 13:1189–1196
93. Kitamura H, Kawata H, Takahashi F, Higuchi Y, Furuichi T, Ohkawa H (1995) Bone marrow neutrophilia and suppressed bone turnover in human interleukin-6 transgenic mice. A cellular relationship among hematopoietic cells, osteoblasts, and osteoclasts mediated by stromal cells in bone marrow. Am J Pathol 147:1682–1692
94. Jilka RL, Hangoc G, Girasole G, Passeri G, Williams DC, Abrams JS, Boyce B, Broxmeyer H, Manolagas SC (1992) Increased osteoclast development after estrogen loss: mediation by interleukin-6. Science 257:88–91
95. Jones DH, Kong YY, Penninger JM (2002) Role of RANKL and RANK in bone loss and arthritis. Ann Rheum Dis 61(Suppl 2):ii32–ii39
96. Hofbauer LC (1999) Osteoprotegerin ligand and osteoprotegerin: novel implications for osteoclast biology and bone metabolism. Eur J Endocrinol 141:195–210
97. Shevde NK, Bendixen AC, Dienger KM, Pike JW (2000) Estrogens suppress RANK ligand-induced osteoclast differentiation via a stromal cell independent mechanism involving c-Jun repression. Proc Natl Acad Sci USA 97:7829–7834
98. Srivastava S, Toraldo G, Weitzmann MN, Cenci S, Ross FP, Pacifici R (2001) Estrogen decreases osteoclast formation by down-regulating receptor activator of NF-kappa B ligand (RANKL)-induced JNK activation. J Biol Chem 276:8836–8840
99. Takayanagi H, Ogasawara K, Hida S, Chiba T, Murata S, Sato K, Takaoka A, Yokochi T, Oda H, Tanaka K, Nakamura K, Taniguchi T (2000) T-cell-mediated regulation of osteoclastogenesis by signalling cross-talk between RANKL and IFN-gamma. Nature 408:600–605
100. Gao Y, Qian WP, Dark K, Toraldo G, Lin AS, Guldberg RE, Flavell RA, Weitzmann MN, Pacifici R (2004) Estrogen prevents bone loss through transforming growth factor beta signaling in T cells. Proc Natl Acad Sci USA 101:16618–16623
101. Kehrl JH, Wakefield LM, Roberts AB, Jakowlew S, Alvarez-Mon M, Derynck R, Sporn MB, Fauci AS (1986) Production of transforming growth factor beta by human T lymphocytes and its potential role in the regulation of T cell growth. J Exp Med 163:1037–1050
102. Gorelik L, Flavell RA (2002) Transforming growth factor-beta in T-cell biology. Nat Rev Immunol 2:46–53
103. Vidal O, Kindblom LG, Ohlsson C (1999) Expression and localization of estrogen receptor-beta in murine and human bone. J Bone Miner Res 14:923–929
104. Spelsberg TC, Subramaniam M, Riggs BL, Khosla S (1999) The actions and interactions of sex steroids and growth factors/cytokines on the skeleton. Mol Endocrinol 13:819–828
105. Kimble RB, Srivastava S, Ross FP, Matayoshi A, Pacifici R (1996) Estrogen deficiency increases the ability of stromal cells to support murine osteoclastogenesis via an interleukin-1and tumor necrosis factor-mediated stimulation of macrophage colony-stimulating factor production. J Biol Chem 271:28890–28897

106. Stein B, Yang MX (1995) Repression of the interleukin-6 promoter by estrogen receptor is mediated by NF-kappa B and C/EBP beta. Mol Cell Biol 15:4971–4979
107. Tau KR, Hefferan TE, Waters KM, Robinson JA, Subramaniam M, Riggs BL, Spelsberg TC (1998) Estrogen regulation of a transforming growth factor-beta inducible early gene that inhibits deoxyribonucleic acid synthesis in human osteoblasts. Endocrinology 139:1346–1353
108. Rickard DJ, Hofbauer LC, Bonde SK, Gori F, Spelsberg TC, Riggs BL (1998) Bone morphogenetic protein-6 production in human osteoblastic cell lines. Selective regulation by estrogen. J Clin Invest 101:413–422
109. Kameda T, Mano H, Yuasa T, Mori Y, Miyazawa K, Shiokawa M, Nakamaru Y, Hiroi E, Hiura K, Kameda A, Yang NN, Hakeda Y, Kumegawa M (1997) Estrogen inhibits bone resorption by directly inducing apoptosis of the bone-resorbing osteoclasts. J Exp Med 186:489–495
110. Sunyer T, Lewis J, Collin-Osdoby P, Osdoby P (1999) Estrogen's bone-protective effects may involve differential IL-1 receptor regulation in human osteoclast-like cells. J Clin Invest 103:1409–1418
111. Srivastava S, Weitzmann MN, Cenci S, Ross FP, Adler S, Pacifici R (1999) Estrogen decreases TNF gene expression by blocking JNK activity and the resulting production of c-Jun and JunD. J Clin Invest 104:503–513
112. Chow J, Tobias JH, Colston KW, Chambers TJ (1992) Estrogen maintains trabecular bone volume in rats not only by suppression of bone resorption but also by stimulation of bone formation. J Clin Invest 89:74–78
113. Gohel A, McCarthy MB, Gronowicz G (1999) Estrogen prevents glucocorticoid-induced apoptosis in osteoblasts in vivo and in vitro. Endocrinology 140:5339–5347
114. Kousteni S, Bellido T, Plotkin LI, O'Brien CA, Bodenner DL, Han L, Han K, DiGregorio GB, Katzenellenbogen JA, Katzenellenbogen BS, Roberson PK, Weinstein RS, Jilka RL, Manolagas SC (2001) Nongenotropic, sex-nonspecific signaling through the estrogen or androgen receptors: dissociation from transcriptional activity. Cell 104:719–730
115. Kousteni S, Chen JR, Bellido T, Han L, Ali AA, O'Brien CA, Plotkin L, Fu Q, Mancino AT, Wen Y, Vertino AM, Powers CC, Stewart SA, Ebert R, Parfitt AM, Weinstein RS, Jilka RL, Manolagas SC (2002) Reversal of bone loss in mice by nongenotropic signaling of sex steroids. Science 298:843–846
116. Kousteni S, Han L, Chen JR, Almeida M, Plotkin LI, Bellido T, Manolagas SC (2003) Kinase-mediated regulation of common transcription factors accounts for the bone-protective effects of sex steroids. J Clin Invest 111:1651–1664
117. Manolagas SC, Kousteni S, Jilka RL (2002) Sex steroids and bone. Recent Prog Horm Res 57:385–409
118. Nelson HD, Humphrey LL, Nygren P, Teutsch SM, Allan JD (2002) Postmenopausal hormone replacement therapy: scientific review. J Am Med Assoc 288:872–881
119. Wells G, Tugwell P, Shea B, Guyatt G, Peterson J, Zytaruk N, Robinson V, Henry D, O'Connell D, Cranney A (2002) Meta-analyses of therapies for postmenopausal osteoporosis. V. Meta-analysis of the efficacy of hormone replacement therapy in treating and preventing osteoporosis in postmenopausal women. Endocr Rev 23: 529–539
120. Rossouw JE, Anderson GL, Prentice RL, LaCroix AZ, Kooperberg C, Stefanick ML, Jackson RD, Beresford SA, Howard BV, Johnson KC, Kotchen JM, Ockene J (2002) Risks and benefits of estrogen plus progestin in healthy postmenopausal women: principal results From the Women's Health Initiative randomized controlled trial. J Am Med Assoc 288:321–333

121. Delmas PD, Bjarnason NH, Mitlak BH, Ravoux AC, Shah AS, Huster WJ, Draper M, Christiansen C (1997) Effects of raloxifene on bone mineral density, serum cholesterol concentrations, and uterine endometrium in postmenopausal women. N Engl J Med 337:1641–1647
122. Ettinger B, Black DM, Mitlak BH, Knickerbocker RK, Nickelsen T, Genant HK, Christiansen C, Delmas PD, Zanchetta JR, Stakkestad J, Gluer CC, Krueger K, Cohen FJ, Eckert S, Ensrud KE, Avioli LV, Lips P, Cummings SR (1999) Reduction of vertebral fracture risk in postmenopausal women with osteoporosis treated with raloxifene: results from a 3-year randomized clinical trial. Multiple Outcomes of Raloxifene Evaluation (MORE) investigators. J Am Med Assoc 282: 637–645
123. Cummings SR, Eckert S, Krueger KA, Grady D, Powles TJ, Cauley JA, Norton L, Nickelsen T, Bjarnason NH, Morrow M, Lippman ME, Black D, Glusman JE, Costa A, Jordan VC (1999) The effect of raloxifene on risk of breast cancer in postmenopausal women: results from the MORE randomized trial. Multiple Outcomes of Raloxifene Evaluation. J Am Med Assoc 281:2189–2197
124. Barrett-Connor E, Grady D, Sashegyi A, Anderson PW, Cox DA, Hoszowski K, Rautaharju P, Harper KD (2002) Raloxifene and cardiovascular events in osteoporotic postmenopausal women: four-year results from the MORE (Multiple Outcomes of Raloxifene Evaluation) randomized trial. J Am Med Assoc 287: 847–857
125. Gianni W, Ricci A, Gazzaniga P, Brama M, Pietropaolo M, Votano S, Patane F, Agliano AM, Spera G, Marigliano V, Ammendola S, Agnusdei D, Migliaccio S, Scandurra R (2004) Raloxifene modulates interleukin-6 and tumor necrosis factor-alpha synthesis in vivo: results from a pilot clinical study. J Clin Endocrinol Metab 89:6097–6099
126. Taranta A, Brama M, Teti A, De l, V, Scandurra R, Spera G, Agnusdei D, Termine JD, Migliaccio S (2002) The selective estrogen receptor modulator raloxifene regulates osteoclast and osteoblast activity in vitro. Bone 30:368–376
127. Tou L, Quibria N, Alexander JM (2001) Regulation of human cbfa1 gene transcription in osteoblasts by selective estrogen receptor modulators (SERMs). Mol Cell Endocrinol 183:71–79
128. Yang NN, Bryant HU, Hardikar S, Sato M, Galvin RJ, Glasebrook AL, Termine JD (1996) Estrogen and raloxifene stimulate transforming growth factor-beta 3 gene expression in rat bone: a potential mechanism for estroge- or raloxifene-mediated bone maintenance. Endocrinology 137:2075–2084
129. Cheung J, Mak YT, Papaioannou S, Evans BA, Fogelman I, Hampson G (2003) Interleukin-6 (IL-6), IL-1, receptor activator of nuclear factor kappaB ligand (RANKL) and osteoprotegerin production by human osteoblastic cells: comparison of the effects of 17-beta oestradiol and raloxifene. J Endocrinol 177:423–433
130. Viereck V, Grundker C, Blaschke S, Niederkleine B, Siggelkow H, Frosch KH, Raddatz D, Emons G, Hofbauer LC (2003) Raloxifene concurrently stimulates osteoprotegerin and inhibits interleukin-6 production by human trabecular osteoblasts. J Clin Endocrinol Metab 88:4206–4213
131. Qu Q, Harkonen PL, Vaananen HK (1999) Comparative effects of estrogen and antiestrogens on differentiation of osteoblasts in mouse bone marrow culture. J Cell BioChem 73:500–507
132. Saintier D, Burde MA, Rey JM, Maudelonde T, de Vernejoul MC, Cohen-Solal ME (2004) 17beta-estradiol downregulates beta3-integrin expression in differentiating and mature human osteoclasts. J Cell Physiol 198:269–276

133. Onoe Y, Miyaura C, Ito M, Ohta H, Nozawa S, Suda T (2000) Comparative effects of estrogen and raloxifene on B lymphopoiesis and bone loss induced by sex steroid deficiency in mice. J Bone Miner Res 15:541–549
134. Lee MY, Eyre DR, Osborne WR (1991) Isolation of a murine osteoclast colony-stimulating factor. Proc Natl Acad Sci USA 88:8500–8504
135. Hofbauer LC, Dunstan CR, Spelsberg TC, Riggs BL, Khosla S (1998) Osteoprotegerin production by human osteoblast lineage cells is stimulated by vitamin D, bone morphogenetic protein-2, and cytokines. BioChem Biophys Res Commun 250:776–781
136. Ahlen J, Andersson S, Mukohyama H, Roth C, Backman A, Conaway HH, Lerner UH (2002) Characterization of the bone-resorptive effect of interleukin-11 in cultured mouse calvarial bones. Bone 31:242–251
137. Takami M, Takahashi N, Udagawa N, Miyaura C, Suda K, Woo JT, Martin TJ, Nagai K, Suda T (2000) Intracellular calcium and protein kinase C mediate expression of receptor activator of nuclear factor-kappaB ligand and osteoprotegerin in osteoblasts. Endocrinology 141:4711–4719
138. Gao YH, Shinki T, Yuasa T, Kataoka-Enomoto H, Komori T, Suda T, Yamaguchi A (1998) Potential role of cbfa1, an essential transcriptional factor for osteoblast differentiation, in osteoclastogenesis: regulation of mRNA expression of osteoclast differentiation factor (ODF). BioChem Biophys Res Commun 252:697–702
139. Palmqvist P, Persson E, Conaway HH, Lerner UH (2002) IL-6, leukemia inhibitory factor, and oncostatin M stimulate bone resorption and regulate the expression of receptor activator of NF-kappa B ligand, osteoprotegerin, and receptor activator of NF-kappa B in mouse calvariae. J Immunol 169:3353–3362
140. Nakashima T, Kobayashi Y, Yamasaki S, Kawakami A, Eguchi K, Sasaki H, Sakai H (2000) Protein expression and functional difference of membrane-bound and soluble receptor activator of NF-kappaB ligand: modulation of the expression by osteotropic factors and cytokines. Biochem Biophys Res Commun 275:768–775
141. Murakami T, Yamamoto M, Ono K, Nishikawa M, Nagata N, Motoyoshi K, Akatsu T (1998) Transforming growth factor-beta1 increases mRNA levels of osteoclastogenesis inhibitory factor in osteoblastic/stromal cells and inhibits the survival of murine osteoclast-like cells. Biochem Biophys Res Commun 252:747–752
142. Quinn JM, Itoh K, Udagawa N, Hausler K, Yasuda H, Shima N, Mizuno A, Higashio K, Takahashi N, Suda T, Martin TJ, Gillespie MT (2001) Transforming growth factor beta affects osteoclast differentiation via direct and indirect actions. J Bone Miner Res 16:1787–1794
143. Hofbauer LC, Shui C, Riggs BL, Dunstan CR, Spelsberg TC, O'Brien T, Khosla S (2001) Effects of immunosuppressants on receptor activator of NF-kappaB ligand and osteoprotegerin production by human osteoblastic and coronary artery smooth muscle cells. Biochem Biophys Res Commun 280:334–339

Chapter 8

The Role of SERMs in the Treatment of Osteoporosis

Adolfo Díez-Pérez · José Luis Dueñas-Díez

8.1
Introduction

Osteoporosis is currently defined as "a skeletal disorder characterized by compromised bone strength predisposing to an increased risk of fracture. Bone strength reflects the integration of two main features: bone density and bone quality" (NIH Consensus 2001). Thus, osteoporosis is a debilitating condition of the skeleton that propends to fractures and is associated with advanced age. The disease has a high prevalence in western countries, as it is a condition associated with advanced age, and it is on the rise since life expectancy has risen dramatically in the last several decades. It is, therefore, a major public health problem because it not only induces morbidity (fractures and chronic sequelae) with a substantial impact on health-related quality of life, but is also associated with increased mortality (Badia et al. 2001, 2004).

Although osteoporosis affects both men and women, the ratio of female to male patients is as high as 6 to 1. This is related not only to the lower total bone acquisition in women during development but also to the abrupt estrogen deficiency as a result of menopause. It has been demonstrated that estrogens play an important role in female bone homeostasis, and their deficiency increases bone resorption. Thus, in recent years the administration of estrogens has been extensively used as the main therapy to prevent osteoporosis in women. Estrogens not only reduce the rate of bone remodeling, acting as an antiresorptive agent, but also offer positive effects on the undesirable symptoms of menopause. There is still much discussion, however, on the overall benefits of an exclusive hormone replacement therapy (HT) either with estrogens alone or combining estrogens and progestogens, because these therapies increase the risk of serious health disorders, such as breast cancer (Writing Group for the Women's Health Initiative Investigators 2002; Million Women Study Collaborators 2003).

Some years ago breast cancer patients treated with tamoxifen showed protection against loss of bone in postmenopausal women (Powles et al. 1996). This clinical result led to a revision of the traditionally accepted role of tamoxifen as an antiestrogen. It is clear that a number of substances can act in some organs or tissues as estrogen agonists and be antagonists in others. As a result of these observations and a better knowledge of the molecular features of estrogen receptors (ERs), the term selective estrogen receptor modulator (SERM) was coined. Tamoxifen and raloxifene belong to this group of substances. This chapter will review the scientific evidence supporting the role of SERMs as bone antiresorptive agents.

8.2 Experimental Results

8.2.1 Tamoxifen

The most extensively used animal model to evaluate the action of SERMs on bone has been the ovariectomized (OVX) rat. In rats, tamoxifen antagonizes bone resorption and uterine growth (Turner et al. 1987, 1988) and reduces the number and size of osteoclasts. The inhibitory effect on bone resorption of tamoxifen has also been reported in dogs and immobilized male rats (Wakley et al. 1988; Waters et al. 1991). As an antiresorptive agent, however, tamoxifen is less effective than 17β-estradiol (17βE2) (Williams et al. 1991) and has no effect when the endogenous production of estrogens is normal (Evans et al. 1994).

8.2.2 Raloxifene

Initial studies of the effects of raloxifene on bone metabolism were also carried out in OVX rats. Animals treated with raloxifene showed significantly lower rates of bone remodeling markers (Black et al. 1994) while bone mineral density (BMD) remained unchanged. The BMD was measured by single photon absorptiometry (Frolik et al. 1996) in distal femur metaphysis and in proximal tibia and by dual-energy X-ray absorptiometry (Sato et al. 1994) in lumbar vertebrae and femur. Research has demonstrated that raloxifene is an efficient drug to prevent the loss of bone mass, which is maintained homogeneously at levels significantly higher than those obtained in OVX rats without treatment and similar to those obtained in animals treated with ethinyl-estradiol (EE) (Sato et al. 1994; Turner et al. 1994). Measurements of BMD, however, shed no light on the dynamics of the bone formation and resorption processes. In order to evaluate these aspects, some investigators (Turner et al. 1994; Evans et al. 1995) carried out histomorphometric analyses after tetracycline labeling in OVX rats. The reduction of the bone resorption area in the trabecular surfaces of the animals treated with raloxifene paralleled the reduction seen in rats treated with EE.

Turner et al. (1994) have estimated bone strength by measuring the minimal effective force required to produce fractures in femoral neck and vertebrae. These researchers found that this force was significantly higher in rats treated with raloxifene and EE than in control rats. In a four-arm comparative trial, Frolik et al. (1996) evaluated the role of raloxifene, EE, tamoxifen, and alendronate as bone-protecting agents. With the exception of the group treated with tamoxifen, all the groups under experimental treatment showed a statistically significant higher protection rate than control animals. Perhaps this result can be partially explained by the finding that the treatment with raloxifene induces a decrease in the density of microcracks (Burr 2003). Moreover, a raloxifene analog, LY 117018, inhibits the osteocytic apoptosis induced by oophorectomy in a rat model (Colishaw et al. 2003).

One of the most valuable experimental findings has been the partial elucidation of the mechanism whereby raloxifene regulates bone homeostasis. By performing transient cotransfection experiments using a transforming growth factor–β promoter-chloramphenicol acetyltransferase reporter construct (TGFβ promoter-CAT reporter) and an ER expression plasmid in human MG63 osteosarcoma cells, Yang et al. (1996) have shown that the TGFβCAT expression was significantly upregulated by raloxifene, with a sevenfold increase, and by 17β-estradiol or tamoxifen, with twofold increases. These authors suggest that raloxifene regulates TGFβ3 gene expression with two fundamental consequences: the production of osteoblasts is promoted and osteoclast differentiation is inhibited (Yang et al. 1996).

Different SERMs (as well as the natural ligand estradiol) can activate more predominantly one of the other estrogen receptors (alpha or beta) . The conformational changes of the ER–ligand complex can vary for different ligands (Katzenellenbogen 2002). Furthermore, the various ligands can activate different intracellular pathways combining with different response elements (Nuttall et al. 2000). Altogether, the genomic responses differ for each compound. With respect to estradiol, the two receptor subtypes elicit different responses. Moreover, diverse activating or repressing genes express themselves in discrete ways for different SERMs (Kian et al. 2004).

8.3 Other SERMs

Levormeloxifene induces an increase in lumbar and tibial bone mass in a rat model and is associated with a decrease in osteocalcin and cholesterol levels, while it has a neutral effect on the uterus (Bain et al. 1997; Nowak et al. 1998). In monkeys, a decrease in bone remodeling with prevention of bone loss has also been demonstrated (Stavisky et al. 1998). Idoxifene is another SERM that activates the ER through the classical estradiol pathway. Its effect on bone is similar, acting as a full antagonist on mammary and uterine tissue (Nuttall et al. 1997, 1998). Droloxifene is efficacious in the prevention of bone loss in OVX rats as well as in the reduction of serum cholesterol levels. Unlike estrogens and tamoxifen, it has no deleterious effects on the uterus. The drug inhibits bone remodeling very much as estrogens do, resulting in a positive effect on bone mass (Ke et al., 1995a,b, 1997a,b; Chen et al. 1995). Ormeloxifene can also prevent bone loss in animal models (Bain et al. 1994; Arshad et al. 2004).

Lasofoxifene is a SERM that also protects from bone loss, reduces cholesterol levels, and exerts a positive effect on bone strength in rats, specifically in male models (Ma et al. 2002). This compound is in the final stages of clinical development. Two other SERMs also in advanced phase III trials are bazedoxifene and arzoxifene, both with protective effects against ovariectomy-induced bone loss. Arzoxifene has shown both bone remodeling reduction with positive effects on bone quality as well as a reduction in cholesterol levels in oophorectomized rats (Biskobing 2003).

Other SERMs are currently under development. Díaz Curiel et al. (1998) have proved that a raloxifene analog, LY117018 HCl, is effective in reducing bone loss in OVX rats. In addition, the administration of the substance permits a significant reduction in the minimal effective dose of human parathyroid hormone (PTHh) required in the treatment of osteopenic rats (Hodsman et al. 1999a,b). Two more compounds, FC1271a 41 and HMR-3339 (Ammann et al. 2004), show promising results in preclinical studies.

8.4 Clinical Effects of SERMs

Research in humans has been mainly focused either in the prevention of osteoporosis in healthy postmenopausal women or in the treatment of already osteoporotic women. Some research programs have extensively used estimates of biochemical markers of bone remodeling, while others have mostly relied on evaluations of BMD, histomorphometry, and fracture incidence.

8.4.1 Tamoxifen

The effects of tamoxifen on bone have been evaluated mainly in breast cancer patients who received the product as an adjuvant agent to other therapies. A number of surveys (Love et al. 1992; Kristensen et al. 1994; Wright et al. 1994; Grey et al. 1995; Kenni et al. 1995) have shown a decrease in some serum biochemical markers related to bone formation, such as osteocalcin (Love et al. 1992; Wright et al. 1994; Kenni et al. 1995) and total alkaline phosphatase (Love et al. 1992; Kenni et al. 1995). Similar data for bone resorption biochemical markers, such as urinary hydroxyproline (Grey et al. 1995; Cozick et al. 1992), urinary C-telopeptide (Grey et al. 1995), urinary pyridinolines (Grey et al. 1995), and type I procollagen peptide (Kenni et al. 1995), have been recorded.

Data on the effect of tamoxifen on bone mass have been obtained from numerous trials carried out on both premenopausal as well as postmenopausal women. Retrospective surveys (Cozick et al. 1992) and the first prospective studies (Gotfredsen et al. 1984; Fentiman et al. 1989) comparing tamoxifen-treated women against the placebo group found no significant differences in BMD at the lumbar spine and femoral neck. In contrast, prospective and randomized surveys carried out with breast cancer patients (Love et al. 1992; Kristensen et al. 1994) revealed a significant, long-term (3-year) prevention of bone loss in women treated with tamoxifen. The effect of tamoxifen on the BMD in healthy, late postmenopausal women (11 years after menopause on average) has been studied by Grey et al. (1995). These researchers found no significant difference in the hip, but the BMD in the lumbar spine of tamoxifen-treated women had certainly increased. In a 3-year survey for the prevention of breast cancer in premenopausal healthy women, however, Powles et al. (1996) found a progressive decrease in the BMD in the tamoxifen-treated group. Likewise, Wright et al. (1994, 1993) found no difference with the control group when evaluating the effect of tamoxifen on cancellous bone by histomorphometry. In the treatment group, though, the bone formation rate had significantly decreased, the total bone remodeling span was longer, and the trabecular connectivity indices were increased.

In the Breast Cancer Prevention Trial (Fisher et al. 1998) a clinical survey aimed at determining the potential of tamoxifen for breast cancer prevention in women at increased risk, 13,338 pre- or postmenopausal women were monitored over 5 years. After randomization, women in the treatment group (n = 6681) were given a 20-mg daily dose of tamoxifen, while the remaining (n = 6707) received a placebo. Although the overall rate of fractures was about the same in both groups, tamoxifen-treated women sustained fewer hip, spine, and Colles fractures. Nevertheless, relevant data may have been biased, since in this trial there was an indiscriminate inclusion of pre- and postmenopausal women and no spinal radiographs were carried out.

In summary, available scientific evidence on the effects of tamoxifen on human bone seems to parallel data collected in animal trials. Tamoxifen, acting as a partial estrogen agonist, seems to have beneficial effects on the preservation of bone mass in postmenopausal women, while in premenopausal women it might act as an estrogen antagonist. An alternative explanation could be that the weaker agonistic effect with respect to estrogens might cause bone loss in estrogen-replete women.

8.4.2 Raloxifene

Early studies indicate that raloxifene has an effect on bone homeostasis similar to that of estrogens. In a survey by Draper et al. (1996) that monitored 251 postmenopausal women aged 45–60 for 8 weeks, subjects were randomized in two treatment groups (treated either with raloxifene or CEE) and a placebo group. Treated women showed a significant decrease when compared with the placebo group in osteocalcin, serum alkaline phosphatase, urinary piridinoline crosslinks, and urinary calcium excretion. The European survey (Delmas et al. 1997), which has already monitored 601 postmenopausal women over 24 months, has revealed a significant reduction against the placebo group for three of the biochemical markers of bone remodeling under study (osteocalcin, bone-specific alkaline phosphatase, and type I collagen C-telopeptide). Lufkin et al. (1998) recorded similar data in a 1-year clinical treatment study of 143 postmenopausal women with osteoporosis.

The effect of raloxifene on bone mass has been assessed in American, European, and international prevention studies. After 24 months of treatment, there was a significant increase in BMD in all the monitored skeletal sites in raloxifene-treated patients against the placebo group. This increase was detected after 12 months of treatment and was maintained over the following 12 months. The first study published was carried out in Europe by Delmas et al. (1997). The American study also researched healthy postmenopausal women and had very similar results, while the international trial assessed the effects of the drug in hysterectomized women (Cosman 1999). A total of 1764 women were monitored in these prevention trials, measuring the biochemical markers of bone remodeling and the BMD of lumbar spine and femoral neck. All three were concealed randomized placebo-controlled studies. In the European and American surveys three treatment doses were tested (30, 60, and 150 mg daily), while the international trial had two treatment groups (with daily 60- and 150-mg doses) and a third group that received conjugated equine estrogens (CEE) 0.625 mg daily. Other studies have evaluated the effect of the drug in Asian women with similar results (Kung et al. 2003; Liu et al. 2004). A recent metaanalysis has evaluated the overall efficacy of the drug across the different trials showing homogeneity in the drug effect and a consistent risk reduction for vertebral fracture (Seeman et al. 2003).

Yet the pivotal study on raloxifene has been the Multiple Outcomes of Raloxifene Evaluation (MORE), a randomized, double-blind, placebo-controlled trial aimed at evaluating the effect of raloxifene on both bone mass as well as on the occurrence of vertebral fractures in a cohort of 7705 women with osteoporosis (Ettinger et al. 1998, 1999; Delmas et al. 2002). After 4 years of treatment, the results showed an increase in bone density both at lumbar spine and femoral neck (Delmas et al. 2002). This positive effect is extended for up to 7 years of treatment (Lufkin et al. 2001). The most important outcome, however, has been the significant risk reduction in the occurrence of new vertebral fractures. Women included in substudy 1 (cases with at least one prevalent vertebral fracture at baseline) had a significant reduction in the risk of sustaining new (incident) vertebral fractures after 3 (Ettinger et al. 1999) and 4 years (Delmas et al. 2002) of treatment of 34% [RR0.66 (95% CI = 0.55, 0.81)] (Fig. 8.1). Women enrolled in substudy 2 (no baseline vertebral fracture) showed a risk reduction of 49% at the end of the 4-year treatment [RR0.51 (95% CI = 0.35, 0.73)] (Delmas et al. 2002). These figures represent the number needed to treat (NNT) value to prevent an event after 4 years of treatment of 12 for patients with prevalent vertebral fracture and 34 for those without. Subgroup exploratory analyses showed a 93% reduction in the risk of suffering multiple vertebral fractures (Lufkin et al. 2001) with sustained efficacy during the fourth year. Other post hoc analyses have also suggested an early efficacy on clinical vertebral fracture after 12 months of treatment (Maricic et al. 2002) and fracture reduction in women with previous treatment with estrogens or estrogen-progestagens (Johnell et al. 2004) (Table 8.1). Perhaps more interesting for the prevention strategy is that in cases with osteopenia (no fracture and BMD in this range), another exploratory analysis demonstrated not only BMD improvement but also sig-

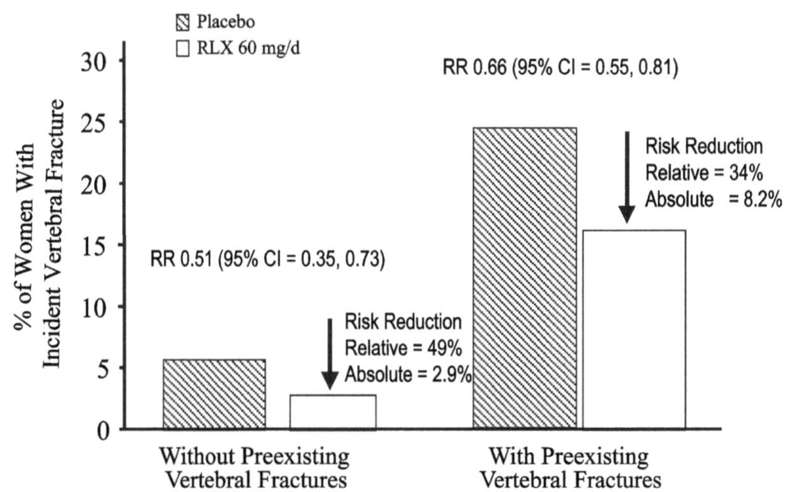

Fig. 8.1. Effect of raloxifene in women with or without preexisting fractures. MORE trial – 4 years (Delmas et al. 2002). RR = relative risk

Table 8.1. Main antifracture results of raloxifene (60 mg daily dose)

	Relative risk reduction
Treatment for 3 years*	
Baseline vertebral fracture	30%
No baseline vertebral fracture	55%
Treatment for 4 years*	
Baseline vertebral fracture	34%
No baseline vertebral fracture	49%
Multiple vertebral fractures ($\geq$ 2)	93%
Clinical vertebral fractures (1 year treatment)	68%
Women with osteopenia*	45%
Fractures during fourth year of treatment*♠	
Baseline vertebral fracture	38%
No baseline vertebral fracture	50%
Moderate or severe vertebral fracture	
Baseline vertebral fracture	37%
No baseline vertebral fracture	61%
Nonvertebral fracture after 3 years (overall population)	N.S.
Nonvertebral fracture after 3 years (high-risk patients)	47%
Nonvertebral fracture after 8 years (overall population)	N.S.
Nonvertebral fracture after 8 years (high-risk patients)	36%

* Vertebral fracture as outcome; ♠ denotes risk reduction during fourth year of treatment only (sustained efficacy). N.S. = no risk reduction

nificant fracture risk reduction (Kanis et al. 2003). However, the drug did not show any reduction in nonvertebral fracture risk after 3 (Cozick et al. 1992) and 8 years of treatment (Siris et al. 2004).

To test the bone formation rate and the activation frequency, Heaney and Draper (1997) carried out a comparative histomorphometric survey. Ten women received a 60-mg daily dose of raloxifene while 8 received a 0.625-mg daily dose of CEE. Biopsies carried out before and after 6 months of treatment revealed a decrease in both parameters, especially in the group treated with estrogens.

The effects of raloxifene on bone histomorphometry were analyzed by Ott et al. (2002). In a group of 54 women enrolled in the MORE study, two transiliac bone biopsies were obtained at baseline and after 2 years of treatment. The results confirmed the safety of the drug on bone tissue since no woven bone, mineralization defect, cell toxicity, or medullary fibrosis was observed. Moreover, the number of empty osteocytic lacunae also suggested an antiapoptotic effect on the osteocyte. More recent experimental data further confirm this antiapoptotic effect of raloxifene on osteoblastic and osteocytic cells (Taranta et al. 2002).

8.5 Bone Quality and Its Relevance

For years osteoporosis has been defined as a disease induced by a decrease in bone mass. This definition was quite simplistic since only one of the components of bone, quantity, is taken into account. A National Institute of Health Consensus Panel Ref. 1 has redefined the disease as a skeletal disorder characterized by an alteration in bone strength that predisposes a person to an increased risk of fracture. This concept of bone strength permits a multidimensional view of the disease and represents a new paradigm in our conception of the disease (Heaney 2003; Bouxsein 2003; Van Rietbergen et al. 2000). The new definition adds a large number of aspects related to the quality of the bony tissue: geometry, microarchitecture, remodeling rate, mineralization degree, and homogeneity and fatigue damage, among others (Sato et al. 1994; Kung et al 2003; Heaney 2002; Bouxsein 2003; Van Rietbergen et al. 2000; Hodgskinson et al. 1993; Hou et al. 1998; Schaffler et al. 1995; Akkus et al. 2003; Ahlborg et al. 2003). The aspects of bone quality are of great relevance to a better understanding of the action of SERMs on bone.

The relationship between the decrease in BMD and an increased fracture risk has been widely demonstrated, in all the measured skeletal regions and by different techniques (Melton et al. 1993; Marshall et al. 1996; Cummings et al. 1993). Marshall et al. (1996) demonstrated in a metaanalysis that one standard deviation decrease in BMD in lumbar spine, hip, or proximal radius increased the risk of fracture in these locations by 50 to 60% (Fig. 8.2). A different picture is seen, however, when the effects on BMD of the different antiresorptives and their relationship with the fracture risk reduction are analyzed.

Antifracture efficacy of drugs that inhibit bone remodeling has been firmly established in a large number of controlled clinical trials. Yet when the results of the different studies are analyzed together, there is a clear discrepancy between the magnitude of the increase in bone density and the associated fracture risk reduction for the different drugs. Figure 8.3 depicts the gains in lumbar spine BMD vs. placebo and the corresponding vertebral fracture risk reduction observed in different trials (Ettinger et al. 1999; Chesnut et al. 2000; Harris et al. 1999; Reginster et al. 2000; Black et al. 1996; Cummings et al. 1998). The BMD gains up to 7%, induced by alendronate in the FIT trial (Cummings et al. 1998), and is accompanied by a fracture risk reduction figure similar to those described for other antiresorptives, risedronate (Harris et al. 1999; Reginster et al. 2000) and raloxifene (Ettinger et al. 1999), that produce less pronounced gains in bone density. Therefore, the limited BMD gain does not explain the dramatic decrease in fracture risk induced by these agents.

Sarkar et al. (2002) analyzed the relationship between the observed increase in BMD in the placebo and in the raloxifene-treated patients of the MORE trial.

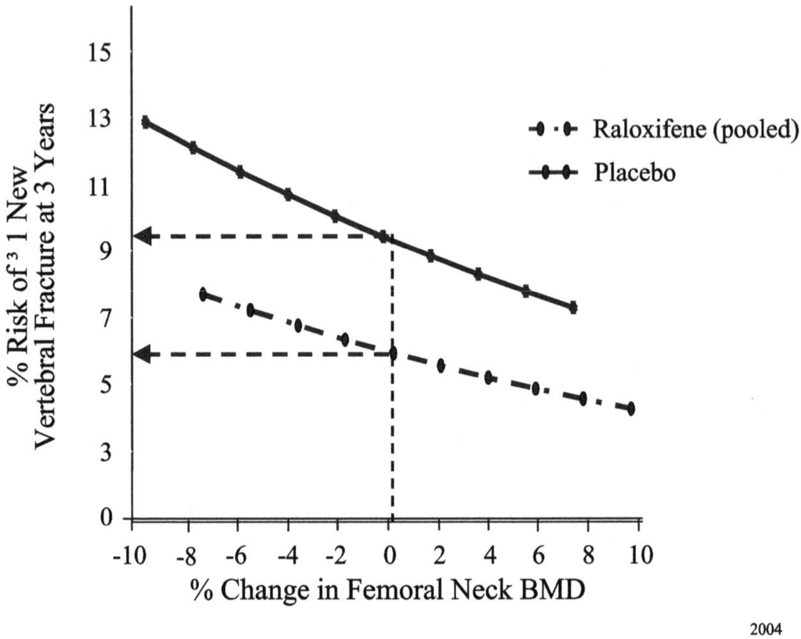

Fig. 8.2. Relationship between change in femoral neck BMD and vertebral fracture risk. MORE trial – 3 years. Similar changes in BMD (*dotted line*) are related to different fracture risks (*arrows*) for the raloxifene- and placebo-treated patients. Adapted from (Lufkin et al. 2001)

Only 4% of the fracture reduction is explained by the changes in bone density for the treated group. Moreover, the curves for the placebo- and raloxifene-treated cases are quite different (Fig. 8.2) (Lufkin et al. 2001, with different slopes and no overlap between them (including the 95% confidence intervals). In other words, the bone intrinsic properties, well beyond the changes observed in BMD, account for the vast majority (96%) of the antifracture efficacy of the drug. Similar variations in bone density are accompanied by very different risks of fracture during the 3-year observation period in the two groups.

Table 8.2. Relative risk of fracture for every standard deviation in BMD (adjusted by age)

BMD measurement	Type of fracture Forearm	Hip	Spine	All fractures
Lumbar spine	1.5	1.6	2.3	1.5
Hip	1.4	2.6	1.8	1.6
Proximal radius	1.8	2.1	2.2	1.5

Metaanalysis of several measurement methods except ultrasound (Cosman 1999)

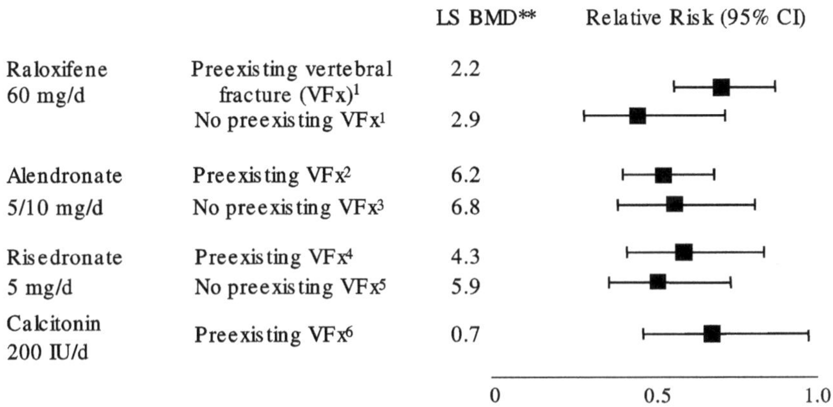

Fig. 8.3. Randomized studies of antiresorptives in postmenopausal women with osteoporosis. Risk of vertebral fractures. Not head-to-head comparison. ** Increase in lumbar spine BMD vs. placebo (Wright et al. 1994; Liu et al. 2004; Seeman et al. 2003; Ettinger et al. 1998, 1999; Delmas et al. 2002)

From these data one can conclude that antiresorptives are capable of inducing striking reductions in fracture risk with limited changes in bone density. Therefore, other factors than bone density should explain their efficacy. Bone quality is the term that encompasses all the non-bone-density elements implied in bone strength, as previously discussed.

From an operational point of view, bone-quality elements can be grouped in three different categories: bone architecture, bone turnover, and intrinsic material properties (Turner 2002; Seeman 2002). Bone architecture could be divided into macroscopic and microscopic architecture. The macroarchitecture, also denominated bone geometry, is genetically determined, and some of its elements are well known. Bone shape and distribution of the mineral material are behind such factors as diameter, moment of inertia, and torsion strength, which are related to the mechanical properties of bone and fracture propensity. Different imaging techniques, from simple radiographs to DXA or CT measurements, can be used to analyze these factors (Beck et al. 2000; Gómez-Alonso et al. 2000; Genant et al. 2004).

The objective of bone turnover is to replace old bone containing impaired material properties with fresh, new bone that is able to offer full strength again. This is the so-called targeted remodeling, and in zones where structural damage (microcracks) has been produced, the resorption is initiated and followed by a formation that completes the replacement cycle. The equilibrium between resorption and formation maintains a neutral bone balance with preservation of the bone mass and microarchitecture. Nevertheless, in situations in which resorption exceeds formation, associated with increased bone remodeling, we can observe negative effects on this microarchitecture. Horizontal struts disappear and the vertical elements of the trabecular network suffer a notching process that greatly impairs the mechanical competence of the trabeculae (Heaney 2003; Parfitt 2004). Bone remodeling is, therefore, a determining element of the microarchitectural integrity of the skeleton. The rapid reduction in the fracture risk observed a few months after starting antiresorptive therapies can be explained largely by the positive effects on this notching process, well before any improvement in bone density is observed (Heaney 2003; Parfitt 2004).

The bone remodeling rate is another determinant of the intrinsic material properties of bony tissue. Bone tissue is composed of two major components, a mineral matrix and an organic matrix, mainly collagen. The mineral component is predominantly hydroxyapatite in normal bone, although different mineral elements can be induced when calcium is replaced by fluoride or strontium. Newly formed bone is mineralized up to approximately 70% in a few months' process (primary mineralization). Full mineralization of each bone remodeling unit requires years (secondary mineralization) and induces several effects: on the one hand, it increases the mean degree of mineralization of bone tissue, and on the other, it increases the homogeneity of the tissue (Seeman 2002). Both factors have been related to decreased bone toughness since, although stiffer, the tissue is more brittle, offering less resistance to the propagation of microcracks (Turner 2002). Data on raloxifene-treated patients demonstrate that the drug preserves a normal degree of mineralization and homogeneity (Boivin et al. 2003), in accordance with the preclinical data supporting a positive effect on microcrack density. Collagen composition is also modulated by the remodeling rate since the crosslinking of the molecules influences the mechanical competence and can vary with aging (Wang et al. 2002).

There is considerable debate on what the normal remodeling rate is. Excessive bone turnover is, as mentioned, negative for microarchitecture integrity. An extremely low turnover, though, can also be deleterious since the normal mechanism of microdamage repair could be impaired (Compston et al. 2002). Microdamage increases with age but negatively correlates with the rate of bone remodeling (Mashiba et al. 2000, 2001). Some experiments with high doses of antiresorptives have shown increased numbers of microcracks in experimental animals (Mashiba et al. 2000, 2001). Therefore, the theoretical concern is the possible depression of remodeling until a level so low (Chavassieux et al. 1997) that the replacement of old bone by fresh new units, albeit mechanically more competent, would be insufficient. Despite no clinical data supporting this theory, SERMs depress turnover to an intermediate degree, safe enough to maintain a sufficient rate of repair. Clinical data support the notion that raloxifene restores bone turnover to premenopausal levels (Johnell et al. 2002; Stepan et al. 2003), and experimental data show that the drug actually decreases microcrack density in bone tissue.

Several additional clinical considerations about antiresorptives in general and SERMs in particular could be discussed. Can they be used in combination with such anabolic agents as PTH, either concomitantly or sequentially? It has been demonstrated that the simultaneous use of a bisphosphonate with PTH decreases bone-forming response (Black et al. 2003; Finkelstein et al. 2003), but preliminary data suggest the opposite when the combined drug is raloxifene (Deal et al. 2004). It is known that drugs that strongly suppress turnover induce a delay in the response to anabolic therapy, while in patients previously treated with raloxifene a full response is observed (Ettinger et al. 2004). Therefore, the practical message is that SERMs appear to be better partners for anabolic agents and that in younger postmenopausal women, SERMs will not jeopardize the anabolic effect if PTH is needed in posterior phases of the disease. Indeed, associations of two antiresorptives are generally useless, can add side effects, have no demonstrated superior efficacy, and are not suitable (Compston et al. 2002). Last but not least, extraskeletal effects of SERMs have enormous potential for the future when ad hoc trials (RUTH, STAR) yield their final results. What is known today is that raloxifene is safe for the breast and the cardiovascular system even after 8 years of treatment (Martino et al. 2004).

8.6 Future SERMs

A large number of compounds selectively regulating ERs are under development and have been briefly reviewed in the preclinical stage. Some have reached clinical research stages. Levormeloxifene (Skrumsager et al. 1997; Bjarnason et al. 1997) has been studied for pharmacokinetics, safety, dosing, and antiresorptive effects. Its development, however, was stopped after the phase II trials when uterine safety problems were detected even though there were positive skeletal effects (Warmig et al. 2003). Idoxifene has demonstrated positive effects on both bone density after 12 months of treatment (Chesnut et al. 1998) as well as on decreased turnover in osteopenic postmenopausal women (Delmas et al. 1998).

In advanced (phase III) stages of their clinical development, three SERMs are currently on the horizon: bazedoxifene, lasofoxifene, and arzoxifene. What these new molecules can offer will be known shortly in a field – the selective regulation of hormone receptor – that has opened unsuspected perspectives for the better management of patients.

References

1. Ahlborg HG, Johnell O, Turner CH, Rannevik G, Karlsson MK (2003) Bone loss and bone size after menopause. N Engl J Med 349:327–334

2. Akkus O, Polyakova-Akkus A, Adar F, Schaffler MB (2003) Aging of microstructural compartments in human compact bone. J Bone Miner Res 18:1012–1019
3. Ammann P, Bourrin S, Brunner F, Meyer JM, Clement-Lacroix P, Baron R, Gaillard M, Rizzoli R (2004) A new selective estrogen receptor modulator HMR-3339 fully corrects bone alterations induced by ovariectomy in adult rats. Bone 35:153–161
4. Arshad M, Sengupta S, Sharma S, Ghosh R, Sawlani V, Singh MM (2004) In vitro anti-resorptive activity and prevention of ovariectomy-induced osteoporosis in female Sprague-Dawley rats by ormeloxifene, a selective estrogen receptor modulator. J Steroid Biochem Mol Biol 91(1–2):67–78
5. Badia X, Diez-Perez A, Alvarez-Sanz C, Diaz Lopez B, Diaz-Curiel M, Guillén F, González-Macias J and the Spanish GRECO Study Group (2001) Measuring quality of life in women with vertebral fractures due to osteoporosis: a comparison of the OQLQ and QUALEFFO. Qual Life Res 10:307–317
6. Badia X, Diez-Perez A, Lahoz R, Lizan L, Nogues X, Iborra J (2004) The ECOS-16 questionnaire for the evaluation of health related quality of life in post-menopausal women with osteoporosis. Health Qual Life Outcomes 2(1):41
7. Bain SD, Edwards MW, Celino DL, Bailey MC, Stachan MJ, Piggott JR, Labroo VM (1994) Centtochroman is a bone specific estrogen in ovariectomized rat. J Bone Min Res 9:394
8. Bain S, Greenspan D, Kurman R, Shalmi M, Guldhammer B, Korsgard N (1997) Levormeloxifene, a non-steroidal, partial estrogen agonist, prevents bone loss, reduces serum cholesterol, and exerts a non-proliferative action on uterine tissues in the ovariectomized rat. In: ASBMR 19th annual meeting, Cincinnati, OH, September, 10–14, 1997. J Bone Miner Res 12(Suppl 1):S347
9. Beck TJ, Looker AC, Ruff CB, Sievanen H, Wahner HW (2000) Structural trends in the aging femoral neck and proximal shaft: analysis of the Third National Health and Nutrition Examination Survey dual-energy X-ray absorptiometry data. J Bone Miner Res 15:2297–2304
10. Biskobing DM (2003) Novel therapies for osteoporosis. Expert Opin Invest Drugs 12:611–621
11. Bjarnason K, Skrumsager BK, Kiehr B (1997) Levormeloxifene: a new partial estrogen receptor agonist demonstrates antiresorptive and antiatherogenic properties in postmenopausal women. In: ASBMR 19th annual meeting, Cincinnati, OH, September, 10–14, 1997. J Bone Miner Res 12(Suppl 1):S346
12. Black LJ, Sato M, Rowley ER, et al. (1994) Raloxifene (LY 139481 HCl) prevents bone loss and reduces serum cholesterol without causing uterine hypertropy in ovariectomized rats. J Clin Invest 93:63–69
13. Black DM, Cummings SR, Karpf DB, Cauley JA, Thompson DE, Nevitt MC, Bauer DC for the FIT trial Research Group (1996) Randomised trial of effect of alendronate on risk of fracture in women with existing vertebral fractures. Lancet 348:1535–1541
14. Black DM, Greenspan SL, Ensrud KE, Palermo L, McGowan JA, Lang TF, et al. (2003) The effects of parathyroid hormone and alendronate alone or in combination in postmenopausal osteoporosis. N Engl J Med 349:1207–1215
15. Boivin G, Lips P, Ott SM, Harper KD, Sarkar S, Pinette KV, et al. (2003) Contribution of raloxifene and calcium and vitamin D3 supplementation to the increase of the degree of mineralization of bone in postmenopausal women. J Clin Endocrinol Metab 88:4199–4205
16. Bouxsein ML (2003) Bone quality: an old concept revisited. Osteoporos Int 14(Suppl 5):S1–S2
17. Burr DB (2003) Microdamage and bone strength. Osteoporos Int 14(Suppl 5):67–72

18. Chavassieux PM, Arlot ME, Reda C, Wei L, Yates J, Meunier PJ (1997) Histomorphometric assessement of the long term effects of alendronate on bone quality and remodelling in patients with osteoporosis. J Clin Invest 100:1475–1480
19. Chen HK, Ke HZ, Jee WS, Ma YZ, Pirie CM, Simmons HA, et al. (1995) Droloxifene prevents ovariectomy-induced bone loss in tibiae and femora of aged female rats: a dual absorptiometric and histomorphometric study. J Bone Miner Res 10:1256–1262
20. Chesnut C, Weiss S, Mulder H, Wasnich R, Greenwald M, Eastell R, et al. (1998) Idoxifene increases bone mineral density in osteopenic postmenopausal women. In: ASBMR IBMS joint meeting, San Francisco, December 1998. Bone 23(Suppl):S389
21. Chesnut III CH, Silverman S, Andriano K, Genant H, Gimona A, Harris S, Kiel D (2000) A randomised trial of nasal spray salmon calcitonin in postmenopausal women with established osteoporosis: the prevent recurrence of osteoporotic fractures study. Am J Med 109:267–276
22. Colishaw S, Reeve J (2003) Effects of SERM LY117018 on bone microdamage. J Bone Miner Res 18:S293
23. Compston JE, Watts NB (2002) Combination therapy for postmenopausal ostoporosis. Clin Endocrinol 56:565–569
24. Cosman F (1999) Skeletal effects of selective estrogen recptor modulators. Am J Man Care 5(Suppl):S168–S179
25. Cozick J, Allen D, Baum M, et al. (1992) Long term effects of Tamoxifen: biological effects of Tamoxifen working party. Eur J Cancer 29:15–21
26. Cummings SR, Black DM, Nevitt MC, Browner W, Cauley J, Ensrud K, Genant HK (1993) Bone density at various sites for prediction of hip fractures. The study of osteoporotic fractures research group. Lancet 341:72–75
27. Cummings SR, Black DM, Thompson DE, Applegate WB, Barret-Connor E, Musliner TA, Palermo L (1998) Alendronate reduces the risk of vertebral fractures in women witout pre-existing vertebral fractures: results of the fracture intervention Trial. J Am Med Assoc 280:2077–2078
28. Deal C, Omizo M, Schwartz EN, Eriksen EF, Cantor P, Wang J, et al. (2004) Raloxifene in combination with teriparatide reduces teriparatide-induced stimulation of bone resorption but not formation in postmenopausal women with osteoporosis. J Bone Min Res 19(Suppl 1):1169
29. Delmas PJ, Bjarnason NH, Mitlak BH, et al. (1997) Effects of Raloxifene on bone mineral density, serum cholesterol concentration and uterine endometrium in postmenopausal women. N Engl J Med 337:1641–1647
30. Delmas P, Garnero P, MacDonald B (1998) Idoxifene reduces bone turnover in osteopenic postmenopausal women. In: ASBMR IBMS joint meeting, San Francisco, December 1998. Bone 23(Suppl):S494–S495
31. Delmas PD, Ensrud KE, Adachi JD, Harper KD, Sarkar S, Gennari C, Reginster JY, Pols HAP, Recker RR, Harris ST, Wu W, Genant HK, Black DM, Eastell R for the Multiple Outcomes of Raloxifene Evaluation (MORE) Investigators (2002) Efficacy of raloxifene on vertebral fracture risk reduction in postmenopausal women with osteoporosis: four-year results from a randomized clinical trial. J Clin Endocrinol Metab 87:3609–3617
32. Díaz Curiel M, Calero JA, Guerrero R, et al. (1998) Effects of LY 117018 HCl on bone remodeling and mineral density in the oophorectomized rat. Am J Obstet Gynecol 178:320–325
33. Draper MW, Flowers DE, Huster WJ, et al. (1996) A controlled trial of Raloxifene (LY 139481) HCl: impact on bone turnover and serum lipid profile in healthy postmenopausal women. J Bone Miner Res 11:835–842

34. Ettinger B, Black D, Cummnings S (1998) Raloxifene reduces the risk of incident vertebral fractures: 24 month interim analyses. Osteoporos Int 8(Suppl 3):11 (abstract)
35. Ettinger B, Black DM, Mitlak BH, Knickerbocker RK, Nickelsen T, Genant H, et al. (1999) Reduction of vertebral fracture risk in postmenopausal women with osteoporosis treated with raloxifene: results from a 3-year randomized clinical trial. Multiple Outcomes of Raloxifene Evaluation (MORE) Investigators. J Am Med Assoc 282:637–645
36. Ettinger B, San Martin J, Crans G, Pavo I (2004) Differential effects of teriparatide on BMD after treatment with raloxifene or alendronate. J Bone Miner Res 19:745–751
37. Evans GL, Turner NY (1995) Tissue selective actions of estrogens analogs. Bone 17(Suppl 4):181S–190S
38. Evans G, Bryant HU, Magee D, et al. (1994) The effects of Raloxifene on tibia histomorphometry in ovariectomized rats. Endocrinology 134:2283–2288
39. Fentiman ES, Caleffi M, Rodin A, et al. (1989) Bone mineral content of women receiving Tamoxifen for mastalgia. Br J Cancer 60:262–264
40. Finkelstein JS, Hayes A, Hunzelman JL, Wyland JJ, Lee H, Neer RM (2003) The effects of parathyroid hormone, alendronate, or both in men with osteoporosis. N Engl J Med 349:1216–1226
41. Fisher B, Costantino JP, Wickerman DL, et al. (1998) Tamoxifen for prevention of breast cancer: report of the National Surgical Adjuvant Breast and Bowel Project P-1 Study. J Natl Cancer Inst 90:1371–1388
42. Frolik CA, Bryant HU, Black EC, et al. (1996) Time-dependent changes in biochemical bone markers and serum cholesterol in ovariectomized rats: effects of raloxifene HCl, tamoxifen, estrogen and alendronate. Bone 18:621–627
43. Genant HK, Lang T, Fuerst T, Pinette KV, Zhou C, Thiebaud D, Díez-Perez A (2004) Treatment with raloxifene for two years increases vertebral bone mineral density as measured by volumetric quantitative computed tomography. Bone 35:1164–1168
44. Gómez-Alonso C, Díaz Curiel M, Hawkins Carranza F, Pérez Cano R, Díez-Perez A (2000) Femoral neck bone mineral density, neck-shaft angle and mean femoral neck width as predictors of hip fracture in men and women. Osteoporos Int 11:714–720
45. Gotfredsen A, Christiansen C, Palshof T (1984) The effect of Tamoxifen on bone mineral content in premenopausal women with breast cancer. Cancer 53:853–857
46. Grey AB, Stapleton JP, Evans MC, et al. (1995) The effect of antiestrogen Tamoxifen on bone mineral density in normal late postmenopausal women. Am J Med 99:636–641
47. Harris ST, Watts NB, Genant HK, McKeever CD, Hangartner T, Keller M, Chesnut III CH, Brown J, Eriksen EF, Hoseyni MS, Axelrod DW, Miller PD for the VERT Study Group (1999) Effects of risedronate treatment on vertebral and non vertebral fractures in women with postmenopausal osteoporosis: a randomised controlled trial. J Am Med Assoc 282:1344–1352
48. Heaney R (2003) Is the paradigm shifting? Bone 33:457–464
49. Heaney RP, Draper MW (1997) Raloxifene and estrogen: comparative bone remodeling kinetics. J Clin Endocrinol Metab 82:3425–3429
50. Hodgskinson R, Currey JD (1993) Separate effects of osteoporosis and density on the strength and stiffness of human cancellous bone. Clin Biomech 8:262–268
51. Hodsman AB, Drost D, Fraher LJ, et al. (1999a) The addition of a Raloxifene analog (LY 117018) allows for reduced PTH (1–34) dosing during reversal of osteopenia in ovariectomized rats. J Bone Miner Res 14:675–679
52. Hodsman AB, Watson PH, Drost D, et al. (1999b) Assessement of maintenance therapy with reduced doses of PTH (1–34) in combination with a Raloxifene analogue (LY 117018) following anabolic therapy in the ovariectomized rat. Bone 24:451–455

53. Hou FJ, Lang SM, Hoshaw SJ, et al. (1998) Human vertebral body apparent and hard tissue stiffness. J Biomech 31:1009–1015
54. Johnell O, Scheele WH, Lu Y, Reginster JY, Need AG, Seeman E (2002) Additive effects of raloxifene and alendronate on bone density and biochemical markers of bone remodeling in postmenopausal women with osteoporosis. J Clin Endocrinol Metab 87:985–992
55. Johnell O, Cauley JA, Kulkarni PM, Wong M, Stock JL (2004) Raloxifene reduces risk of vertebral fractures and breast cancer in postmenopausal women regardless of prior hormone therapy. J Fam Pract 53:789–796
56. Kanis JA, Johnell O, Black DM, Downs RW Jr, Sarkar S, Fuerst T, et al. (2003) Effect of raloxifene on the risk of new vertebral fracture in postmenopausal women with osteopenia or osteoporosis: a reanalysis of the Multiple Outcomes of Raloxifene Evaluation trial. Bone 33:293–300
57. Katzenellenbogen BS (2002) Defining the "S" in SERMs. Science 295(5564):2380–2381
58. Ke HZ, Chen HK, Qi H, Pirie CM, Simmons HA, Ma YF, et al. (1995a) Effects of droloxifene on prevention of cancellous bone loss and bone turnover in the axial skeleton of aged, ovariectomized rats. Bone 17:491–496
59. Ke HZ, Simmons HA, Pirie CM, Crawford DT, Thompson DD (1995b) Droloxifene, a new estrogen antagonist/agonist, prevents bone loss in ovariectomized rats. Endocrinology 136:2435–2441
60. Ke HZ, Chen HK, Simmons HA, Qi H, Crawford DT, Pirie CM, et al. (1997a) Comparative effects of droloxifene, tamoxifen, and estrogen on bone, serum cholesterol, and uterine histology in the ovariectomized rat model. Bone 20:31–39
61. Ke HZ, Chidsey-FrinK L, Qi H, Crawford DT, Pirie CM, Simmons HA et al (1997b) Droloxifene increases bone mass in ovariectomized rats with established osteopenia. In: ASBMR 19th annual meeting, Cincinnati, OH, September, 10–14, 1997. J Bone Miner Res 12(Suppl 1)
62. Kenni AM, Prestwood KM, Pilbeam CC, et al. (1995) The short term effects of Tamoxifen on bone turnover in older women. J Clin Endocrinol Metab 80:3287–3291
63. Kian Tee M, Rogatsky I, Tzagarakis-Foster C, et al. (2004) Estradiol and selective estrogen receptor modulators differentially regulate target genes with estrogen receptors alpha and beta. Mol Biol Cell 15:1262–1272
64. Kristensen B, Ejlertsen B, Dalgaard P, et al. (1994) Tamoxifen and bone metabolism in postmenopausal low risk breast cancer patients: a randomized study. J Clin Oncol 12:992–997
65. Kung AW, Chao HT, Huang KE, Need AG, Taechakraichana N, Loh FH, et al. (2003) Efficacy and safety of raloxifene 60 milligrams/day in postmenopausal Asian women. J Clin Endocrinol Metab 88:3130–3136
66. Liu J, Zhu H, Huang Q, Zhang Z, Li H, Qin Y, Zhang Y, Wei D, Lu J, Liu H, Xen X, Liu Y, Ekangaki A, Zheng Y, Diez-Perez A, Harper K (2004) Effects of raloxifene hydrochloride on bone mineral density, bone metabolism and serum lipids in Chinese postmenopausal women with osteoporosis: a multi-center, randomized, placebo-controlled clinical trial. Chin Med J 117:1029–1035 (in English)
67. Love RR, Mazeis RB, Barden HS, et al. (1992) Effects of Tamoxifen on bone mineral density in postmenopausal women with breast cancer. N Engl J Med 326:852–856
68. Lufkin EG, Whitaker MD, Nickelsen T, et al. (1998) Treatment of stablished postmenopausal osteoporosis with Raloxifene: a randomized trial. J Bone Miner Res 13:1747–1754
69. Lufkin E, et al. (2001) North American Menopause Society 12th annual meeting program and abstract book, 4–6 October 2001, p 21, 70

70. Ma YL, Bryant HU, Zeng Q, Palkowitz A, Jee WS, Turner CH, Sato M (2002) Long-term dosing of arzoxifene lowers cholesterol, reduces bone turnover, and preserves bone quality in ovariectomized rats. J Bone Miner Res 17:2256–2264
71. Maricic M, Adachi JD, Sarkar S, Wu W, Wong M, Harper KD (2002) Early effects of raloxifene on clinical vertebral fractures at 12 months in postmenopausal women with osteoporosis. Arch Intern Med 162:1140–1143
72. Marshall D, Johnell O, Wedel H (1996) Meta-analysis of how well measures of bone mineral density predict occurrence of osteoporotic fractures. Br Med J 312:1254–1259
73. Martino S, Cauley JA, Barrett-Connor E, Powles TJ, Mershon J, Disch D et al (2004) Continuing outcomes relevant to Evista: breast cancer incidence in postmenopausal osteoporotic women in a randomized trial of raloxifene. J Natl Cancer Inst 96:1751–1761
74. Gómez-Alonso Mashiba T, Hirano T, Turner C, Forwood MR, Johnston CC, Burr D (2000) Suppressed bone turnover by biphosphonates increases microamage accumulation and reduces some biomechanical properties in dog rib. J Bone Miner Res 15:613–620
75. Mashiba T, Turner C, Hirano T, Forwood MR, Johnston CC, Burr D (2001) Effects of suppressed bone turnover by biphosphonates on microdamage accumulation and biomechanical properties in clinically relevant skeletal sites in beagles. Bone 28:524–531
76. Melton LJ III, Atkinson EJ, O'Fallon WM, Wahner HW, Riggs BL (1993) Long term fracture prediction by bone mineral assessed at different skeletal sites. J Bone Miner Res 8:1227–1233
77. Million Women Study Collaborators (2003) Breast cancer and hormone-replacement therapy in the Million Women Study. Lancet 362:419–427
78. NIH Consensus Development Panel on Osteoporosis, Prevention, Diagnosis and Therapy (2001) J Am Med Assoc 285:785–795
79. Nowak J, Hornby SB, Andersen A, Siogren T, Feslersen U, Christiensen ND (1998) Effect of 12 month treatment with levormeloxifene on bone, serum cholesterol, osteocalcin and uterus in ovariectomized rat. In: ASBMR IBMS joint meeting, San Francisco, December 1998. Bone 23(Suppl):S610
80. Nuttall ME, Nadeau D, Prichett WP, Gowen M (1997) Idoxifene, a tissue selective estrogen agonist/antagonist has a mechanism of action in bone similar to estrogen and distinct from raloxifene. In: ASBMR 19th annual meeting, Cincinnati, OH, September, 10–14, 1997. J Bone Miner Res 12(Suppl 1):S170
81. Nuttall ME, Nadeau D, Stroup G, Hoffman S, Vasko-Moser J, Gowen M (1998) Idoxifene antagonizes the effects of estrogen in the breast and endometrium: a therapeutically favorable profile over estrogen in reproductive tissues. In: ASBMR IBMS joint meeting, San Francisco, December 1998. Bone 23(Suppl):S611
82. Nuttall ME, Stroup GB, Fisher PW, et al. (2000) Distinct mechanisms of action of selective estrogen receptor modulators in breast and osteoblastic cells. Am J Physiol Cell Physiol 279:C1550–C1557
83. Ott SM, Oleksik A, Lu Y, Harper K, Lips P (2002) Bone histomorphometric and biochemical marker results of a 2-year placebo-controlled trial of raloxifene in postmenopausal women. J Bone Miner Res 17:341–348
84. Parfitt AM (2004) What is the normal rate of bone remodeling? Bone 35:1–3
85. Powles TS, Hickish T, Kanis JA, et al. (1996) Effect of tamoxifene on bone mineral density measured by dual energy X-ray absorciometry in healthy premenopausal and postmenopausal women. J Clin Oncol 14:78–84

86. Qu Q, Zheng H, Dahllund J, Laine A, Cockcroft N, Peng Z, Koskinen M, Hemminki K, Kangas L, Väänänen K, Härkönen P (2000) Selective estrogenic effects of a novel triphenylethylene compound, FC1271a, on bone, cholesterol level, and reproductive tissues in intact and ovariectomized rats. Endocrinology 141:809–820
87. Reginster J-Y, Minne HW, Sorensen OH, Hooper M, Roux C, Brandi ML, Lund B for the VERT Study Group (2000) Randomized trial of the effects of risedronate on vertebral fractures in women with established postmenopausal osteoporosis. Osteoporos Int 11:83–91
88. Sarkar S, Mitlack B, Wong M, Stock JL, Black DM, Harper K (2002) Relationships between bone mineral density and incident vertebral fracture risk with raloxifene therapy. J Bone Miner Res 17:1–10
89. Sato M, McClintock C, Kim J, et al. (1994) Dual-energy X-ray absorptiometry of Raloxifene effects on the lumbar vertebrae and femora of ovariectomized rats. J Bone Miner Res 9:715–724
90. Schaffler MB, Choi K, Milgrom C (1995) Aging and microdamage accumulation in human compact bone. Bone 17:521–525
91. Seeman E (2002) Pathogenesis of bone fragility in women and men. Lancet 359:1841–1850
92. Seeman E, Crans G, Diez-Perez A, Cummings S (2003) Meta-analysis of the efficacy of raloxifene on reduction of vertebral fracture risk. J Bone Min Res 18(Suppl 2):SU164
93. Siris ES, Harris ST, Eastell R, Zanchetta J, Goemaere S, Diez-Perez A et al (2004) Effect of raloxifene on the risk of nonvertebral fractures after 8 years: results from the Continuous Outcomes Relevant to Evista (CORE) study. J Bone Miner Res 19(Suppl 1): F428
94. Skrumsager BK, Kiehr B, Bjarnason K (1997) Levormeloxifene: safety and pharmacokinetics after multiple dosing of fifty-six postmenopausal women. In: ASBMR 19th annual meeting, Cincinnati, OH, September, 10–14, 1997. J Bone Miner Res 12(Suppl 1):S346
95. Stavisky R, Hotchkiss C, Nowak J, Kaplan J (1998) Levormeloxifene prevents bone loss and decreases bone turnover in ovariectomized cynomologus macaques. In: ASBMR IBMS joint meeting, San Francisco, December 1998. Bone 23(Suppl):S610
96. Stepan JJ, Alenfeld F, Boivin G, Feyen JH, Lakatos P (2003) Mechanisms of action of antiresorptive therapies of postmenopausal osteoporosis. Endocr Regul 37:225–238
97. Taranta A, Brama M, Teti A, De luca V, Scandurra R, Spera G, Agnusdei D, Termine JD, Migliaccio S (2002) The selective estrogen receptor modulator raloxifene regulates osteoclast and osteoblast activity in vitro. Bone 30(2):368–376
98. Turner CH (2002) Biomechanics of bone: Determinants of skeletal fragility and bone quality. Osteoporos Int 13:97–104
99. Turner RT, Wakley GK, Hannon KS, et al. (1987) Tamoxifen presents the altered bone turnover resulting from ovarian hormone deficiency. J Bone Miner Res 2:449–456
100. Turner RT, Wakley GK, Hannon KS, et al. (1988) Tamoxifen inhibits osteoclast mediated reabsortion of trabecular bone in ovarian deficient rat. Endocrinology 122:1146–1150
101. Turner CH, Sato M, Bryant HU (1994) Raloxifene preserve bone strenght and bone mass in ovariectomized rats. Endocrinology 135:2001–2005
102. Van Rietbergen B, Eckstein F, Koller B, et al. (2000) Trabecular bone tissue strains in the healthy and osteoporotic human femur. Orthopaed Res Soc 46:33
103. Wakley GK, Baum RL, Hannon KS, et al. (1988) Tamoxifen treatment reduces osteopenia induced by inmovilization in the rat. Calcif Tissue Int 43:383–388
104. Wang X, Shen X, Li X, Mauli Agrawal C (2002) Age-related changes in the collagen network and toughness of bone. Bone 31:1–7

105. Warmig L, Christoffersen C, Riis BJ, Stakkestad JA, Delmas PD, Christiansen C (2003) Adverse effects of a SERM (levormeloxifene). Safety parameters and bone mineral density after treatment withdrawal. Maturitas 44:189–199
106. Waters DJ, Caywood DD, Turner RT (1991) Effect of tamoxifen citrate on canine inmobilization osteoporosis. Vet Surg 20:392–396
107. Williams DC, Paul DC, Black LJ (1991) Effects of estrogen and tamoxifen on serum osteocalcin levels in ovariectomized rats. Bone Miner 14:205–220
108. Wright CDP, Mansell RE, Gazet JC, et al. (1993) Effect of long term Tamoxifen treatment on bone turnover in women with breast cancer. Br Med J 306:429–430
109. Wright CD, Garrahan NJ, Stanton M, et al. (1994) Effect of long term Tamoxifen therapy on cancellous bone remodeling and structure in women with breast cancer. J Bone Miner Res 9:153–159
110. Writing Group for the Women's Health Initiative Investigators (2002) Risks and benefits of estrogen plus progestin in healthy postmenopausal women: principal results from the Women's Health Initiative randomized controlled trial. J Am Med Assoc 288:321–333
111. Yang NN, Bryant HU, Hardikar S, et al. (1996) Estrogen and Raloxifene stimulate transforming growth factor β_3 gene expression in rat bone: a potential mechanism for estrogen or Raloxifene mediated bone maintenance. Endocrinology 137:2075–2084

Chapter 9

Cardiovascular Disease and SERMs

Antonio Cano

A wealth of epidemiological, clinical, and experimental studies link estrogens with cardiovascular disease (CVD). This evidence has promoted CVD as a key area within the extragenital effects of estrogens. The question is of interest because it directly affects the wide clinical use of estrogens as contraceptive agents or as principal constituents of hormonal therapy (HT) formulations in postmenopausal women. The significance of the subject is further reinforced by the relevance of CVD as a cause of mortality and morbidity in both women and men.

CVD is a generic denomination mainly integrated by coronary heart disease (CHD) and stroke. Although not considered as a form of CVD in some instances, venous thromboembolic disease (VTED) shares with the other forms of CVD the territorial assignment, the vascular tree, although clear differences exist in the main pathophysiological mechanisms. In most CVD forms, however, thrombus formation plays a crucial role.

All forms of CVD are serious disorders, although CHD is the most prevalent and lethal. Global data in the USA attribute 54% of deaths from CVD to C HD and 18% to stroke (http://www.americanheart.org). Figures for Europe are similar, where about half of deaths from CVD correspond to CHD and nearly one third to stroke (British Heart Foundation 2000). The burden of the disease is also shared by developing countries where it is estimated that CVD will be the leading cause of death by 2010 (World Health Organization Web site www.who.int/ncd/cvd). Specific gender patterns have been detected for both the prevalence as well as the behavior of CHD, further suggesting a relevant role for reproductive hormones. Fewer differences have been found for stroke.

VTED has a lower prevalence (approximately 1/1000 persons per year), but it rises exponentially with age from $<$ 5 cases per 100,000 persons $<$ 15 years old to $\cong$ 500 cases per 100,000 (0.5%) at age 80 years (White 2003). Against the strong gender differences found in CHD statistics, no convincing difference between men and women have been detected for VTED (Silverstein et al. 1998).

The observation that, compared with men, women maintain some level of protection against CHD has nourished the debate about a possible favorable effect associated with exposure to estrogens. Furthermore, most of the information gathered in the latter years has confirmed the association of estrogens with many benefits both in experimental as well as in clinical models at the level of intermediate indicators. Consequently, HT was proposed not only for control of symptoms but also for primary and secondary CHD prevention in postmenopausal women. Contrary to the beneficial effects found in the first, observational studies, three more recent randomized controlled trials have found that HT is neutral (Hulley et al. 1998; Anderson et al. 2004) or even prejudicial (Rossouw et al. 2002) when administered to women for the purpose of CVD prevention. The data yielded by these studies affect not only CHD but also stroke and VTED, where HT has been shown to be detrimental, too. Following this evidence, scientific societies, such as the American Heart Association, have advised against the use of HT for the prevention of CVD in women (Mosca et al. 2004). The mixture of protective effects, mainly at the level of risk factors and of data gathered from experimental models, as well as of neutral or prejudicial clinical outcomes defines the present picture. It is one where the confirmation of estrogens as important regulators of CVD pathophysiology emerges as a main conclusion. Consequently, selective estrogen receptor modulators (SERMs) offer a unique opportunity to achieve cardiovascular outcome profiles that might improve those attained by conventional HT.

This chapter will analyze some specific traits of CVD that will be used to review the principal variables that have exhibited sensitivity to estrogen agonism. Then, current information on the particular actions of SERMs will be presented.

9.1 The Focal Phenotype of CVD

The vascular tree is divided into two main, well-demarcated areas composed of the arterial and the venous trees. They both define different microenvironments that create the conditions for the development of focal episodes determining the occurrence of obstructive phenomena that are at the base of CVD. Arterial episodes (CHD and stroke) occur at sites of inflamed arteries, while VTED or venous stroke episodes develop as a result of thrombus formation at discrete locations in the venous tree.

Atherosclerosis, a disease of the vascular wall, is the substrate for the arterial forms of CVD. Atherosclerotic plaques exhibit a focal distribution along the arterial tree as a consequence of local conditions that favor their initiation and progression. Low or reversed shear stress, for example, contributes to plaque development, a process in which the regulation of several genes may be involved (Resnick and Gimbrone 1995).

Thrombosis is the other phenomenon that crucially contributes to both the arterial and the venous forms of CVD, although the type of thrombus,

Table 9.1. Risk factors for coronary heart disease and venous thromboembolic disease [adapted from Friedewald (1996) and Rosendaal (1999)]

Coronary heart disease		Venous thromboembolic disease		
Unmodifiable	Modifiable	Genetic	Acquired	Mixed genetic and acquired
Age	Cigarette smoking	Protein C deficiency	Immobilization	Increased concentration of prothrombin
Male gender	High blood pressure	Protein S deficiency	Surgery	Increased concentration of factor VIII
Family history of premature disease	High blood cholesterol	Antithrombin deficiency	Trauma	Hyper-homocystinemia
	Physical inactivity	Factor V Leiden	Pregnancy	
	Diabetes	Prothrombin 20210 A	Puerperium	
	Overweight	Increased concentration of factor IX	Lupus anticoagulant	
	Psychological conditions		Malignant disease Female hormones	
			Diseases affecting liver, endothelium, or other organs producing clotting factors	
			Abnormal dietary intake of substrates or vitamins (vitamin K)	

its biological determinants, and consequently the corresponding risk factors differ for each form (Table 9.1). There is a list of factors that are involved in the increased thrombotic risk within the arterial tree (Table 9.2). Some of them directly depend on the altered focal environment, while others are systemic. The interaction between platelets and the arterial wall is one critical step. Platelet adhesion and deposition is strongly determined by local wall

Table 9.2. Factors affecting thrombogenicity in coronary heart disease [from Badimon et al. (1999)]

Local factors	Systemic factors
Degree of plaque disruption (i.e., erosion, ulcer)	Cholesterol, Lp(a)
Degree of stenosis (i.e., change in geometry)	Catecholamines (i.e., smoking, stress, cocaine)
Tissue substrate (i.e., lipid-rich plaque)	Fibrinogen, impaired fibrinolysis (i.e., PMI-1), activated platelets and clotting (i.e., factor VII, thrombin generation, F1 + 2)
Surface of residual thrombus (i.e., recurrence)	Infections (C. Pneumoniae, CMV, H. Pylori)
Vasoconstriction (i.e., platelets, thrombin)	Diabetes

phenomena, essentially inflammation, with or without the substrate of an atheromatous plaque. The activation of platelets is followed by the induction of platelet coagulation activity, a process in which there is close collaboration with leukocytes adhering to the initial plug (Cano and Van Baal 2001). Liberation of tissue factor is another mechanism that participates in the generation of a thrombus.

Hypercoagulable states, in turn, have been traditionally associated with venous thrombosis. Consequently, attention has been paid to alterations of the hemostatic balance. Although this is a systemic variable, focality is favored due to the contribution of decreased blood flow, as confirmed by the preferential development of venous thrombi at the level of valves, an area of stasis where low-velocity flow is moderately turbulent.

In conclusion, hemostasia intervenes in distinct critical steps of both the arterial and venous forms of CVD. The particulars, however, differ in each case, as confirmed by the different array of risk factors for CHD and VTED. The participation of the vascular wall is pivotal in explaining the focality of these processes. Within the vascular wall, the role of the endothelium is critical given its involvement in the origin of atherosclerosis and its influence on the development of VTED (for review see Cano and Van Baal 2001; Cano 2003).

9.1.1 The Crucial Role of the Endothelium

The vascular wall is an organ composed of an endothelium, smooth muscle, and fibroblasts. The endothelium has a privileged position to act as both a sensor and an effector. The endothelium governs remodeling by releasing growth factors and vasoactive substances that regulate cellular growth and apoptosis. The key role of endothelium in the plasticity of the vascular wall helps to better understand the modern hypotheses that root the initiation and development of atherosclerosis in endothelial dysfunction (Ross 1999). The rupture of the coordinated equilibrium of checks and balances that is at the base of endothelial homeostasis is followed by a well-described sequence of events starting with the increase of adhesiveness of the endothelium to leukocytes or platelets and leading to an atherosclerotic plaque (Ross 1999) (Fig. 1). The progression of the plaque follows several steps represented by lesions I to IV (Fuster et al. 1992a,b).

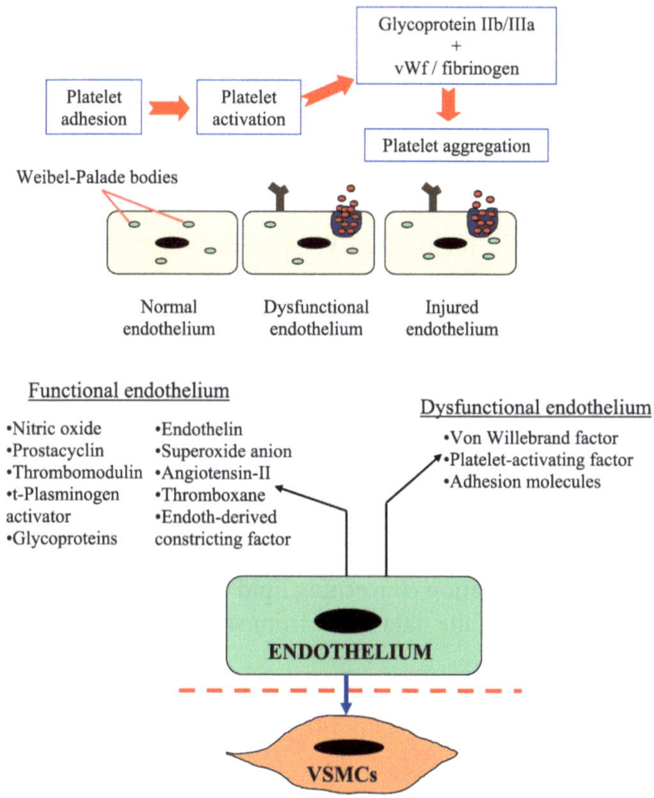

Fig. 9.1. A dysfunctional or injured endothelium is at the basis for initiation of and progression to atherosclerosis. Several mechanisms, such as adhesion molecules or liberation of von Willebrand factor (vWf, *upper panel*), determine a series of phenomena, including platelet activation and aggregation. This participation of platelets involves the implication of molecules like glycoprotein IIb/IIIa, fibrinogen, and von Willebrand factor. The endothelium also acts as a source of signals that regulate local functions, including VSMCs (*lower panel*). A list of the most relevant messengers produced by a functional and a dysfunctonal endothelium is presented in the *lower panel*

A very innovative area of research has focused on the determinants of plaque stability. An important role seems to be played by enzymes involved in the degradation of the extracellular matrix. The rupture of unstable plaques induces platelet activation, too. Acute thrombus formation under these conditions seems fundamental to the onset of acute ischemic events.

A key concept inferred from the ideas discussed above is the difference between the development of conditions that favor the clinical eruption of any form of CVD (i.e., atherosclerosis) and the proper occurrence of the clinical event, since the inductors do not necessarily have to be the same. Furthermore, the possibility exists that a concrete factor may be protective at several stages of the silent form of the disease, but once it is sufficiently advanced, it may act as a trigger. This distinction is pivotal when considering the role of hormones, which have been shown to differentially regulate atherosclerosis and proper clinical events.

9.2 Estrogen Agonism and CVD

Some crucial steps in the biology of CVD have demonstrated sensitivity to estrogen agonists. Some of these actions have shown to be mediated by the classical pathway of estrogen receptors (ERs), though in other cases the involved mechanisms seem more complex and require the consideration of alternative options (Mendelsohn 2002). The available evidence concentrates on actions on lipids or on direct actions on the vascular wall.

9.2.1 Lipids

There is plenty of information concerning lipid changes as a result of estrogen agonistic effects. Most of the data come from studies with either synthetic or natural estrogens.

A protective lipid profile, with reduction of total cholesterol and LDL and a modest increase in high-density lipoprotein (HDL), has been associated with oral estrogen therapy (Writing Group for the PEPI Trial 1995). This effect, however, has been considered negligible when compared with the benefits traditionally ascribed to estrogens (Marsh et al. 1999).

More interest has been generated by the potential effects of estrogens as modulators of LDL oxidation, a mechanism considered to be the authentic mediator of the detrimental action of LDL particles in atherosclerosis. Oxidized LDL becomes trapped in an artery and is then internalized by macrophages (Steinberg 1997; Navab et al. 1996; Morel et al. 1983; Griendling and Alexander 1997). This internalization leads to the formation of lipid peroxides resulting in the formation of foam cells. Additionally, oxidized LDL is an agent that by itself promotes vasoconstriction and platelet activation (Kugiyama et al. 1990; Chin et al. 1992; Chen et al. 1996).

Estrogens have been shown to limit LDL susceptibility to oxidation, although this action is under discussion at present. Only supraphysiological doses have demonstrated this effect in the laboratory (Hermenegildo et al. 2001; Santanam et al. 1998). Some indirect evidence favoring protection, such as the reduction of antibodies to oxidized LDL, has been proposed (Hoogerbrugge et al. 1998), but, again, there is no general consensus on the subject (Uint et al. 2003; Heikkinen et al. 1998). More recent research has found that estrogens reduce the production of $F_{2\alpha}$-isoprostanes, a product of a nonenzymatic, free radical catalyzed peroxidation of arachidonic acid (Liu et al. 1998) that has been recognized as a stable, good biomarker of in vivo oxidative stress (de Zwart et al. 1999; Pratico 1999). Moreover, increased $F_{2\alpha}$-isoprostane levels have been found in human atherosclerotic lesions (Oguogho et al. 2001) and are being considered as a reliable biomarker of both atherosclerosis (Gross et al. 2005) and coronary events (Vassalle et al. 2003) (Fig. 9.2).

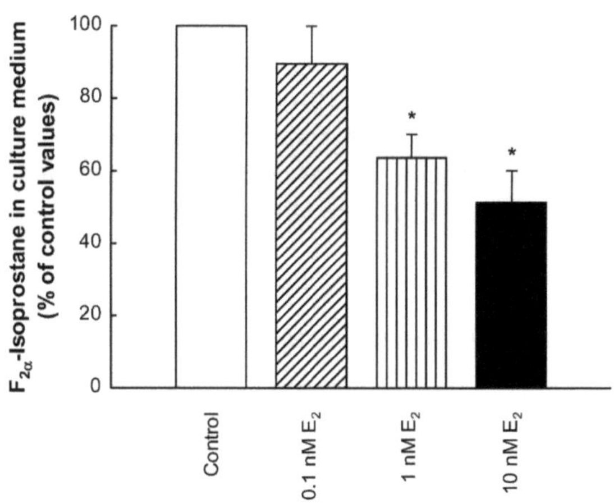

Fig. 9.2. Physiological concentrations of estradiol decrease the production of $F_{2\alpha}$-isoprostanes in medium from cultured human umbilical vein endothelial cells in culture. (From Hermenegildo et al. 2002)

9.2.2 Vascular Wall

The vascular wall is a target for sexual hormones. In the particular case of estrogens, specific receptors have been found in both endothelium and vascular smooth muscle cells (VSMC) (Venkov et al. 1996; Karas et al. 1994). The trophic effects of estrogens on the endothelium have been advocated as crucial against initiation and promotion of atherosclerosis. Thus, cellular and animal models, as well as clinical observation with doppler techniques, confirm that estrogens promote vasodilation. This effect is maintained for years in menopausal women subjected to HT (Jokela et al. 2003). Nitric oxide (NO) and prostacyclin (PGI), two main locally produced antiaggregant and vasodilatory mediators, are the principal agents in this myorelaxant effect of estrogens (Couzin 2004). In agreement with current concepts, their effects have been demonstrated as protective against atherosclerosis in animal models (Perrault et al. 2003; Niebauer et al. 2003; Todaka et al. 1999). Together with the protection associated with these mediators, the inhibition of TNF-alpha-induced endothelial cell apoptosis in a dose-dependent manner has been an additional beneficial effect linked with estrogens (Spyridopoulos et al. 1997).

Proliferation and migration of VSMC follows endothelial dysfunction. Limitation of this activity in VSMC has been understood to be protective against atherosclerosis. The effect of estrogens on VSMC proliferation is controversial. Some studies have reported a reduced proliferative capacity by estrogens in a dose-dependent manner (Bhalla et al. 1997; Moraghan et al. 1996; Espinosa et al. 1996; Akishita et al. 1997) and through activation of ER (Vargas et al. 1996). In contrast, other investigators have found induction of VSMC proliferation with estrogens (Ricciardelli et al. 1994; Song et al. 1998).

Experiments in monkeys have shown that estrogens alone, or in association with progestogens, protect against diet-induced atherosclerosis (Clarkson 1994). There has been some discussion on whether or not this is the case in humans, although HT was unable to have a significant effect on the progression of the disease in women with established atherosclerosis (Hodis et al. 2003).

9.3 SERMs as an Alternative to Estrogens in CVD

The expectations created for estrogens faded as a result of the publication of randomized clinical studies, which failed to show any protection against any of the CVD forms in postmenopausal women receiving hormones (Hulley et al. 1998; Rossouw et al. 2002). The clear opposition between these trials and most of the experimental and previous clinical studies has raised much discussion in the literature (Speroff 2002). Despite the many criticisms against distinct details of the discrepant studies, there is consensus on the appreciable regulatory effects of the hormone on the vascular wall. This conception, together with the significant advances experienced by the knowledge on the molecular details of estrogen action, has created a great opportunity for investigating alternative agonists with a potentially better profile than estrogens themselves.

In one *a priori* analysis the versatility of ER modulation offers a wide array of options. These include the selective activation of either the ERα or the ERβ isoform, or the use of compounds sufficiently similar to estrogens so as to bind to the ER, yet different enough to generate a ligand–receptor complex with a 3D conformation capable of activating cell functions with a profile distinct to estrogens (Fig. 9.3). The interesting observation that ERβ can interact with ERα, together with the varied distribution of each ER isoform in different tissues, has raised attractive possibilities associated with selective binding to one or another isoform. Despite the recent availability of compounds with selective agonism for either ERα or ERβ (Harrington et al. 2003; Muthyala et al. 2003; Ghosh et al. 2003), there is no clear proof to date associating the selective action of any of the available SERMs in the vascular system with preferential binding to one of the two ER isoforms. Consequently, the most consistent data on cardiovascular effects of SERMs have been obtained in studies with compounds that have been approved for use in patients, particularly tamoxifen, raloxifene, and toremifene.

Another important point to keep in mind when reviewing the cardiovascular effects of SERMs is that, in the absence of clinical studies of consistency comparable to estrogens, most of the available evidence has been obtained in experimental models. The work has concentrated on the selective areas of vascular physiology that have shown susceptibility to ER activation and, therefore, has followed steps that often overlap with those taken in research with estrogens.

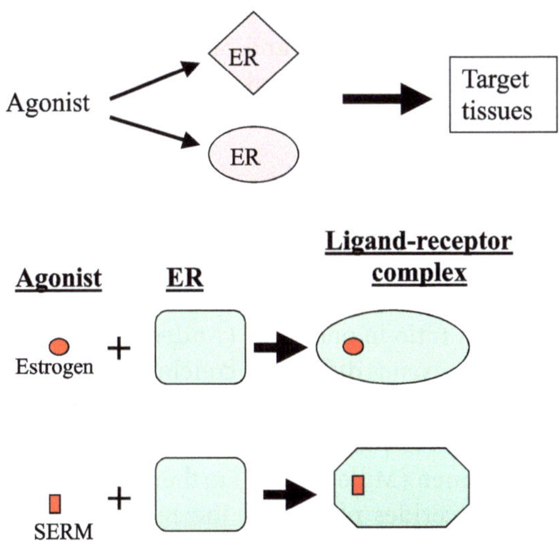

Fig. 9.3. Several mechanisms underlie the functional versatility of the ER. The different distributions of the alpha and beta isotypes of ER conditions a first step that warrants distinct functional profiles depending on the higher or lower affinity of the ligand for one or another isotype (*upper panel*). Then, different ligands generate distinct 3D conformations in the ligand–receptor complex that condition different interaction profiles with the promoters of target genes (*lower panel*)

9.4 Actions of SERMs

9.4.1 Arterial Disease

Most of the forms of arterial disease result from atherosclerosis and its complications. The evidence against protection refers not only to CHD but also against stroke (Hulley et al. 1998; Rossouw et al. 2002; Bath and Gray 2005).

9.4.1.1 *Lipids and Lipid Peroxidation*

Changes in the lipid profile, which exhibits small differences from that associated with oral estrogens, have been described for tamoxifen, toremifene, and raloxifene. One common finding has been the decrease in the circulating concentration of cholesterol and LDL cholesterol, an effect with a magnitude that seems directly related to pretreatment levels (Walsh et al. 1998; Delmas et al. 1997; Saarto et al. 1996; Decensi et al. 2003; Joensuu et al. 2000; Herrington et al. 2000). Contrary to the increase in triglycerides described for estrogens, a more beneficial neutral response appears associated with SERMs. Slight increases in triglycerides, however, have been found in women treated with raloxifene (Mosca et al. 2001b; Reid et al. 2004), and cases of acute triglyceridemia have been associated with tamoxifen (Hozumi et al. 1997; Kanel et al. 1997). Only toremifene has achieved increases in the levels of high-density lipoprotein (HDL) (Saarto et al. 1996).

More refined analyses have focused on changes in the ratio of serum concentration of apolipoprotein B, the common constituent in all lipoproteins comprising non-HDL cholesterol, to apoliprotein A, the apolipoprotein associated with HDL. Raloxifene was equivalent to HT in lowering the apolipoprotein B/apolipoprotein A ratio in one study (Anderson et al. 2001).

Because of the similarity, it is difficult to conclude whether the lipid changes induced by SERMs offer any advantage over the profile determined by HT. Triglyceride levels have been proposed as an independent risk factor for CVD in postmenopausal women (Miller 1998). Further, there are some indications that increases in triglycerides may favor the reduction in the size of LDL particles. Smaller LDL particles are more susceptible to oxidation and have been associated with a higher risk potential (Austin et al. 1988), but whether this observation confers any clinical prejudice to hypertriglyceridemia has not been proven at present.

There is fragmentary information concerning the behavior of some more recent SERMs. Whereas ospemifene showed a neutral effect (Ylikorkala et al.

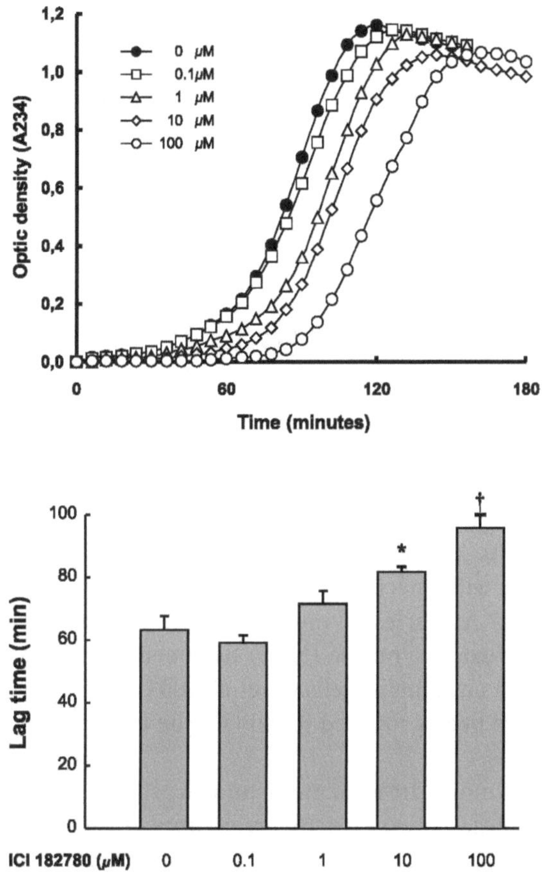

Fig. 9.4. One pure antiestrogen, ICI 182780, increased the resistance of LDL particles to oxidation. Isolated LDL particles were subjected to oxidation by copper, and the lag time to oxidation, as measured by changes in optical density, increased as a function of the concentration of ICI 182780 (*upper panel*). The increase in the lag time (min) determined by the different concentrations of ICI 182780 is shown in the *lower panel*

2003), HMR 3339, a newly designed molecule that binds to human recombinant ER and shows selective agonistic and antagonistic activity in vitro and in vivo, rapidly decreased cholesterol and LDL in a dose-dependent manner (Vogelvang et al. 2004). It seems, therefore, that the decrease in non-HDL cholesterol is a hepatic effect quite accessible to compounds that, despite differences in chemical structure, are capable of exerting some type of SERM activity.

The relevance attributed to oxidized lipids, and particularly oxidized LDL, in atherogenesis has precipitated interest in the ability of SERMs to this regard. Ex vivo experiments have confirmed that both tamoxifen and raloxifene exert some protection against the oxidation of LDL particles (Arteaga et al. 2003; Zuckerman and Bryan 1996) and that, interestingly, raloxifene is a more powerful antioxidant than tamoxifen or estradiol. It seems that this antioxidant effect is not mediated by the activation of the ER since pure antiestrogens like ICI 182780 and other SERMs like EM 652 have proven to have similar protective effects on LDL (Hermenegildo et al. 2002) (Fig. 9.4).

Little evidence exists concerning alternative actions on oxidative stress, such as modulation of the circulating levels of isoprostanes or myeloperoxidase. Some interference with the actions of myeloperoxidase, however, was found in one study (Zuckerman and Bryan 1996). Antioxidant properties have been described for other types of SERMs, thus confirming the wide extension of this potential in the different families of these compounds (Baumer et al. 2001).

9.4.1.2
Direct Actions on Vascular Wall

9.4.1.2.1
Endothelium

The idea that the endothelium is a target organ for estrogens derives from more than just the identification of both isoforms of ER in this tissue (Mendelsohn 2000). There is ample evidence showing rapid responses that are compatible with mechanisms distinct from the classical pathway for estrogen action. A species of membrane ER that determines a rapid activation of nitric oxide synthase (NOS) has been described recently in immortalized human endothelial cells (Li et al. 2003). Both genomic and nongenomic actions have been proposed to explain the estrogenic regulation of endothelial functions.

Among the local mediators directly produced by endothelium, NO and PGI emerge as two principal regulators of vascular tone and platelet aggregation. Both are sensitive to estrogenic stimuli, and, as mentioned in a previous section, their role is crucial in atherogenesis. How their production is modulated by SERMs is, consequently, an important test of vascular protection.

Much of the data concerning the effects of SERMs on these endothelial mediators refer to raloxifene, given its wide therapeutical use in women free of malignancies. Raloxifene has demonstrated the induction of NOS and NO production in endothelial cells in culture. Furthermore, this effect occurs in seconds and involves nongenomic mechanisms where NOS is phosphorylated in a process implicating Akt and extracellular signal-regulated protein kinase with the participation of ER alpha and reduction of oxidative stress (Simoncini and Genazzani 2000; Wassmann et al. 2002). In agreement with this agonistic action, experiments on the same cellular model have confirmed an activation of cyclooxygenase-1 and -2 at both the protein and the gene level, leading to increased prostacyclin production (Oviedo et al. 2004, 2005). Selective blockade of both isoforms of ER has confirmed the involvement of both ERα and ERβ as well as the likely participation of a mechanism distinct to the classical ER-dependent pathway.

Experiments with isolated vessels have confirmed the enhancing effect of raloxifene on endothelial NOS (Rahimian et al. 2002) with a similar behavior for tamoxifen (Hutchison et al. 2001).

The data with cells and isolated organs have been corroborated in animal models. An increase in endothelial NOS expression and activity was observed in spontaneously hypertensive rats (Wassmann et al. 2002), whereas in ovariectomized ewes the vasodilating effect of raloxifene surpassed that of estrogens (Gaynor et al. 2000). Endothelium-dependent vasodilation was observed for rabbit coronary arteries in vitro, an effect that agrees with some vascular relaxing properties described for toremifene, tamoxifen, idoxifene, and EM 652 in rat vessels (Gonzalez-Perez and Crespo 2003; Thorin et al. 2003; Figtree et al. 2000; Christopher et al. 2002; Tatchum-Talom et al. 2003).

Mixed evidence, however, has been described in women. Raloxifene improved flow-mediated, endothelium-dependent vasodilation in postmenopausal women (Sarrel et al. 2003) to an extent similar to that of HT (Colacurci et al. 2003; Saitta et al. 2001). Other investigators, however, have been unable to detect any effect of raloxifene (Ceresini et al. 2003; Griffiths et al. 2003). Flow-mediated vasodilation has been described for droloxifene (Herrington et al. 2000), while a neutral effect on vascular reactivity has been described for ospemifene, a more recent SERM (Ylikorkala et al. 2003).

One early sign of endothelial dysfunction consists of the expression of cell adhesion molecules at the endothelial surface. These molecules facilitate leukocyte and platelet binding. Further, endothelial permeability is dependent on interendothelial junctions, where the participation of cadherin, a transmembrane, endothelium-specific glycoprotein, exerts an important level of control (Bobryshev et al. 1999; Fulimoto et al. 1998). Once expressed, adhesion molecules may be shed from the endothelial surface. An increase in adhesion molecules in plasma, therefore, is understood as a sign of endothelial dysfunction and permeability. Furthermore, raised levels of cell adhesion molecules in blood have been associated with increased risk for CHD (Blankenberg et al. 2001; Hwang et al. 1997). A well-established effect of estrogens has been the reduction of the circulating concentration of cell adhesion molecules (Koh et al. 1997), an effect paralleled by raloxifene (Blum et al. 2000; Sbarouni et al. 2003; Colacurci et al. 2003). Different actions have been found for other SERMs in the sparse literature available. Tamoxifen had a neutral effect in one study (Simoncini et al. 1999), whereas in another study droloxifene had a mixed effect, with a decrease in E-selectin and an increase in vascular cell-adhesion molecule-1 (VCAM-1) (Herrington et al. 2001).

Finally, a new area of research has concentrated on monocyte chemotactic protein-1 (MCP-1), a 76-amino acid peptide that is one of the best-studied members of the C–C chemokine subfamily. Recent human and animal studies indicate that the recruitment of macrophages to the arterial lesion is predominantly mediated by MCP-1. There are preliminary data showing that both tamoxifen and raloxifene parallel estradiol in reducing the expression of MCP-1 in a model of endothelial cells in culture (Seli et al. 2002).

9.4.1.2.2
VSMC

Indirect evidence suggests that the blockade of VSMC proliferation is associated with ER agonism (Lavigne et al. 1999). The data obtained with SERMs are still sparse and mainly restricted to raloxifene. In experiments in vitro, raloxifene exhibited an effect similar to estrogens in inducing arrest and apoptosis in VSMC (Takahashi et al. 2003; Mori-Abe et al. 2003). Consistent with this observation, raloxifene was equivalent to estradiol in limiting intimal thickening in a model of ovariectomized senile ewes (Selzman et al. 2002). Some evidence favors a similar protective effect for other SERMs, like idoxifene (Yue et al. 2000) and tamoxifen (Dubey et al. 1999; Somjen et al. 1998; Grainger et al. 1993).

9.4.1.2.3
Atherosclerotic Plaque

The biological effects that have been described above, i.e., reduction of LDL and its oxidation, the protection of endothelial function, and the limitation of VSMC proliferation, globally suggest a protective effect against atherosclerosis. This hypothesis has been assayed with the use of distinct animal models with diet-induced atherosclerosis. Some experiments have been carried out in genetically modified mice that have been subjected to targeted inactivation of the apolipoprotein E (apo E) and LDL receptor (LDLR) genes. These animals respond to moderate amounts of dietary cholesterol with severe hypercholesterolemia and develop lipid-rich vascular lesions resembling human atherosclerotic plaques. An atheroprotective effect has been confirmed for estrogens in rabbits (Haines et al. 1999; Haarbo et al. 1991; Bjarnason et al. 1997, 2001; Hough and Zilversmit 1986) and monkeys (Adams et al. 1990; Wagner et al. 1991) subjected to an atherogenic diet. Experiments with LDLR- and apoE-null mice further confirmed that the extent of atheroprotection by estradiol was greater than could be explained solely by the change in lipid levels (Hodgin et al. 2001; Tangirala et al. 1995; Elhage et al. 1997; Marsh et al. 1999).

The data obtained with SERMs are more mixed. Tamoxifen attenuated atheroma development in apoE-null mice, an effect that correlated with changes in the lipoprotein profile and with elevated levels of transforming growth factor-β (Reckless et al. 1997). The accumulation of cholesterol in atherosclerotic lesions (Bjarnason et al. 1997) in the aorta was limited by raloxifene in a model of cholesterol-fed rabbits. Subsequent experiments with the same model confirmed that raloxifene reduced atherosclerosis (Bjarnason et al. 2000), an effect similar to that of estrogens in another study where progression of advanced atherosclerosis was limited (Bjarnason et al. 2001) (Fig. 9.5). In a primate model, however, in which a tête-a-tête comparison between estrogens and raloxifene was carried out, only estrogens, but not raloxifene, effectively limited atherosclerosis (Clarkson et al. 1998). Protection against VSMC proliferation in culture as well as in experimental models of atherogenesis in rats has been described for idoxifene (Yue et al. 2000). A more active reendothelialization was observed in treated animals in the same study.

Only fragmentary information exists in the human. In a study on 27 postmenopausal women with breast cancer, tamoxifen slightly slowed the progression of atherosclerosis as assessed by changes in carotid intima-media thickness (Stamatelopoulos et al. 2004).

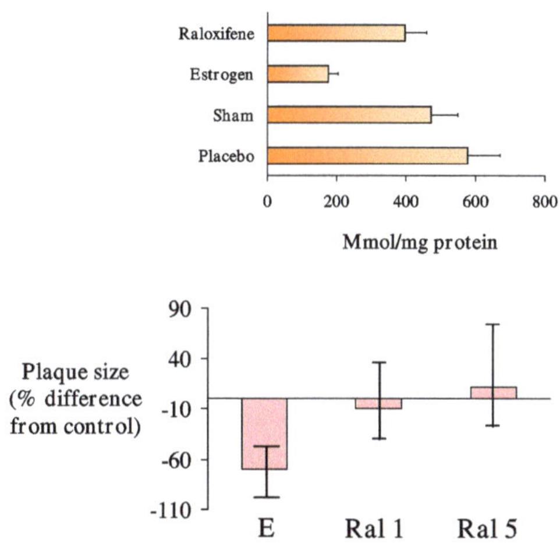

Fig. 9.5. Protection by SERMs against atherosclerosis has been researched in animals. In a model of ovariectomized rabbits, raloxifene reduced the cholesterol content in the inner part of the aorta more than placebo did (*upper panel*). This effect was more intense in animals treated with estradiol (Bjarnason et al. 1997). In contrast, in a different model of oophorectomized monkeys (*lower panel*), estradiol, and not raloxifene at two different dosages, significantly decreased the size of atherosclerotic plaques (Clarkson et al. 1998)

9.4.1.3
Inflammatory Markers and Mediators

The results of both the WHI and HERS studies have contributed decisively to clarifying the difference between atherogenesis itself and the rupture of one atheromatous plaque as the concrete phenomenon leading to an occlusive vascular event. Although necessarily interrelated, the slow progression of a stable plaque, with its consequent reduction of the arterial lumen, may have its ischemic effects limited by the adaptive response including the concurrent development of collateral circulation (Fuster et al. 1992a,b). The concatenation of acute thrombosis as a result of either plaque disruption or severe erosion of the endothelial surface is, however, at the base of most acute coronary syndromes. This concept defines the support of the most widely accepted hypothesis on the action of hormones. As a result of this conception, much interest has arisen in the study of inflammatory mechanisms that underlie disruption of the cap of a lipid-rich plaque, the characteristic form of so-called unstable plaques. It has been shown that estrogens may modify local inflammatory processes and promote the expression and activity of metalloproteinases, a group of enzymes active in the digestion of the matrix (Zanger et al. 2000).

In this new scenario much attention is being paid to the investigation of a series of markers of inflammation as reliable indicators of coronary risk. Their value is stressed by the observation that up to one third of events occurs in subjects without traditional risk factors. The C-reactive protein (CRP) seems to provide the strongest risk prediction for CHD in women (Albert 2000; Ridker 2001), although homocysteine, interleukin-6 (IL-6), and lipoprotein (a) [Lp(a)], among others, have each been independently associated with increased risk for CHD in women (for a review see Davison and Davis 2003; Rader 2000).

As for lipids, the effects of SERMs do not overlap exactly those of HT. Oral estrogens increase the circulating levels of CRP (Writing Group for the PEPI Trial 1995), while this is not the case for raloxifene (Walsh et al. 2000). A better profile was observed for droloxifene as well as for tamoxifen, which achieved a diminution of CRP (Herrington et al. 2001; Cushman et al. 2001).

Slight, yet similar, range decreases were observed for oral estrogens and raloxifene when studied for changes in homocysteine (Walsh et al. 2000; Smolders et al. 2002; Mijatovic et al. 1998; De Leo et al. 2001), a molecule that may have damaging effects on endothelium. A reduction was found for Lp(a), too, although in this case the decrease achieved for estrogens was of a higher magnitude in one study (– 19% vs. – 7%) (Walsh et al. 2001). Droloxifene, however, was more efficient than estrogens in reducing Lp(a) levels (Herrington et al. 2000).

IL-6 participates in both atherogenesis and inflammatory processes. In one interesting mouse model that was double deficient at the apoE and IL-6 loci, animals displayed similar hypercholesterolemia compared to apoE-null mice, but disclosed larger and more calcified lesions at 1 year of age (Klinge 2001). Thus, IL-6 appears to be involved at the fibrous plaque stage of the atherosclerotic process. Moreover, IL-6 is a key factor in the generation of the hepatic acute-phase response and so increases the levels of CRP, fibrinogen, platelet

Table 9.3. Effects of SERMs on inflammatory markers in postmenopausal women

Marker	Author (year)	Intervention Type of drug and dose per day	Type of study	Number of subjects	Effect of SERM
CRP	Walsh (2000)	Raloxifene 60/120 mg vs. Placebo vs. HT	RCT	390	⇔
	Herrington (2001)	Droloxifene 60 mg vs. CEE 0.625 mg	RCT	35	⇓
	Cushman (2001)	Tamoxifen 20 mg vs. placebo	RCT	111	⇓
IL-6	Walsh (2001)	Raloxifene 60 mg vs. placebo vs CEE 0.625 mg + MPA 2.5 mg	RCT	184	⇔
	Gianni (2004)	Raloxifene 60 mg	Observational	14	⇓
Homocysteine	Mijatovic(1998)	Raloxifene 60/120 mg vs. CEE	RCT	52	⇓
	Walsh (2000)	Raloxifene 60/120 mg vs. placebo vs. HT	RCT	390	⇓
	De Leo (2001)	Raloxifene 60 mg vs. placebo	RCT	45	⇓
	Smolders (2002)	Raloxifene 60 mg or 150 mg vs. placebo vs. HT	RCT	95	⇓
TNFα	Walsh (2001)	Raloxifene 60 mg vs. placebo vs. CEE0.625 mg + MPA 2.5 mg	RCT	184	⇓
Lp(a)	Herrington (2000)	Droloxifene 60 mg vs. CEE 0.625 mg	RCT	24	⇓
	Walsh (2001)	Raloxifene 60 mg vs. placebo vs. CEE 0.625 mg + MPA 2.5 mg	RCT	184	⇓

number and activity, and blood viscosity. Only raloxifene has been tested for IL-6, which did not change in one study (Walsh et al. 2001) and decreased by 35% in another study after 24 months of treatment (Gianni et al. 2004). Tumor necrosis factor α (TNFα) is another cytokine associated with cardiovascular risk in epidemiological studies (Ridker et al. 2000). Similar decreases for TNFα have been found in a study comparing HT and raloxifene (Walsh et al. 2001).

In conclusion, SERMs exhibit changes in inflammatory markers that do not match those found with oral HT. Some variability exists within HT itself, depending on the compound (estrogens or tibolone) and on the administration route (oral vs. transdermal). There is sufficient background to hold the value of inflammatory markers as strong indicators of coronary risk, but whether interventions modifying their circulating levels have an influence in risk is still uncertain. A summary of the effects of SERMs on inflammatory markers may be found in Table 9.3.

9.4.1.4
Hemostasia

The apparent protection conferred to the endothelium by estrogens in healthy women operates in favor of platelet stabilization. This interpretation agrees with studies on platelet aggregation that is diminished in response to different stimulants while under exposure to estrogens (Bar et al. 1993, 2000; Nakano et al. 1998; Chen et al. 1998). Nonetheless, in women with advanced atherosclerosis and unstable plaques the picture may be different. Furthermore, little is known about the mechanisms involved in platelet activation, and the sparse evidence is not always favorable to estrogens (García-Martínez et al. 2004). Whether a different profile is imposed by SERMs is not totally clear. Recent work has demonstrated that raloxifene shares with estradiol some protective effects on platelet aggregation induced by ovariectomy (Jayachandran et al. 2005). In a flow chamber model tamoxifen has shown no effect on platelet aggregation (Miller et al. 1994), an effect that agrees with experiments on platelets subjected to different endocrine environments since, unlike hormonal contraceptives, tamoxifen reduced intracellular calcium and release (Miller et al. 1995).

Additionally, attention has been focused on some factors that, operating in the hemostatic balance, have been attributed the role of risk markers of clinical events. Thus, increased plasma concentration of factor VII, fibrinogen, plasminogen activator inhibitor type 1 (PAI-1), and the already mentioned Lp(a) have been associated with the occurrence of CHD. Much work has been done on the modulation of these factors by HT (for a review see Cano and Van Baal 2001), and both similarities and differences have been found in the sparse literature on SERM action. Raloxifene and droloxifene decrease fibrinogen more actively than does HT (Walsh et al. 1998; Herrington et al. 2000). In contrast, the effective reduction demonstrated for PAI-1 with oral HT was not confirmed for raloxifene or droloxifene (Walsh et al. 1998; de Valk-de Roo et al. 1999; Herrington et al. 2000).

9.4.1.5
Clinical Data

There are no randomized clinical trials on the efficacy of SERMs in either the primary or the secondary prevention of CHD. The Raloxifene Use for the Heart

(RUTH) study is a trial specifically designed to clarify the effect of raloxifene on the risk of CHD. The study had included 10,101 women from 26 countries at the closure of the inclusion period, August 2000 (Mosca et al. 2001a). Results from the trial remain to be reported.

Indirect evidence favoring protection has been obtained from a post hoc analysis of the data from the Multiple Outcomes of Raloxifene Evaluation (MORE) study in the subgroup of women who were at increased risk. Using the same scoring system as in the RUTH study to stratify women, a total of 1035 women were assessed as being at significant coronary risk (Barrett-Connor et al. 2002). When women within the group that had been randomized to raloxifene were separated from those randomized to placebo it came up that treatment was associated with protection against new clinical events, and that the higher the score, the greater the protection (Fig. 9.6).

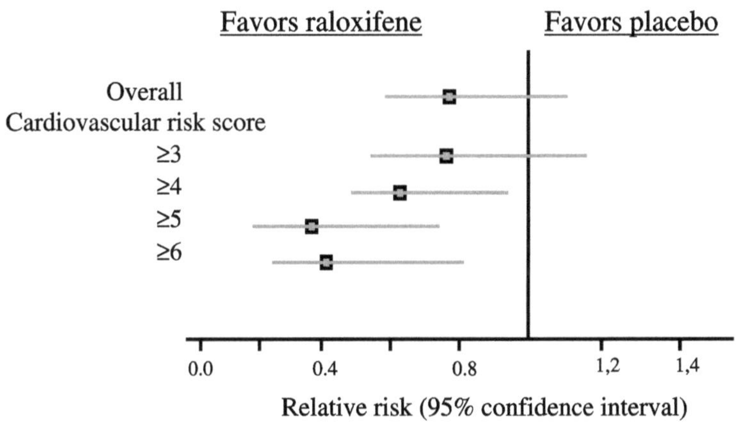

Fig. 9.6. Relative risk (±95% confidence intervals) for any cardiovascular event in the group treated with raloxifene or placebo. The information was obtained from the subgroup of women at increased cardiovascular risk in the MORE study. The overall data seem to favor raloxifene, but this effect is clearer when women were grouped according to their risk as assessed by the previously defined severity score (from Barrett-Connor et al. 2002)

The effects of tamoxifen in women with and without CHD have been analyzed in the National Surgical Adjuvant Breast and Bowel Project Breast Cancer Prevention Trial (BCPT). This randomized, placebo-controlled study included 13,388 women at increased risk for breast cancer. The conclusions of the trial are somewhat limited by the fact that it was designed to investigate the effect of tamoxifen as a chemopreventive for breast cancer, and not its effect on CVD risk. There was no indication that tamoxifen would modify the risk of CHD in women with or without heart disease (Reis et al. 2001).

9.4.2 VTED

A consistent observation linked with estrogen agonism has been the increased risk of VTED. Both hormonal contraceptives and HT determine increased risk oscillating from 2- to 11-fold for contraceptives (Hannaford and Owen-Smith 1998) and from 2- to 4-fold for HT (Daly et al. 1996; Jick et al. 1996; Grodstein et al. 1996; Pérez-Gutthan et al. 1997; Varas-Lorenzo et al. 1998). The risk has been associated with estrogens, but particularly in the case of some third-generation molecules used in contraception, also with the progestogenic component (Vandenbroucke et al. 2001). Interestingly, and despite intensive research, there is not a sufficiently clear understanding of the mechanisms set in motion by hormones to promote risk (Cano and Van Baal 2001). Venous thrombogenesis seems influenced by both hypercoagulable states and flow disturbances, including the independent or collaborative effects of decreased flow and local turbulence (Cano 2003). Much of the research has focused on the inhibitory action that some studies have detected for hormones on the natural anticoagulant system. It is intriguing, however, that increased risk associated with exogenous hormones is not reproduced by endogenous hormones. As mentioned above, age and not gender determines the increase in risk in the general population. Some data find an even slightly higher risk for men during aging (Silverstein et al. 1998).

It is remarkable that most of the data collected from the available SERMs are unanimous in reproducing an estrogen agonistic profile in venous thrombogenesis. The vast clinical experience acquired with tamoxifen confirms an augmented risk for both deep venous thrombosis and pulmonary embolism. This increase, however, did not presuppose increased mortality in the overview of randomized trials of adjuvant tamoxifen for early breast cancer, where the one extra death per 5000 woman-years of tamoxifen attributed to pulmonary embolus was not statistically significant (Early Breast Cancer Trialists' Collaborative Group 1998).

The main source of data for raloxifene derives from the MORE study. A twofold increased risk for VTED was observed through 4 years of followup (Delmas et al. 2002), and, as for HT and tamoxifen, an accumulation of events occurred during the first year.

There is discussion on the adequacy of tests to identify the hypercoagulable states underlying susceptibility to VTED. The complexity of factors and interactions involved in the hemostatic equilibrium has favored the use of functional tests. Among the several options available the measurement of fragments 1 + 2 (F 1 + 2), the amino terminus fragment split during the activation of prothrombin has been widely considered the test of choice. The sparse information available for SERMs, however, is unclear. Raloxifene did not modify

F 1 + 2 fragments in one study where HT was also neutral (Walsh et al. 1998). Other investigators, however, detected slight increases in F 1 + 2 fragments for HT in another direct comparison with raloxifene (de Valk-de Roo et al. 1999).

9.5 Conclusion and Outlook for the Future

The different profiles of the diseases integrated within CVD make their sensitivity to the modulation of ER or, in a more general view encompassing other alternative agonistic pathways, of estrogen action rather variable. There is a clear gender influence on CHD only, but, and of interest, the administration of hormones affects the risk for other forms of CVD, like VTED or stroke. This reality, together with the vast amount of experimental data confirming the action of estrogens on several mechanisms crucial in the pathogenesis of each form of CVD, has reinforced the concept of the important regulatory potential of estrogens. Advances in the knowledge of estrogen action have opened up the field of SERMs, which in one *a priori* analysis should accomplish a peculiar profile of actions. The data obtained to date confirm this assumption.

The greatest amount of information has been compiled for CHD. The most widely used SERMs, like tamoxifen and raloxifene, seem to behave acceptably concerning the mechanisms underlying the disruption of atherosclerotic plaques. This may be an advantage over estrogens, and some preliminary clinical data seem to favor this interpretation. In contrast, it seems estrogens might perform better in protecting against atherosclerosis development. There is very little information on whether SERMs may offer advantages against arterial stroke, although the increase associated with estrogens in recent randomized, placebo-controlled clinical trials have not been detected for SERMs. Although it only offered data on mortality and did not clearly separate the distinct CVD forms, the important overview of randomized trials of adjuvant tamoxifen could not find increased mortality for the aggregate of all cardiac or vascular deaths (Early Breast Cancer Trialists' Collaborative Group 1998).

Venous thrombosis defines a field where there is a strong parallel performance of estrogens and of the SERMs presently developed. This adds to the still mysterious mechanisms underlying the increase in risk that has been found. There is plenty of evidence in favor of an antagonism of hormones on the anticoagulant pathway of hemostatic equilibrium, but very poor data have been obtained with functional tests of coagulation. The dearth of information on the mechanisms by which estrogens/SERMs interfere with anticoagulation further impairs the finding of successful research options.

In conclusion, we are at a very preliminary step on what is probably a long but promising path. The modulation of estrogen action seems a powerful mechanism in the control of CVD risk. Additional advances in the knowledge of estrogen action as well as in the improvement in the design process of new SERMs should offer substantial progress in this area. The concomitant acquisition of clinical data, as is expected from the RUTH study, will consolidate research developments.

References

1. Adams MR, Kaplan JR, Manuck SB, Koritnik DR, Parks JS, Wolfe MS, Clarkson TB (1990) Inhibition of coronary artery atherosclerosis by 17-beta estradiol in ovariectomized monkeys. Lack of an effect of added progesterone. Arteriosclerosis 10:1051–1057
2. Akishita M, Ouchi Y, Miyoshi H, Kozaki K, Inoue S, Ishikawa M, Eto M, Toba K, Orimo H (1997) Estrogen inhibits cuff-induced intimal thickening of rat femoral artery: effects on migration and proliferation of vascular smooth muscle cells. Atherosclerosis 130:1–10
3. Albert MA (2000) The role of C-reactive protein in cardiovascular disease risk. Curr Cardiol Rep 2:274–279
4. Anderson PW, Cox DA, Sashegyi A, Paul S, Silfen SL, Walsh BW (2001) Effects of raloxifene and hormone replacement therapy on markers of serum atherogenicity in healthy postmenopausal women. Maturitas 39:71–77
5. Anderson GL, Limacher M, Assaf AR, Bassford T, Beresford SA, Black H, Bonds D, Brunner R, Brzyski R, Caan B, Chlebowski R, Curb D, Gass M, Hays J, Heiss G, Hendrix S, Howard BV, Hsia J, Hubbell A, Jackson R, Johnson KC, Judd H, Kotchen JM, Kuller L, LaCroix AZ, Lane D, Langer RD, Lasser N, Lewis CE, Manson J, Margolis K, Ockene J, O'Sullivan MJ, Phillips L, Prentice RL, Ritenbaugh C, Robbins J, Rossouw JE, Sarto G, Stefanick ML, Van Horn L, Wactawski-Wende J, Wallace R, Wassertheil-Smoller S, Women's Health Initiative Steering Committee (2004) Effects of conjugated equine estrogen in postmenopausal women with hysterectomy: the Women's Health Initiative randomized controlled trial. J Am Med Assoc 291:1701–1712
6. Arteaga E, Villaseca P, Bianchi M, Rojas A, Marshall G (2003) Raloxifene is a better antioxidant of low-density lipoprotein than estradiol or tamoxifen in postmenopausal women in vitro. Menopause 10:142–146
7. Austin MA, Breslow JL, Hennekens CH, Buring JE, Willett WC, Krauss RM (1988) Low-density lipoprotein subclass patterns and risk of myocardial infarction. J Am Med Assoc 260:1917–1921
8. Badimon JJ, Zaman A, Helft G, Fayad Z, Fuster V (1999) Acute coronary syndromes: pathophysiology and preventive priorities. Thromb Haemost 82:997–1004
9. Bar J, Tepper R, Fuchs J, Pardo J, Goldberger S, Ovadia J (1993) The effect of estrogen replacement therapy on platelet aggregation and adenosine triphosphate release in postmenopausal women. Obstet Gynecol 81:261–264
10. Bar J, Lahav J, Hod M, Ben-Rafael Z, Weinberger I, Brosens J (2000) Regulation of platelet aggregation and adenosine triphosphate release in vitro by 17beta-estradiol and medroxyprogesterone acetate in postmenopausal women. Thromb Haemost 84:695–700
11. Barrett-Connor E, Grady D, Sashegyi A, Anderson PW, Cox DA, Hoszowski K, Rautaharju P, Harper KD, MORE Investigators (Multiple Outcomes of Raloxifene Evaluation) (2002) Raloxifene and cardiovascular events in osteoporotic postmenopausal women: four-year results from the MORE (Multiple Outcomes of Raloxifene Evaluation) randomized trial. J Am Med Assoc 287:847–857

12. Bath PMW, Gray LJ (2005) Association between hormone replacement therapy and subsequent stroke: a meta-analysis. Br Med J DOI:10.1136/BMJ.38331.655347.8F
13. Baumer AT, Wassmann S, Ahlbory K, Strehlow K, Muller C, Sauer H, Bohm M, Nickenig G (2001) Reduction of oxidative stress and AT1 receptor expression by the selective oestrogen receptor modulator idoxifene. Br J Pharmacol 134:579–584
14. Bhalla RC, Toth KF, Bhatty RA, Thompson LP, Sharma RV (1997) Estrogen reduces proliferation and agonist-induced calcium increase in coronary artery smooth muscle cells. Am J Physiol 272:H1996–2003
15. Bjarnason NH, Haarbo J, Byrjalsen I, Kauffman RF, Christiansen C (1997) Raloxifene inhibits aortic accumulation of cholesterol in ovariectomized, cholesterol-fed rabbits. Circulation 96:1964–1969
16. Bjarnason NH, Haarbo J, Byrjalsen I, Kauffman RF, Knadler MP, Christiansen C (2000) Raloxifene reduces atherosclerosis: studies of optimized raloxifene doses in ovariectomized, cholesterol-fed rabbits. Clin Endocrinol 52:225–233
17. Bjarnason NH, Haarbo J, Byrjalsen I, Alexandersen P, Kauffman RF, Christiansen C (2001) Raloxifene and estrogen reduces progression of advanced atherosclerosis – a study in ovariectomized, cholesterol-fed rabbits. Atherosclerosis 154:97–102
18. Blankenberg S, Rupprecht HJ, Bickel C, Peetz D, Hafner G, Tiret L, Meyer J (2001) Circulating cell adhesion molecules and death in patients with coronary artery disease. Circulation 104:1336–1342
19. Blum A, Schenke WH, Hathaway L, Mincemoyer R, Csako G, Waclawiw MA, Cannon RO III (2000) Effects of estrogen and the selective estrogen receptor modulator raloxifene on markers of inflammation in postmenopausal women. Am J Cardiol 86: 892–895
20. Bobryshev YV, Cherian SM, Inder SJ, Lord RSA (1999) Neovascular expression of VE-cadherin in human atherosclerotic arteries in its relation to intimal inflammation. Cardiovasc Res 43:1003–1017
21. British Heart Foundation (2000) European cardiovascular disease statistics
22. Cano A (2003) Blood flow and hemostasis. In: Schneider HPG (ed) Menopause: The State of the Art in Research and Management. Parthenon, London, pp 139–145
23. Cano A, Van Baal WM (2001) The mechanisms of thrombotic risk induced by hormone replacement therapy. Maturitas 40:17–38
24. Ceresini G, Marchini L, Rebecchi I, Morganti S, Bertone L, Montanari I, Bacchi-Modena A, Sgarabotto M, Baldini M, Denti L, Ablondi F, Ceda GP, Valenti G (2003) Effects of raloxifene on carotid blood flow resistance and endothelium-dependent vasodilation in postmenopausal women. Atherosclerosis 167:121–127
25. Chen LY, Mehta P, Mehta JL (1996) Oxidized LDL decreases L-arginine uptake and nitric oxide synthase protein expression in human platelets: relevance of the effect of oxidized LDL on platelet function. Circulation 93: 1740–1746
26. Chen FPL, Lee N, Wang CH, Soong YK (1998) Effects of hormone replacement therapy on cardiovascular risk factors in postmenopausal women. Fertil Steril 69:267–273
27. Chin JH, Azhar S, Hoffman BB (1992) Inactivation of endothelial derived relaxing factor by oxidized lipoproteins. J Clin Invest 89(1):10–18
28. Christopher TA, Lopez BL, Stillwagon JC, Gao F, Gao E, Ma XL, Ohlstein EH, Yue TL (2002) Idoxifene causes endothelium-dependent, nitric oxide-mediated vasorelaxation in male rats. Eur J Pharmacol 446:139–143
29. Clarkson TB (1994) Estrogens, progestins, and coronary heart disease in cynomolgus monkeys. Fertil Steril 62(Suppl 2):147S–151S

30. Clarkson TB, Anthony MS, Jerome CP (1998) Lack of effect of raloxifene on coronary artery atherosclerosis of postmenopausal monkeys. J Clin Endocrinol Metab 83:721–726
31. Colacurci N, Manzella D, Fornaro F, Carbonella M, Paolisso G (2003) Endothelial function and menopause: effects of raloxifene administration. J Clin Endocrinol Metab 88:2135–2140
32. Couzin J (2004) Estrogen's ties to COX-2 may explain heart disease gender gap. Science 306:1277
33. Cushman M, Costantino JP, Tracy RP, Song K, Buckley L, Roberts JD, Krag DN (2001) Tamoxifen and cardiac risk factors in healthy women: suggestion of an anti-inflammatory effect. Arterioscler Thromb Vasc Biol 21:255–261
34. Daly E, Vessey MP, Hawkins MM, Carson JL, Gough P, Marsh S (1996) Risk of venous thromboembolism in users of hormone replacement therapy. Lancet 348: 977–980
35. Davison S, Davis SR (2003) New markers for cardiovascular disease risk in women: impact of endogenous estrogen status and exogenous postmenopausal hormone therapy. J Clin Endocrinol Metab 88:2470–2478
36. Decensi A, Robertson C, Viale G, Pigatto F, Johansson H, Kisanga ER, Veronesi P, Torrisi R, Cazzaniga M, Mora S, Sandri MT, Pelosi G, Luini A, Goldhirsch A, Lien, EA, Veronesi U (2003) A randomized trial of low-dose tamoxifen on breast cancer proliferation and blood estrogenic biomarkers. J Natl Cancer Inst 95: 779–790
37. De Leo V, la Marca A, Morgante G, Lanzetta D, Setacci C, Petraglia F (2001) Randomized control study of the effects of raloxifene on serum lipids and homocysteine in older women. Am J Obstet Gynecol 184:350–353.
38. Delmas PD, Bjarnason NH, Mitlak BH, Ravoux AC, Shah AS, Huster WJ, Draper M, Christiansen C (1997) Effects of raloxifene on bone mineral density, serum cholesterol concentrations, and uterine endometrium in postmenopausal women. N Engl J Med 337:1641–1647
39. Delmas PD, Ensrud KE, Adachi JD, Harper KD, Sarkar S, Gennari C, Reginster JY, Pols HA, Recker RR, Harris ST, Wu W, Genant HK, Black DM, Eastell R (2002) Multiple Outcomes of Raloxifene Evaluation Investigators Efficacy of raloxifene on vertebral fracture risk reduction in postmenopausal women with osteoporosis: four-year results from a randomized clinical trial. J Clin Endocrinol Metab 87: 3609–3617
40. de Valk-de Roo GW, Stehouwer CD, Meijer P, Mijatovic V, Kluft C, Kenemans P, Cohen F, Watts S, Netelenbos C (1999) Both raloxifene and estrogen reduce major cardiovascular risk factors in healthy postmenopausal women: a 2-year, placebo-controlled study. Arterioscler Thromb Vasc Biol 19:2993–3000
41. de Zwart LL, Meerman JH, Commandeur JN, Vermeulen NP (1999) Biomarkers of free radical damage applications in experimental animals and in humans. Free Radic Biol Med 26:202–226
42. Dubey RK, Tyurina YY, Tyurin VA, Gillespie DG, Branch RA, Jackson EK, Kagan VE (1999) Estrogen and tamoxifen metabolites protect smooth muscle cell membrane phospholipids against peroxidation and inhibit cell growth. Circ Res 84:229–239
43. Early Breast Cancer Trialists' Collaborative Group (1998) Tamoxifen for early breast cancer: an overview of the randomised trials. Lancet 351:1451–1467
44. Elhage R, Arnal JF, Pieraggi MT, Duverger N, Fievet C, Faye JC, Bayard F (1997) 17 beta-estradiol prevents fatty streak formation in apolipoprotein E-deficient mice. Arterioscler Thromb Vasc Biol 17:2679–2684

45. Espinosa E, Oemar BS, Luscher TF (1996) 17 beta-Estradiol and smooth muscle cell proliferation in aortic cells of male and female rats. Biochem Biophys Res Commun 221:8–14
46. European Cardiovascular disease statistics. 2000 edition. British Heart Foundation
47. Figtree GA, Webb CM, Collins P (2000) Tamoxifen acutely relaxes coronary arteries by an endothelium-, nitric oxide-, and estrogen receptor-dependent mechanism. J Pharmacol Exp Ther 295:519–523
48. Friedewald WT (1996) Epidemiology of cardiovascular diseases. In: Bennett JC, Plum F (eds) Cecil Textbook of Medicine. Saunders, Philadelphia, pp 170–173
49. Fulimoto J, Sakaguchi H, Hirose R, Tamaya T (1998) Sex steroidal regulation of vessel permeability associated with vessel endothelial cadherin (v-cadherin). J Steroid Biochem Mol Biol 67:25–32
50. Fuster V, Badimon L, Badimon JJ, et al. (1992a) The pathogenesis of coronary artery disease and the acute coronary syndromes. N Engl J Med 326:242–250
51. Fuster V, Badimon L, Badimon JJ, et al. (1992b) The pathogenesis of coronary artery disease and the acute coronary syndromes. N Engl J Med 326:310–318
52. García-Martínez MC, Labiós M, Hermenegildo C, Tarín JJ, O'Connor E, Cano A (2004) The effect of hormone replacement therapy on Ca2+ mobilization and P-selectin (CD62P) expression in platelets examined under flow cytometry. Blood Coagul Fibrinolysis 15:1–8
53. Gaynor JS, Monnet E, Selzman C, Parker D, Kaufman L, Bryant HU, Mallinckrodt C, Wrigley R, Whitehill T, Turner AS (2000) The effect of raloxifene on coronary arteries in aged ovariectomized ewes. J Vet Pharmacol Ther 23:175–179
54. Ghosh U, Ganessunker D, Sattigeri VJ, Carlson KE, Mortensen DJ, Katzenellenbogen BS, Katzenellenbogen JA (2003) Estrogenic diazenes: heterocyclic non-steroidal estrogens of unusual structure with selectivity for estrogen receptor subtypes. Bioorg Med Chem 11:629–657
55. Gianni W, Ricci A, Gazzaniga P, Brama M, Pietropaolo M, Votano S, Patane F, Agliano AM, Spera G, Marigliano V, Ammendola S, Agnusdei D, Migliaccio S, Scandurra R (2004) Raloxifene modulates interleukin-6 and tumor necrosis factor-alpha synthesis in vivo: results from a pilot clinical study. J Clin Endocrinol Metab 89:6097–6099
56. Gonzalez-Perez J, Crespo MJ (2003) Chronic effects of toremifene on the vasculature of menopause-induced rats. Vasc Pharmacol 40:261–268
57. Grainger DJ, Weissberg PL, Metcalfe JC (1993) Tamoxifen decreases the rate of proliferation of rat vascular smooth-muscle cells in culture by inducing production of transforming growth factor beta. Biochem J 294:109–112
58. Griendling KK, Alexander RW (1997) Oxidative stress and cardiovascular disease. Circulation 96:3264–3265
59. Griffiths KA, Sader MA, Skilton MR, Harmer JA, Celermajer DS (2003) Effects of raloxifene on endothelium-dependent dilation, lipoproteins, and markers of vascular function in postmenopausal women with coronary artery disease. J Am Coll Cardiol 42:698–704
60. Grodstein F, Stampfer MJ, Goldhaber SZ, Goldhaber SZ, Manson JE, Colditz GA, Speizer FE, et al. (1996) Prospective study of exogenous hormones and risk of pulmonary embolism in women. Lancet 348:983–987
61. Gross M, Steffes M, Jacobs DR Jr, Yu X, Lewis L, Lewis CE, Loria CM (2005) Plasma F2-isoprostanes and coronary artery calcification: the CARDIA study. Clin Chem 51:125–131

62. Haarbo J, Hansen BF, Christiansen C (1991) Hormone replacement therapy prevents coronary artery disease in ovariectomized cholesterol-fed rabbits. APMIS 99: 721–727
63. Haarbo J, Leth-Espensen P, Stender S, Christiansen C (1991) Estrogen monotherapy and combined estrogen-progestogen replacement therapy attenuate aortic accumulation of cholesterol in ovariectomized cholesterol-fed rabbits. J Clin Invest 87:1274–1279
64. Haines CJ, James AE, Panesar NS, Ngai TJ, Sahota DS, Jones RL, Chang AM (1999) The effect of percutaneous oestradiol on atheroma formation in ovariectomized cholesterol-fed rabbits. Atherosclerosis 143:369–375
65. Hannaford PC, Owen-Smith V (1998) Using epidemiological data to guide clinical practice: review of studies on cardiovascular disease and use of combined oral contraceptives. Br Med J 316:984–987
66. Harrington WR, Sheng S, Barnett DH, Petz LN, Katzenellenbogen JA, Katzenellenbogen BS (2003) Activities of estrogen receptor alpha- and beta-selective ligands at diverse estrogen responsive gene sites mediating transactivation or transrepression. Mol Cell Endocrinol 206:13–22
67. Heikkinen AM, Niskanen L, Yla-Herttuala S, Luoma J, Tuppurainen MT, Komulainen M, Saarikoski S (1998) Postmenopausal hormone replacement therapy and autoantibodies against oxidized LDL. Maturitas 29:155–161
68. Hermenegildo C, García-Martínez MC, Tarín JJ, Llácer A, Cano A (2001) The effect of oral hormone replacement therapy on lipoprotein profile, resistance of LDL to oxidation and LDL particle size. Maturitas 38:287–295
69. Hermenegildo C, García-Martínez MC, Tarín JJ, Cano A (2002) Inhibition of low-density lipoprotein oxidation by the pure antiestrogens ICI 182780 and EM-652 (SCH 57068). Menopause 9:430–435
70. Herrington DM, Pusser BE, Riley WA, Thuren TY, Brosnihan KB, Brinton EA, MacLean DB (2000) Cardiovascular effects of droloxifene, a new selective estrogen receptor modulator, in healthy postmenopausal women. Arterioscler Thromb Vasc Biol 20:1606–1612
71. Herrington DM, Brosnihan KB, Pusser BE, Seely EW, Ridker PM, Rifai N, MacLean DB (2001) Differential effects of E and droloxifene on C-reactive protein and other markers of inflammation in healthy postmenopausal women. J Clin Endocrinol Metab 86:4216–4222
72. Hodgin JB, Krege JH, Reddick RL, Korach KS, Smithies O, Maeda N (2001) Estrogen receptor alpha is a major mediator of 17beta-estradiol's atheroprotective effects on lesion size in Apoe-/- mice. J Clin Invest 107:333–340
73. Hodis HN, Mack WJ, Azen SP, Lobo RA, Shoupe D, Mahrer PR, Faxon DP, Cashin-Hemphill L, Sanmarco ME, French WJ, Shook TL, Gaarder TD, Mehra AO, Rabbani R, Sevanian A, Shil AB, Torres M, Vogelbach KH, Selzer RH, Women's Estrogen-Progestin Lipid-Lowering Hormone Atherosclerosis Regression Trial Research Group (2003) Hormone therapy and the progression of coronary-artery atherosclerosis in postmenopausal women. N Engl J Med 349:535–545
74. Hoogerbrugge N, Zillikens MC, Jansen H, Meeter K, Deckers JW, Birkenhager JC (1998) Estrogen replacement decreases the level of antibodies against oxidized low-density lipoprotein in postmenopausal women with coronary heart disease. Metabolism 47:675–680
75. Hough JL, Zilversmit DB (1986) Effect of 17 beta estradiol on aortic cholesterol content and metabolism in cholesterol-fed rabbits. Arteriosclerosis 6:57–63
76. Hozumi Y, Kawano M, Miyata M (1997) Severe hypertriglyceridemia caused by tamoxifen-treatment after breast cancer surgery. Endocr J 44:745–749

77. Hulley S, Grady D, Bush T, Furberg C, Herrington D, Riggs B, Vittinghoff E (1998) Randomized trial of estrogen plus progestin for secondary prevention of coronary heart disease in postmenopausal women. Heart and Estrogen/progestin Replacement Study (HERS) Research Group. J Am Med Assoc 280:605–613
78. Hutchison SJ, Chou TM, Chatterjee K, Sudhir K (2001) Tamoxifen is an acute, estrogen-like, coronary vasodilator of porcine coronary arteries in vitro. J Cardiovasc Pharmacol 38:657–665
79. Hwang SJ, Ballantyne CM, Sharrett AR, Smith LC, Davis CE, Gotto AM Jr, Boerwinkle E (1997) Circulating adhesion molecules VCAM-1, ICAM-1, and E-selectin in carotid atherosclerosis and incident coronary heart disease cases: the Atherosclerosis Risk In Communities (ARIC) study. Circulation 96:4219–4225
80. Jayachandran M, Mukherjee R, Steinkamp T, Labreche P, Bracamonte MP, Okano H, Owen WG, Miller VM (2005) Differential effects of 17{beta}-estradiol, conjugated equine estrogen and raloxifene on mRNA expression, aggregation and secretion in platelets. Am J Physiol Heart Circ Physiol 288:H2355–362
81. Jick H, Derby LE, Myers MW, Vasilakis C, Newton KM (1996) Risk of hospital admission for idiopathic venous thromboembolism among users of postmenopausal oestrogens. Lancet 348:981–983
82. Joensuu H, Holli K, Oksanen H, Valavaara R (2000) Serum lipid levels during and after adjuvant toremifene or tamoxifen therapy for breast cancer. Breast Cancer Res Treat 63:225–234
83. Jokela H, Dastidar P, Rontu R, Salomaki A, Teisala K, Lehtimaki T, Punnonen R (2003) Effects of long-term estrogen replacement therapy versus combined hormone replacement therapy on nitric oxide-dependent vasomotor function. J Clin Endocrinol Metab 88:4348–4354
84. Kanel KT, Wolmark N, Thompson PD (1997) Delayed severe hypertriglyceridemia from tamoxifen. N Engl J Med 337:281
85. Karas RH, Patterson BL, Mendelsohn ME (1994) Human vascular smooth muscle cells contain functional estrogen receptor. Circulation 89:1943–1950
86. Klinge CM (2001) Estrogen receptor interaction with estrogen response elements. Nucleic Acids Res 29:2905
87. Koh KK, Bui MN, Mincemoyer R, Cannon RO III (1997) Effects of hormone therapy on inflammatory cell adhesion molecules in postmenopausal healthy women. Am J Cardiol 80:1505–1507
88. Kugiyama K, Kerns SA, Morrisett JD, Roberts R, Henry PD (1990) Impairment of endothelium-dependent arterial relaxation by lysolecithin in modified low-density lipoproteins. Nature 344:160–162
89. Lavigne MC, Ramwell PW, Clarke R (1999) Inhibition of estrogen receptor function promotes porcine coronary artery smooth muscle cell proliferation. Steroids 64:472–480
90. Li L, Haynes MP, Bender JR (2003) Plasma membrane localization and function of the estrogen receptor alpha variant (ER46) in human endothelial cells. Proc Natl Acad Sci USA 100:4807–4812
91. Liu TZ, Stern A, Morrow JD (1998) The isoprostanes: unique bioactive products of lipid peroxidation: an overview. J Biomed Sci 5:415–420
92. Marsh MM, Walker VR, Curtiss LK, Banka CL (1999) Protection against atherosclerosis by estrogen is independent of plasma cholesterol levels in LDL receptor-deficient mice. J Lipid Res 40:893–900
93. Mendelsohn ME (2000) Mechanisms of estrogen action in the cardiovascular system. J Steroid Biochem Mol Biol 74:337–343

94. Mendelsohn ME (2002) Genomic and nongenomic effects of estrogen in the vasculature. Am J Cardiol 90(1A):3F–6F
95. Mijatovic V, Netelenbos C, van der Mooren MJ, de Valk-de Roo GW, Jakobs C, Kenemans P (1998) Randomized, double-blind, placebo-controlled study of the effects of raloxifene and conjugated equine estrogen on plasma homocysteine levels in healthy postmenopausal women. Fertil Steril 70:1085–1089
96. Miller M (1998) Is hypertriglyceridaemia an independent risk factor for coronary heart disease? The epidemiological evidence. Eur Heart J 19(Suppl H):H18–22
97. Miller ME, Dores GM, Thorpe SL, Akerley WL (1994) Paradoxical influence of estrogenic hormones on platelet-endothelial cell interactions. Thromb Res 74:577–594
98. Miller ME, Thorpe SL, Dores GM (1995) Influence of hormones on platelet intracellular calcium. Thromb Res 77:515–530
99. Moraghan T, Antoniucci DM, Grenert JP, Sieck GC, Johnson C, Miller VM, Fitzpatrick LA (1996) Differential response in cell proliferation to beta estradiol in coronary arterial vascular smooth muscle cells obtained from mature female versus male animals. Endocrinology 137:5174–5177
100. Morel DW, Hessler JR, Chisholm GM (1983) Low density lipoprotein cytotoxicity induced by free radical peroxidation of lipid. J Lipid Res 24:1070–1076
101. Mori-Abe A, Tsutsumi S, Takahashi K, Toya M, Yoshida M, Du B, Kawagoe J, Nakahara K, Takahashi T, Ohmichi M, Kurachi H (2003) Estrogen and raloxifene induce apoptosis by activating p38 mitogen-activated protein kinase cascade in synthetic vascular smooth muscle cells. J Endocrinol 178:417–426
102. Mosca L, Barrett-Connor E, Wenger NK, Collins P, Grady D, Kornitzer M, Moscarelli E, Paul S, Wright TJ, Helterbrand JD, Anderson PW (2001a) Design and methods of the Raloxifene Use for The Heart (RUTH) study. Am J Cardiol 88: 392–395
103. Mosca L, Harper K, Sarkar S, O'Gorman J, Anderson PW, Cox DA, Barrett-Connor E (2001b) Effect of raloxifene on serum triglycerides in postmenopausal women: influence of predisposing factors for hypertriglyceridemia. Clin Ther 23:1552–1565
104. Mosca L, Appel LJ, Benjamin EJ, Berra K, Chandra-Strobos N, Fabunmi RP, Grady D, Haan CK, Hayes SN, Judelson DR, Keenan NL, McBride P, Oparil S, Ouyang P, Oz MC, Mendelsohn ME, Pasternak RC, Pinn VW, Robertson RM, Schenck-Gustafsson K, Sila CA, Smith SC Jr, Sopko G, Taylor AL, Walsh BW, Wenger NK, Williams CL, American Heart Association (2004) Evidence-based guidelines for cardiovascular disease prevention in women. Circulation 109:672–693
105. Muthyala RS, Sheng S, Carlson KE, Katzenellenbogen BS, Katzenellenbogen JA (2003) Bridged bicyclic cores containing a 1,1-diarylethylene motif are high-affinity subtype-selective ligands for the estrogen receptor. J Med Chem 46:1589–1602
106. Nakano Y, Oshima T, Matsuura H, Kajiyama G, Kambe M (1998) Effect of 17beta-estradiol on inhibition of platelet aggregation in vitro is mediated by an increase in NO synthesis. Arterioscler Thromb Vasc Biol 18:961–967
107. Navab M, Berliner JA, Watson AD, et al. (1996) The Yin and Yang of oxidation in the development of the fatty streak: a review based on the 1994 George Lyman Duff Memorial Lecture. Arterioscler Thromb Vasc Biol 16:831–842
108. Niebauer J, Maxwell AJ, Lin PS, Wang D, Tsao PS, Cooke JP (2003) NOS inhibition accelerates atherogenesis: reversal by exercise. Am J Physiol Heart Circ Physiol 285:H535–540
109. Oguogho A, Kritz H, Wagner O, Sinzinger H (2001) 6-oxo-PGF(1 alpha) and 8-epi-PGF(2 alpha) in the arterial wall layers of various species: a comparison between intact and atherosclerotic areas. Prostaglandins Leukot Essent Fatty Acids 64:167–171

110. Oviedo PJ, Hermenegildo C, Cano A (2004) Raloxifene increases the capacity of serum to promote prostacyclin release in human endothelial cells: implication of COX-1 and COX-2. Menopause 11:430–437
111. Oviedo P, Hermenegildo C, Tarín JJ, Cano A (2005) Raloxifene promotes prostacyclin release in human endothelial cells role of COX-1 and COX-2. Fertil Steril 83:1822–1829
112. Pérez-Gutthan S, García-Rodríguez LA, Castellsague J, Duque-Oliart A (1997) Hormone replacement therapy and risk of venous thromboembolism: population based case-control study. Br Med J 314:796–800
113. Perrault LP, Malo O, Bidouard JP, Villeneuve N, Vilaine JP, Vanhoutte PM (2003) Inhibiting the NO pathway with intracoronary L-NAME infusion increases endothelial dysfunction and intimal hyperplasia after heart transplantation. J Heart Lung Transplant 22:439–451
114. Pratico D (1999) F(2)-isoprostanes: sensitive and specific non-invasive indices of lipid peroxidation in vivo. Atherosclerosis 147:1–10
115. Rader DJ (2000) Inflammatory markers of coronary risk. N Engl J Med 343:1179
116. Rahimian R, Dube GP, Toma W, Dos Santos N, McManus BM, van Breemen C (2002) Raloxifene enhances nitric oxide release in rat aorta via increasing endothelial nitric oxide mRNA expression. Eur J Pharmacol 434:141–149
117. Reckless J, Metcalfe JC, Grainger DJ (1997) Tamoxifen decreases cholesterol sevenfold and abolishes lipid lesion development in apolipoprotein E knockout mice. Circulation 95:1542–1548
118. Reid IR, Eastell R, Fogelman I, Adachi JD, Rosen A, Netelenbos C, Watts NB, Seeman E, Ciaccia AV, Draper MW (2004) A comparison of the effects of raloxifene and conjugated equine estrogen on bone and lipids in healthy postmenopausal women. Arch Intern Med 164:871–879
119. Reis SE, Costantino JP, Wickerham DL, Tan-Chiu E, Wang J, Kavanah M (2001) Cardiovascular effects of tamoxifen in women with and without heart disease: breast cancer prevention trial. National Surgical Adjuvant Breast and Bowel Project Breast Cancer Prevention Trial Investigators. J Natl Cancer Inst 93:16–21
120. Resnick N, Gimbrone MA Jr (1995) Hemodynamic forces are complex regulators of endothelial gene expression. FASEB J 9:874–882
121. Ricciardelli C, Horsfall DJ, Sykes PJ, Marshall VR, Tilley WD (1994) Effects of oestradiol-17 beta and 5 alpha-dihydrotestosterone on guinea-pig prostate smooth muscle cell proliferation and steroid receptor expression in vitro. J Endocrinol 140:373–383
122. Ridker PM (2001) High-sensitivity C-reactive protein: potential adjunct for global risk assessment in the primary prevention of cardiovascular disease. Circulation 103:1813–1818
123. Ridker PM, Rifai N, Pfeffer M, Sacks F, Lepage S, Braunwald E (2000) Elevation of tumor necrosis factor-alpha and increased risk of recurrent coronary events after myocardial infarction. Circulation 101:2149–2153
124. Rosendaal FR (1999) Venous thrombosis: a multicausal disease. Lancet 353: 1167–73
125. Ross R (1999) Atherosclerosis – an inflammatory disease. N Engl J Med 340:115–126
126. Rossouw JE, Anderson GL, Prentice RL, LaCroix AZ, Kooperberg C, Stefanick ML, et al. (2002) Risks and benefits of estrogen plus progestin in healthy postmenopausal women: principal results From the Women's Health Initiative randomized controlled trial. J Am Med Assoc 288:321–333
127. Saarto T, Blomqvist C, Ehnholm C, Taskinen MR, Elomaa I (1996) Antiatherogenic effects of adjuvant antiestrogens: a randomized trial comparing the effects of tamoxifen

and toremifene on plasma lipid levels in postmenopausal women with node-positive breast cancer. J Clin Oncol 14:429–433
128. Saitta A, Altavilla D, Cucinotta D, Morabito N, Frisina N, Corrado F, D'Anna R, Lasco A, Squadrito G, Gaudio A, Cancellieri F, Arcoraci V, Squadrito F (2001) Randomized, double-blind, placebo-controlled study on effects of raloxifene and hormone replacement therapy on plasma no concentrations, endothelin-1 levels, and endothelium-dependent vasodilation in postmenopausal women. Arterioscler Thromb Vasc Biol 21:1512–1519
129. Santanam N, Shern-Brewer R, McClatchey R, Castellano PZ, Murphy AA, Voelkel S, Parthasarathy S (1998) Estradiol as an antioxidant: incompatible with its physiological concentrations and function. J Lip Res 39:2111–2118
130. Sarrel PM, Nawaz H, Chan W, Fuchs M, Katz DL (2003) Raloxifene and endothelial function in healthy postmenopausal women. Am J Obstet Gynecol 188:304–309
131. Sbarouni E, Flevari P, Kroupis C, Kyriakides ZS, Koniavitou K, Kremastinos DT (2003) The effects of raloxifene and simvastatin on plasma lipids and endothelium. Cardiovasc Drugs Ther 17:319–323
132. Seli E, Pehlivan T, Selam B, Garcia-Velasco JA, Arici A (2002) Estradiol down-regulates MCP-1 expression in human coronary artery endothelial cells. Fertil Steril 77: 542–547
133. Selzman CH, Turner AS, Gaynor JS, Miller SA, Monnet E, Harken AH (2002) Inhibition of intimal hyperplasia using the selective estrogen receptor modulator raloxifene. Arch Surg 137:333–336
134. Silverstein MD, Heit JA, Mohr DN, et al. (1998) Trends in the incidence of deep vein thrombosis and pulmonary embolism: a 25-year population-based study. Arch Intern Med 158:585–593
135. Simoncini T, Genazzani AR (2000) Raloxifene acutely stimulates nitric oxide release from human endothelial cells via an activation of endothelial nitric oxide synthase. J Clin Endocrinol Metab 85:2966–2969
136. Simoncini T, De Caterina R, Genazzani AR (1999) Selective estrogen receptor modulators: different actions on vascular cell adhesion molecule-1 (VCAM-1) expression in human endothelial cells. J Clin Endocrinol Metab 84:815–818
137. Smolders RG, Vogelvang TE, Mijatovic V, van Baal WM, Neele SJ, Netelenbos JC, Kenemans P, van der Mooren MJ (2002) A 2-year, randomized, comparative, placebo-controlled study on the effects of raloxifene on lipoprotein(a) and homocysteine. Maturitas 41:105–114
138. Somjen D, Kohen F, Jaffe A, Amir-Zaltsman Y, Knoll E, Stern N (1998) Effects of gonadal steroids and their antagonists on DNA synthesis in human vascular cells. Hypertension 32:39–45
139. Song J, Wan Y, Rolfe BE, Campbell JH, Campbell GR (1998) Effect of estrogen on vascular smooth muscle cells is dependent upon cellular phenotype. Atherosclerosis 140:97–104
140. Speroff L (2002) The impact of the Women's Health Initiative on clinical practice. J Soc Gynecol Invest 9:251–253
141. Spyridopoulos I, Sullivan AB, Kearney M, Isner JM, Losordo DW (1997) Estrogen-receptor-mediated inhibition of human endothelial cell apoptosis. Estradiol as a survival factor. Circulation 95:1505–1514
142. Stamatelopoulos KS, Lekakis JP, Poulakaki NA, Papamichael CM, Venetsanou K, Aznaouridis K, Protogerou AD, Papaioannou TG, Kumar S, Stamatelopoulos SF (2004) Tamoxifen improves endothelial function and reduces carotid intima-media thickness in postmenopausal women. Am Heart J 147:1093–1099

143. Steinberg D (1997) Low density lipoprotein oxidation and its pathobiological significance. J Biol Chem 272:20963–20966
144. Takahashi K, Ohmichi M, Yoshida M, Hisamoto K, Mabuchi S, Arimoto-Ishida E, Mori A, Tsutsumi S, Tasaka K, Murata Y, Kurachi H (2003) Both estrogen and raloxifene cause G1 arrest of vascular smooth muscle cells. J Endocrinol 178: 319–329
145. Tangirala RK, Rubin EM, Palinski W (1995) Quantitation of atherosclerosis in murine models: correlation between lesions in the aortic origin and in the entire aorta, and differences in the extent of lesions between sexes in LDL receptor-deficient and apolipoprotein E-deficient mice. J Lipid Res 36:2320–2328
146. Tatchum-Talom R, Martel C, Labrie F, Marette A (2003) Acute vascular effects of the selective estrogen receptor modulator EM-652 (SCH 57068) in the rat mesenteric vascular bed. Cardiovasc Res 57:535–543
147. Thorin E, Pham-Dang M, Clement R, Mercier I, Calderone A (2003) Hyper-reactivity of cerebral arteries from ovariectomized rats: therapeutic benefit of tamoxifen. Br J Pharmacol 140:1187–1192
148. Todaka T, Yokoyama C, Yanamoto H, Hashimoto N, Nagata I, Tsukahara T, Hara S, Hatae T, Morishita R, Aoki M, Ogihara T, Kaneda Y, Tanabe T (1999) Gene transfer of human prostacyclin synthase prevents neointimal formation after carotid balloon injury in rats. Stroke 30:419–426
149. Uint L, Gebara OC, Pinto LB, Wajngarten M, Boschcov P, da Luz PL, Gidlund M (2003) Hormone replacement therapy increases levels of antibodies against heat shock protein 65 and certain species of oxidized low density lipoprotein. Braz J Med Biol Res 36:491–494
150. Vandenbroucke JP, Rosing J, Bloemenkamp KW, Middeldorp S, Helmerhorst FM, Bouma BN, Rosendaal FR (2001) Oral contraceptives and the risk of venous thrombosis. N Engl J Med 344:1527–1535
151. Varas-Lorenzo C, García-Rodríguez LA, Cattaruzzi C, Troncon MG, Agostinis L, Pérez-Gutthann S (1998) Hormone replacement therapyand the risk of hospitalization for venous thromboembolism: a population-based study in southern Europe. Am J Epidemiol 147:387–390
152. Vargas R, Hewes B, Rego A, Farhat MY, Suarez R, Ramwell PW (1996) Estradiol effect on rate of proliferation of rat carotid segments: effect of gender and tamoxifen. J Cardiovasc Pharmacol 27:495–499
153. Vassalle C, Botto N, Andreassi MG, Berti S, Biagini A (2003) Evidence for enhanced 8-isoprostane plasma levels, as index of oxidative stress in vivo, in patients with coronary artery disease. Coron Artery Dis 14:213–218
154. Venkov C, Rankin A, Vaughan D (1996) Identification of authentic estrogen receptor in cultured endothelial cells: a potential mechanism for steroid hormone regulation of endothelial function. Circulation 94:727–733
155. Vogelvang TE, Mijatovic V, Kenemans P, Teerlink T, van der Mooren MJ (2004) HMR 3339, a novel selective estrogen receptor modulator, reduces total cholesterol, low-density lipoprotein cholesterol, and homocysteine in healthy postmenopausal women. Fertil Steril 82:1540–1549
156. Wagner JD, Clarkson TB, St Clair RW, Schwenke DC, Shively CA, Adams MR (1991) Estrogen and progesterone replacement therapy reduces low density lipoprotein accumulation in the coronary arteries of surgically postmenopausal cynomolgus monkeys. J Clin Invest 88:1995–2002
157. Walsh BW, Cox DA, Sashegyi A, Dean RA, Tracy RP, Anderson PW (2001) Role of tumor necrosis factor-alpha and interleukin-6 in the effects of hormone replacement

therapy and raloxifene on C-reactive protein in postmenopausal women. Am J Cardiol 88:825–828
158. Walsh BW, Kuller LH, Wild RA, Paul S, Farmer M, Lawrence JB, et al. (1998) Effects of raloxifene on serum lipids and coagulation factors in healthy postmenopausal women. J Am Med Assoc 279:1445–1451
159. Walsh BW, Paul S, Wild RA, Dean RA, Tracy RP, Cox DA, Anderson PW (2000) The effects of hormone replacement therapy and raloxifene on C-reactive protein and homocysteine in healthy postmenopausal women: a randomized, controlled trial. J Clin Endocrinol Metab 85:214–218
160. Wassmann S, Laufs U, Stamenkovic D, Linz W, Stasch JP, Ahlbory K, Rosen R, Bohm M, Nickenig G (2002) Raloxifene improves endothelial dysfunction in hypertension by reduced oxidative stress and enhanced nitric oxide production. Circulation 105:2083–2091
161. White RH (2003) The epidemiology of venous thromboembolism. Circulation 107(23 Suppl 1):I4–8
162. Writing Group for the PEPI Trial (1995) Effects of estrogen or estrogen/progestin regimens on heart disease risk factors in postmenopausal women. The Postmenopausal Estrogen/Progestin Interventions (PEPI) Trial. J Am Med Assoc 273:199–208
163. Ylikorkala O, Cacciatore B, Halonen K, Lassila R, Lammintausta R, Rutanen EM, Heikkinen J, Komi J (2003) Effects of ospemifene, a novel SERM, on vascular markers and function in healthy, postmenopausal women. Menopause 10:440–447
164. Yue TL, Vickery-Clark L, Louden CS, Gu JL, Ma XL, Narayanan PK, Li X, Chen J, Storer B, Willette R, Gossett KA, Ohlstein EH (2000) Selective estrogen receptor modulator idoxifene inhibits smooth muscle cell proliferation, enhances reendothelialization, and inhibits neointimal formation in vivo after vascular injury. Circulation 102(Suppl 3):III281–288
165. Zanger D, Yang BK, Ardans J, Waclawiw MA, Csako G, Wahl LM, Cannon RO III (2000) Divergent effects of hormone therapy on serum markers of inflammation in postmenopausal women with coronary artery disease on appropriate medical management. J Am Coll Cardiol 36:1797–1802
166. Zuckerman SH, Bryan N (1996) Inhibition of LDL oxidation and myeloperoxidase dependent tyrosyl radical formation by the selective estrogen receptor modulator raloxifene (LY139481 HCL). Atherosclerosis 126:65–75

Chapter 10

SERMs and the Breast

Joaquim Calaf i Alsina · Antonio Cano Sanchez

10.1 Introduction

Lactation is a basic period in mammalian reproduction, and the breast, its function, and pathology have a very important place in medicine and society. In developed countries breast cancer is the most important issue, far more important than nonlactational galactorrhea; it is frequently related to infertility or unsuccessful breastfeeding and is a major health concern among women.

Breast cancer is the most common malignant tumor in women. It comprises 18% of all female cancers, before cervix (15%) and colon (9%) cancer. After lung cancer it is the most frequent malignancy resulting in death (Brinton and Devesa 1996). However, the incidence and mortality vary widely among countries. From 6 per 100,000 women/year in Japan to almost 30 in the UK. Studies in migrants show that the rates of breast cancer tend to be those of the host country within one or two generations and become different from those of the family members remaining in the country of origin. This suggests that nutritional and other environmental factors are more important than genetics.

Age is the most important risk factor. Both the incidence of the disease and related mortality increase with age, and there is a clear slowing after menopause (Fig. 10.1). This alone suggests a relationship between estrogen priming and the incidence of the disease. This is corroborated by the differences in incidence according to the duration of reproductive life. Early menarche or late menopause increases the risk of presenting a breast cancer, and having had an oophorectomy before age 35 lowers the risk of presenting breast cancer to 40% of that presented by women reaching natural menopause at around age 50. Other anthropometric factors like body weight or body mass index are negatively related to breast cancer incidence. Skin and fat tissue are major sites for aromatase, an enzyme converting androgenic precursors to estrogens, and consequently obese women are able to produce more estrogens. Obesity is also negatively related to circulating levels of sex hormone binding globulin (SHBG), a plasmatic protein that binds potent estrogens like estradiol, and thus leaving a higher percentage of circulating estrogens "free" to bind

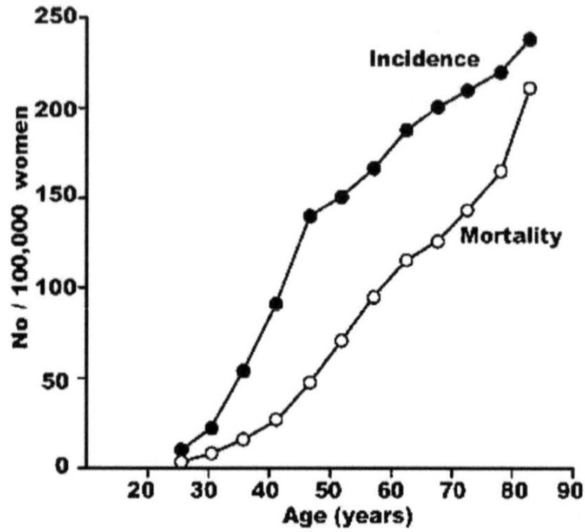

Fig. 10.1. Age-specific incidence and mortality for breast cancer in United Kingdom. Reproduced with permission from McPherson et al. (2000)

to estrogen receptors (ERs). Other risk factors identified, like socioeconomic group, alcohol consumption, and saturated-fat-rich diets, seem to act through an increase in the ability to produce estrogens.

With these evidences in mind the rationality of any attempt at blocking the access of an estrogen molecule to its receptor, and consequently diminishing the risk of breast cancer, seems justified. SERMs, a family of molecules characterized by their ability to bind to ERs with high affinity and competing with genuine estrogens, are in a preferential position to play this role. In fact tamoxifen, the first widely used SERM, has been the major tool for adjuvant therapy in early, ER(+) breast cancer and remains the only drug accepted for preventive intervention in high-risk women. In this battle against breast cancer SERMs have to find their place among new agents also able to minimize the estrogenic stimulation of the breast cell, normal or neoplastic, as aromatase inhibitors or "pure" ER antagonists.

In this chapter we will review the basic aspects of endocrine regulation of breast tissue growth and development. The relationship between genetics, estrogen exposure, and breast cancer risk will be discussed, and preclinical and clinical experience in the use of SERMS for both prevention and adjuvant treatment of ER-positive breast cancer will be reviewed and put in perspective.

10.2 Biology of Breast Development and its Endocrine Regulation

Mammary epithelium is very sensitive to hormonal stimulation. It is where proliferative events take place and where neoplastic transformation begins.

Crucial for the understanding of this process are the studies of Russo (Russo and Russo 1997), according to which any carcinogenetic action takes place in the less differentiated and highly proliferating areas of the breast.

Consequently, breast cancer develops as the result of the synergy between a foreign stimulating agent and an especially sensitive area of the mammary epithelium. According to Russo and coworkers (1992), the mammary ductal tree shows a clear regional specialization. From their studies it can be deduced that, from birth, the mammary gland enters in a continuous branching process giving rise to the lobules. Since this is a dynamic process, lobules can be found in different developmental stages that have been classified in four categories. Type 1 lobule, also called the terminal ductal lobular unit, is the less differentiated structure.

Type 1 lobules evolve into type 2 lobules by incorporating a higher number of ducts. During pregnancy all of them progress to type 3 lobules endowed with a highly dense duct branching system. Lactation is based on type 4 lobules, with an intense secreting activity that regresses to types 2 and 3 after weaning. After menopause the majority of these structures regress to type 1 (Russo et al. 1992). Consequently, pregnancy is a determinant factor for the development of type 3 and 4 lobules and, in nulliparae, type 1 is predominant. It is in this type of lobule where cancer develops more frequently. After age 50 the lobular composition of the breast tissue is predominantly composed of type 1 lobules in both nulliparae and early para women. However, the risk of developing a cancer is higher in nulliparae, and it is plausible that type 1 lobules from the former have a higher malignancy potential since they have never reached type 4 differentiation.

Explaining this higher tendency to malignancy are the observations of a higher proliferating activity in type 1 lobules, especially in nulliparae, and also a higher concentration of estrogen and progesterone receptors. According to this, the majority of the most common breast cancers arise from type 1 lobules, whereas type 2 lobules used to be the place of origin of atypical hyperplasias or in situ carcinomas. Type 3 lobules are the site of fibro-adenomas or cysts (Wellings et al. 1975).

10.3 Framework of Breast Cancer Research

An integrated analysis of the biological, epidemiological, and clinical data recently available has led to a multitarget approach to the investigation of the origins of breast cancer (Wolman et al. 1997). This involves new knowledge in molecular genetics, cellular biology, and endocrine environment.

In the field of molecular genetics, several susceptibility genes for breast cancer have been identified. The genes involved in the regulation of development and differentiation of normal breast tissue and the role of their abnormality in the onset of a tumor are crucial in the understanding of the disease. The isolation of the proteins regulated by these genes open new approaches for tumoral research (McPherson et al. 2000).

Two genes, BRCA1 and BRCA2, have been identified and are present in a relevant proportion of high-risk families. They are located in the long arms of chromosomes 17 and 13, respectively. They are large genes allowing for multiple mutations at different positions and thus making the detection of genetic abnormalities in a given patient technically and time demanding. P53 and PTEN are genes associated with rare familial syndromes including breast cancer, but, together with other unknown genes, they are also involved in an increase in risk above the general population level. They are probably rather common and account for a substantial part of the genetic contribution to breast cancer (Black 1994).

A second element in breast cancer genesis is cellular biology. The availability of cellular models able to reproduce the development of a breast cancer allows the study of the sequential morphologic changes and to test the impact of different manipulations of factors modifying the progression of the disease.

In this field two models contribute especially to the advance of research: the culture of primordial mammary cells, able to grow even as a xenograft, and the transgenic mouse. The mouse hyperplasic alveolar node is the most advanced model of preneoplastic breast tissue. It is a focal lesion related to situations known to be at high risk of developing breast cancer. It has been used to investigate the role of chemical carcinogens, viruses, hormones, and growth factors in its progression to a malignant tumor.

A third basic element is the micro environment of the tumor. The tumoral cells are surrounded by other cellular and acellular components and establish with them a paracrine relationship that determines the ability of the tumor to grow and create metastasis. Relevant in this sense are the members of the family of IGFs and the proteases, cytokines, or factors regulating tumoral angiogenesis like vascular endothelium growth factor. Also very important in clinical terms are the evidences of the high aromatase concentrations in the tumor itself and in the surrounding benign areas, assuring a local contribution of high levels of estrogens to tumor growth (Santner et al. 1997).

Finally, estrogen-dependent tissues are all related by the endocrine information system where the messengers are estrogenic molecules. As has already been mentioned, any modification, positive or negative, in the availability of estrogen to the mammary breast cells has an impact on the future risk of breast cancer. This opens new and interesting research lines in methods to diminish breast tissue estrogenic priming and thus diminish the risk of presenting the disease.

10.4 Relationship Between Estrogens and Breast Cancer

10.4.1 Endogenous Estrogens

The origin of a malignant tumor is a random genetic mutation leading to the loss of mitotic control by the cells. Normal cells experience mutations regularly, and they are necessary mechanisms of adaptation that are strictly controlled. Malignant transformation, however, means a loss of control and a chaotic, uncontrolled growth.

The factors inducing and maintaining mutations leading to malignant growth can be distinguished as inducers or promoters. The former are the genuine carcinogens giving rise to genomic modification, whereas the latter maintain and amplify the lesion. However, both roles can be interconnected. Estrogens, as naturally occurring substances, do not fulfill the criteria of a carcinogen but exert a proliferative effect leading to continuous cellular divisions, a risk situation for the appearance of mutations. The errors, appearing during the process of DNA replication, are corrected by a complex repair system in which cellular proteases and specific genes like P53 are involved.

If the effectiveness of this repair system is overcome by the intense proliferating rate induced by estrogens, a number of abnormally mutated cells will continue to divide and give rise to a malignant tumor, making estrogens both inducers and promoters (Fig. 10.2) (Ames and Gold 1990).

Based on this concept of correlation between high replication rate/high persistent mutation risk, Pike et al. (1983) formulated the hypothesis of "breast tissue age" and developed a mathematical model to predict the effects of exposure to ovarian hormones. This model incorporates reproductive and endocrine items related to breast cancer and is able to predict the relative risk of individual situations with results that are very close to those observed in clinical trials. According to this hypothesis, both the years of exposure and the circulating serum levels of estrogens are associated to short-term breast cancer risk in postmenopausal women (Toniolo et al. 1995).

Consequently, any life event related to an increase in breast tissue exposure to estrogens leads to a higher risk of developing a cancer. Thus early menarche or late menopause increases the risk of presenting a cancer, whereas long periods of hypoestrogenic amenorrhea or early oophorectomy decreases the risk as compared to the general population. Obesity implies a larger amount of skin and fat, both tissues rich in aromatase, the enzyme that converts androgens to estrogens. At the same time high body mass index is an independent factor diminishing the hepatic secretion of sex hormone binding globulin (SHBG), a transport protein binding both to testosterone and estradiol and limiting its

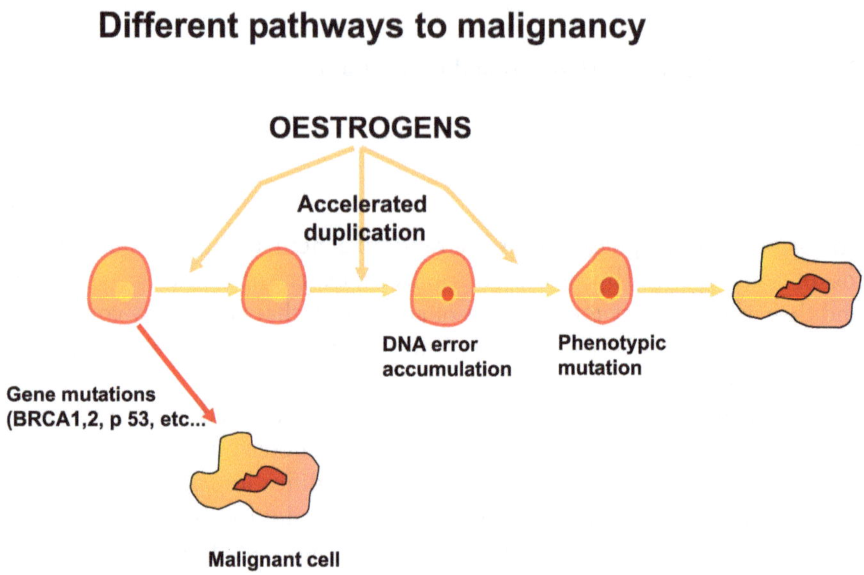

Fig. 10.2. Breast epithelial cells can evolve into a malignant ones either as a consequence of the functioning of the repair system or after repeated replication favored by estrogens. Both mechanisms can coexist and act synergistically

bioavailability (McTiernan et al. 2003). Thus, in obese postmenopausal women the peripheral production of estrogens is higher as compared to lean ones, and those estrogens are more available to the ER. This leads to a higher breast cancer incidence (Endogenous Hormones and Breast Cancer Collaborative Group 2003).

Conversely, circumstances reducing estrogen production such as exercise, reduced alcohol intake, or low-fat diet decrease the risk (Chlebowski et al. 1999; McTiernan et al. 2004). The role of smoking remains controversial because mutagenic substances present in tobacco smoke can cause DNA damage, but current smoking can have an antiestrogenic effect by interfering in estrogen metabolism (Manier et al. 2004). In summary, any anthropometric or behavioral circumstance increasing endogenous production of estrogens and consequently higher circulating concentrations increases the likelihood of presenting a breast cancer in the future.

10.4.2 Exogenous Estrogens

The consequences of the administration of substances with estrogenic activity on brest cancer incidence are probably different before and after menopause. During reproductive age the concentrations of estrogens during the spontaneous cycle or in some anovulatory situations like polycystic ovary syndrome change from woman to woman and cycle to cycle. With the administration of hormonal contraception the synthetic steroids contained in contraceptive preparations block the ovarian function and replace the endogenous hormones. In these circumstances the circulating concentrations of estrogens are relatively homogeneous and not necessarily higher than those present during the natural cycle. At the present time several cohort studies have failed to show any increase in breast cancer among users of hormonal contraception (Marchbanks et al. 2002).

After menopause the exogenous hormones just add to those produced through peripheral metabolization of androgens and mean an increase in estrogen availability to breast epithelium. Until recently the evidences on the effect of hormone therapy (HT) after menopause came from observational or cohort studies. In 1995 an evaluation of this topic among the participants of the Nurse's Health Study (Colditz et al. 1995) detected a small increase in the risk of presenting a breast cancer after the use of HT, either estrogens alone or combined with progestins, for more than 5 years. A reanalysis of the data published in 51 studies comparing the information from 52,705 cases of breast cancer with 108,411 controls (Collaborative Group on Hormonal Factors in Breast Cancer 1997) confirmed an increase in risk among users of HT.

In recent years two large-sample, prospective, double-blind, randomized trials have been performed to evaluate the usefulness of HT as a tool for secondary (Heart and Estrogen/Progestin Replacement Study, HERS) or primary (Women's Health Initiative, WHI) prevention of cardiovascular disease in postmenopausal women (Grady et al. 2002; Rossouw et al. 2002; Anderson et al. 2004). HERS randomized 2763 postmenopausal women with coronary disease to receive a combination of conjugated equine estrogens (CEE) 0.625 mg/d plus 2.5 mg medroxyprogesterone acetate or placebo. Two thousand three hundred twenty-one surviving HERS participants consented to continue the 4-year placebo-controlled period with a subsequent open-label observational study for 2.7 years. It totalized a 6.8-year followup period. Breast cancer was one of the outcomes evaluated in the study, and after nearly 7 years of treatment the difference between hormone and placebo group was insignificant even if the incidence was slightly higher in the treated group (RH = 1.27; 95% CI = 0.84–1.94) (Hulley et al. 2002).

WHI had two different arms. One included postmenopausal women with intact uterus randomly assigned to receive daily (Rossouw 2002). A parallel study randomized postmenopausal hysterectomized women to receive either placebo or 0.625 mg/d of CEE. The two studies included a total of 27,347 women. The study with nonhysterectomized women was interrupted prematurely, after a mean of 5 years of treatment, because health risks exceeded benefits. Among them an increase in invasive breast cancer was observed

Fig. 10.3. Effect of daily treatment with CEE + MPA on breast cancer incidence as compared to placebo. WHI study, nonhysterectomized women. Reproduced with permission from Chlebowski et al. (2003)

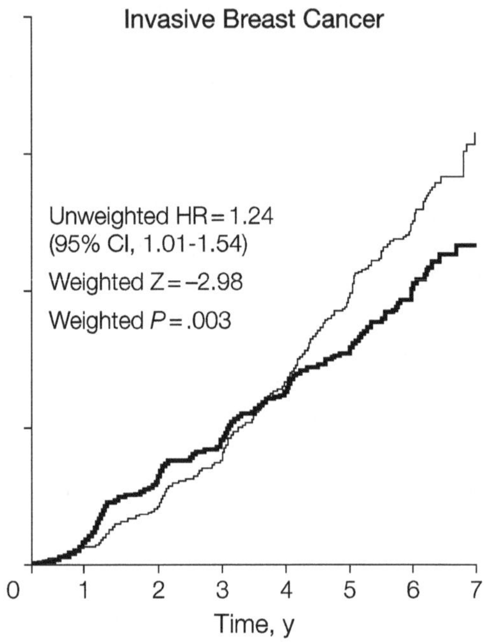

in the treated group up from the fourth year of treatment (HR = 1.24 95% CI = 1.01–1.54) with the intent of treating analysis (Fig. 10.3). When a sensitivity analysis was performed excluding the events in nonadherent women, the observed effect was slightly higher (HR = 1.49) with the possibility of an earlier appearance of the effect. Unlike what had been observed in previous studies (Holli et al. 1997), where tumors were slightly larger (1.7 cm [1.1] vs. 1.5 cm [0.9]), tumors have been diagnosed at a more advanced stage compared to those in the placebo group and were similar in histology (Chlebowski et al. 2003).

The part of the study involving hysterectomized women was also interrupted in February 2004 after nearly 7 years of treatment because there was no protective effect on the risk of heart disease, but the risk of stroke increased at the same rate as for the estrogen plus progestin combination.

It is important to note that the invasive breast cancer rate was 23% lower in the CEE group than in the placebo group (26 vs. 33 cases per 10,000 woman-years) approaching statistical significance (HR = 0.77 95% CI = 0.50–1.01). These results do not support the previously quoted hypothesis on the effects of estrogen exposure and breast cancer incidence, but some aspects must be taken into account. The majority of studies have found a higher effect of HT on breast cancer incidence when progestins were associated to estrogens. At the same time a high percentage of hysterectomized women are also oophorectomized

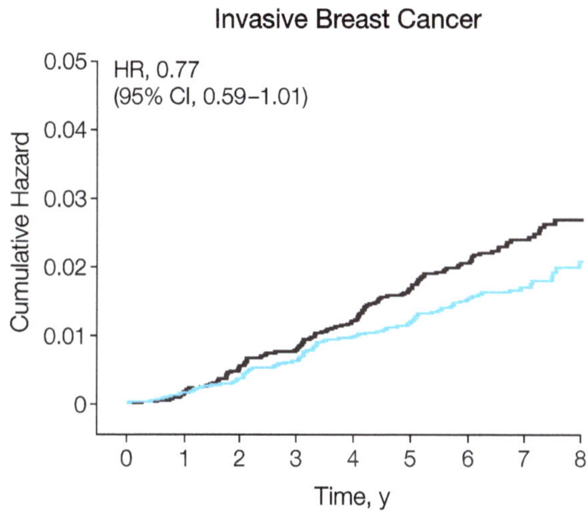

Fig. 10.4. Effect of daily treatment with CEE alone on breast cancer incidence as compared to placebo. WHI study, hysterectomized women. Reproduced with permission from Anderson et al. (2004)

and, consequently, the endogenous contribution of androgen precursors for aromatization is limited to adrenal secretion. Thus these results do not override the general advice of limiting postmenopausal estrogen (Fig. 10.4) administration to symptomatic women at the lowest effective dose (Anderson et al. 2004).

10.5 Pharmacological Blockade of Estrogen Receptors: The Concept of Chemoprophylaxis

The evidence for a negative effect of estrogen exposure on breast cancer risk raises automatically the idea of minimizing the risk by diminishing the binding of estrogens to their receptors. Oophorectomy has been the first measure to show effectiveness in improving the evolution of advanced breast cancer. This alternative was challenged by the discovery of molecules able to bind to ERs competing with estrogens. The substances were called "antiestrogens" and shown to be at least as effective as surgery without invasive measures (Buchanan et al. 1986; Ingle et al. 1986).

The evidence that tamoxifen was able to exert estrogenic effects on several tissues like the bone (Love et al. 1992) opened the door to the concept of SERMs, which is explained in detail in Chaps. 2 and 3 of this book. The mechanisms of action of these substances on ERs is explained in detail in Chap. 3. However, it is pertinent to comment on some special aspects of its action on mammary cancer cells. IGF-1 is a key element in growth control of malignant breast cells through endocrine and paracrine pathways. Tamoxifen and its active metabolite are able to inhibit IGF-1-stimulated growth (Jordan

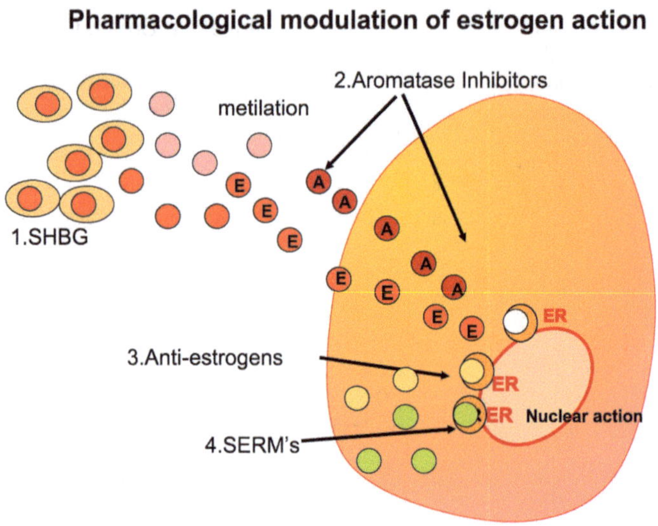

Fig. 10.5. Drugs can impair the estrogenic stimulation of the mammary cell in different ways: 1. Increasing SHBG hepatic secretion and diminishing the amount of free bioavailable hormone. 2. Inhibiting the activity of aromatase and blocking the conversion of weak androgens to estrogens. 3. Pure antiestrogens, like fulvestrant, compete with estrogens to bind to the receptor and blocks its ability to influence on nuclear action. 4. SERMs bind to the receptor but influences selectively on cellualar action depending on the tissue. (A = androgens, E = estrogens, ER = estrogen receptors, SHBG = sex hormone binding globulin)

1994), modulate the expression of IGFBPs (Lee and Yee 1995), reduce the autocrine secretion of IGFs (Huff et al. 1988), and reduce both the plasmatic levels (Colletti et al. 1989) and the receptor population (Freiss et al. 1990) of IGF-1.

Tamoxifen has pioneered the field of primary and secondary chemoprevention of breast cancer, which has been followed by second- and third-generation SERMs and alternative approaches as aromatase inhibitors or "pure antiestrogens", as will be explained below (Fig. 10.5).

10.5.1 Tamoxifen as Adjuvant Therapy in Early ER(+) Breast Cancer

Tamoxifen has been widely used in the adjuvant treatment of invasive breast cancer associated to surgery and chemotherapy. It has been shown to be effective in preventing new contralateral tumors and local or peripheral recurrences (Nolvadex Adjuvant Trial Organization 1983; Cuzick and Baum 1985; Abe et al. 1998). The overview comprised 37,000 women from 55 randomized trials and included events occurring more than 5 years after randomization. The effects of tamoxifen administration in cases with a low or zero level of ER measured in the primary tumor (about 8000 women) appeared to be small, and consequently analysis of recurrence and total mortality have been restricted to patients with ER(+) tumors or untested (around 30,000 cases altogether). Both recurrence and mortality reductions over approx. 10 years of followup had a clear significant trend toward greater effect with longer treatment. After 1, 2, and 5 years of adjuvant treatment, recurrences were reduced by 21, 19, and 47% and mortality by 12, 17, and 26%, respectively. Even if the relative reduction in mortality was similar for both node-negative and node-positive patients, the absolute mortality reductions were greater in node-positive women. The proportional reductions in contralateral breast cancer were 13, 26, and 47%, respectively, for the aforementioned periods of treatment (Fig. 10.6).

Toremifen is a SERM considered a tamoxifen analog characterized by one chlorine atom and is approved for first-line treatment of metastasic breast cancer in postmenopausal women who have tumors that are either ER(+) or of unknown status. In a 3-year face-to-face study with tamoxifen, there were no significant differences between both drugs. The number and profile of adverse events are also similar. Experience with toremifen is limited and far from that accumulated with tamoxifen.

Until recently tamoxifen has been the gold standard for adjuvant therapy in ER(+) early breast cancer. Recent information from controlled trials comparing tamoxifen to aromatase inhibitors has challenged this idea. More research is needed to establish the respective roles of the two families of substances in the hormonal management of breast cancer (Chlebowski et al. 2002).

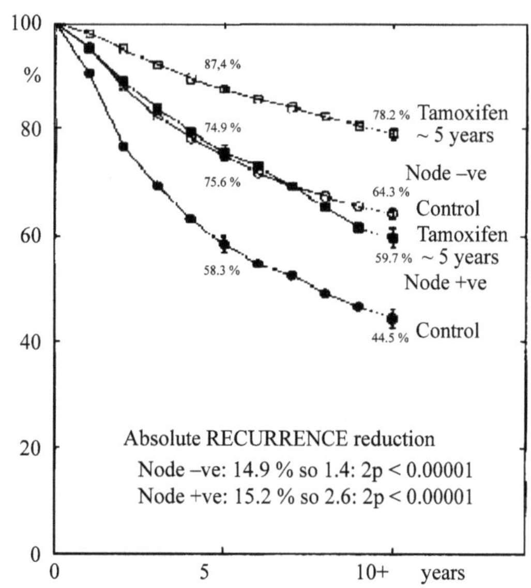

Fig. 10.6. Reduction in the risk of recurrence obtained with the administration of 20 mg/d of tamoxifen and subdivided by nodal status. Reproduced with permission from Abe et al. and the Early Breast Cancer Collaborative Group (1998)

10.5.2 Tamoxifen in Primary Prevention of ER(+) Breast Cancer

Since SERMs are able to block (estrogen-dependent) malignant mammary cell growth, it is logical to deduce that its administration to healthy women should prevent the progression from premalignant to malignant epithelial cells. The administration of tamoxifen to different groups of high-risk women has produced relevant information on the advantages and inconveniences of such an approach (Chlebowski et al. 1999).

The most relevant study is the Breast Cancer Prevention Trial (BCPT, NSABP-P1) (Fisher et al. 1998). Initiated in the USA by the National Surgical Adjuvant Breast and Bowel Project, this study recruited 13,388 women considered at high risk for breast cancer based on Gail's probability algorithm (Gail et al. 1989).

The women were randomized to receive either tamoxifen (6681) or placebo (6707) for 5 years. However, the trial was stopped prematurely because the findings provided strong evidence of a reduction in breast cancer with tamoxifen therapy. The results have been released and made available at http://cancertrials.nci.nih.gov. These are the first available data supporting the hypothesis that breast cancer can be pharmacologically prevented in an at-risk female population. The administration of tamoxifen was effective in reducing by 69% the annual rate of ER(+) tumors, both invasive and in situ, but was ineffective in reducing the occurrence of ER(–) neoplasias (Young 1999).

This prevention was evident in all risk category groups included in Gail's score and with any previous history of breast lesions (atypical hyperplasia, lobular carcinoma in situ, etc.) (Fig. 10.7).

Three other studies were conducted to investigate the preventive potential of tamoxifen. One in Italy (Veronesi et al. 1998), one at the Royal Marsden Hospital, United Kingdom (Powles et al. 1998), and a multicentric international study (IBIS 2002). The British study was the smallest in size (2471 participants) but concentrated on women with a high incidence of family history and consequently presented a higher number of breast cancers. The Italian trial included only women with previous hysterectomy and, accordingly, around 50% had also undergone bilateral oophorectomy. The family risk was low: only 15% had a first-degree relative affected by breast cancer. Both European studies permitted concurrent HRT, and 26% of the participants in the British trial received HRT while on study and 42% had "ever received" HT for menopausal symptoms. Neither of the studies showed any positive effect of the treatment with tamoxifen on the incidence of breast cancer. Reasons for this lack of effect can be different for each trial.

The Italian study included low-risk women, especially as concerns the aspects expected to be protected by tamoxifen, and the sample was too small to

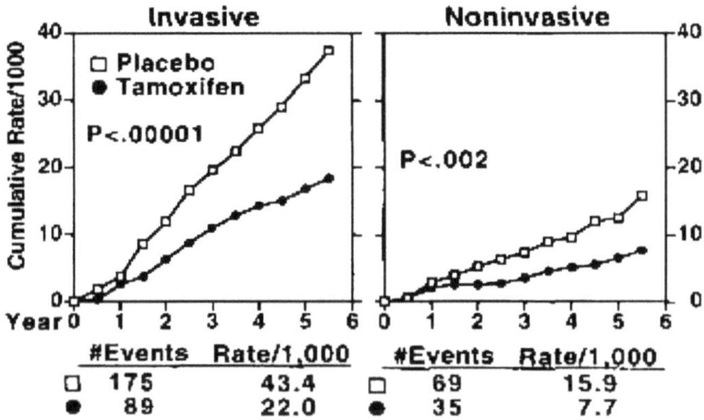

Fig. 10.7. Effect of tamoxifen administration on incidence of invasive (*left panel*) or noninvasive (*right panel*) breast cancer. Reproduced with permission from Fisher et al. and other National Surgical Adjuvant Breast and Bowel Project Investigators (1998)

show differences with the placebo group. The compliance has been reported to be very low since only 149 women completed the expected 5 years of treatment. Two recently published subanalyses of the Italian trial focus on two especially high-risk subgroups: HRT users (Veronesi et al. 2002a) and those fulfilling precise risk criteria for breast cancer (Veronesi 2002b). Both subanalyses show significant protection from tamoxifen administration. As the authors point out, "Tamoxifen's effect appears to be restricted to women who are predicted to be at high risk of the hormone-dependent form of breast cancer. If it proves to be true the same reduction in the absolute numbers of breast cancer could be obtained by restricting treatment to the reduced women at high risk and thus improve the cost effectiveness of the intervention".

The results obtained in the UK trial are more difficult to explain. Since the sample was basically composed of rather young women (62% younger than 50 years old) with increased risk by family history (96% with a first-degree relative affected), it can be postulated that the origin of the majority of cancers was probably more genetic than hormonal. Furthermore, there is no information on the receptor status of the tumor detected in both placebo and treated group.

The IBIS-I study was promoted by the UK Coordinating Committee for Cancer Research and supported by the Imperial Cancer Research Fund. A group of 7152 high-risk women were selected according to criteria related to familial cases of breast cancer, previous atypical biopsies, and parity. The most important group was that of women with two or more first- or second-degree relatives with breast cancer. For this group the yearly frequency of breast cancer, in the absence of any intervention, was calculated to be 7.50 per 1000 women. This proved to be accurate since the actual frequency in the placebo group was 6.74 per 1000, not significantly different from that projected. The study took place predominantly in the UK, Australia, and New Zealand, with testimonial participation of some European countries (Spain, Ireland, Finland, Italy, Belgium, and Switzerland).

After median followup of 50 months a risk reduction of 32% in the tamoxifen-treated group has been observed. This protection was independent of age, degree of risk, and previous or actual use of HRT. The most striking outcome of the study has been the significant increase in the death rate of all causes in the tamoxifen group as compared to that receiving placebo (25 vs. 11 cases). The increases correspond to cancers other than breast cancer (only four deaths were due to breast cancer, two in each study group), pulmonary embolism other vascular causes, and cardiac deaths. The variety of causes of death and the lack of an increase in overall frequency suggests that this may be a chance finding excepting thromboembolic events, which will be discussed in detail later. This increase in overall mortality in the treated group raises the issue of the cost-benefit of these interventions. If the number of breast cancers has been lower than expected, and the reduction in the number of new cases is at the cost of unexpected deaths, the appropriateness of the treatment has to be carefully evaluated. The editorial introduction at the moment of the IBIS publication was entitled "Chemoprevention of breast cancer: a promising idea with an uncertain future" (Kinsinger and Harris 2002). A summary of the data on prevention trials is presented in Table 10.1.

Table 10.1.

Trial	Sample size	Women/years of followup	Cancers/1000 women/year	
			Placebo	Tamoxifen
BCPT	13.388	46.858	6.6	3.6
Powles	2.471	12.355	5.0	4.7
Veronesi	5.408	20.731	2.3	2.1
IBIS	7.152	29.967	101	69

10.5.3 Drawbacks of Tamoxifen as a Preventive Agent

The estrogenicity of tamoxifen at several levels brings both advantages and inconveniences. Among the former we have already mentioned bone quality and vaginal proliferation. However, the inconveniences, especially endometrial polyps and cancer and thrombotic events, are important enough to avoid the systematic use of this drug as a preventive agent except with well-identified high-risk patients. Thus a careful cost-benefit analysis is needed.

A recent review by Cuzick et al. has pooled the information generated by the four randomized prevention trials mentioned above (Cuzick et al. 2003). The observed reduction in breast cancer incidence was 38%, in good agreement with what was expected from the individual trials. When analyzing according to ER status, there was no reduction in the incidence of ER(−) tumors, and a reduction of 48% was observed in the incidence of ER(+) cancers. These figures clearly confirm that tamoxifen can reduce the risk of ER(+) breast cancer.

The rates of endometrial cancer were increased in the tamoxifen group in all trials. The consensus relative risk was 2.4 (1.5–4.0) in the prevention trials, and the hazard ratio was 3.4 (1.8–6.4) in the adjuvant studies. The risk increase is seen almost exclusively after 50 years of age, and the information available suggests that the cancers detected in the tamoxifen-treated women are not of worse prognosis than those detected in the general population. The endometrial action of tamoxifen seems to be exerted mainly through the IGF system rather than by direct binding to ERs. Tamoxifen decreases the synthesis of IGFBPs and potentiates the tisular activity of IGF-1 through tyrosine phosphorylation (Kleinman et al. 1996) (Fig. 10.8).

Besides cancer, tamoxifen induces benign changes in the endometrial and subendometrial structures, which induce a burden of unnecessary examinations (ultrasound, hysteroscopy, biopsy etc.) and surgery (D&Cs, hysterectomies) due to misleading or false positive ultrasonographic reports (Dijkhuizen et al. 1996). Since the absolute incidence of the disease is low

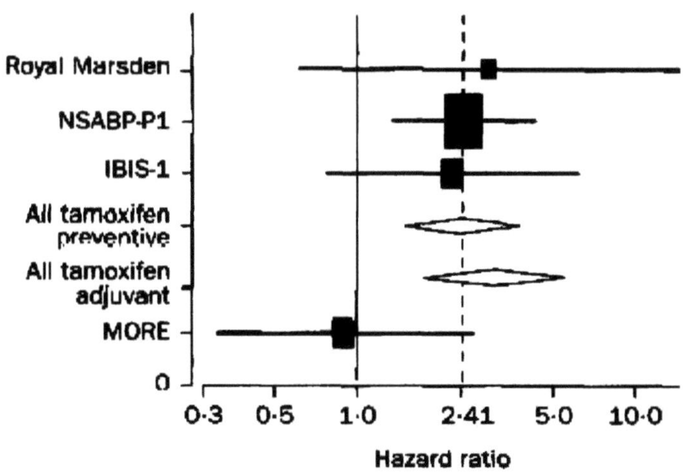

Fig. 10.8. Hazard ratio of presenting an endometrial cancer as the consequence of treatment with tamoxifen or raloxifene (MORE study). Reproduced with permission from Cuzick et al. (2003)

and frequently manifested by abnormal bleeding, the American College of Obstetricians and Gynecologists recommends limiting the endometrial examination of tamoxifen users to those presenting with abnormal bleeding. This situation makes very suitable the availability of new agents devoid of endometrial activity.

Tamoxifen users present also a doubling incidence of deep venous thrombosis (DVT) and pulmonary embolism (PE) (118 vs. 62 cases). This increase is similar to that seen with HRT. There are some aspects of this side effect that should be commented on to improve the management of women eligible for tamoxifen treatment and at risk for DVT (Goldhaber 2005). In the subanalysis of the Italian study (Decensi et al. 2005), the venous thromboembolism definition included DVT, PE, and superficial phlebitis. Most of the VTE that the authors reported were, in fact, cases of superficial phlebitis, whereas the admitted definition of venous thromboembolism excludes this entity. Such conceptual differences, together with differences in age and background characteristics between the four studies, can explain the diversity in the incidences observed.

It is interesting to note that in IBIS, where the rate of thromboembolic events was about 2.5 times higher in the tamoxifen group, the majority of the events took place within 3 months of major surgery or after long-term immobility. Twenty of 25 such events were in women in the tamoxifen group. This is why the authors strongly suggest discontinuing tamoxifen before any surgery or longstanding immobility and providing appropriate antithrombotic measures. The treatment should not be restarted until full mobility is restored.

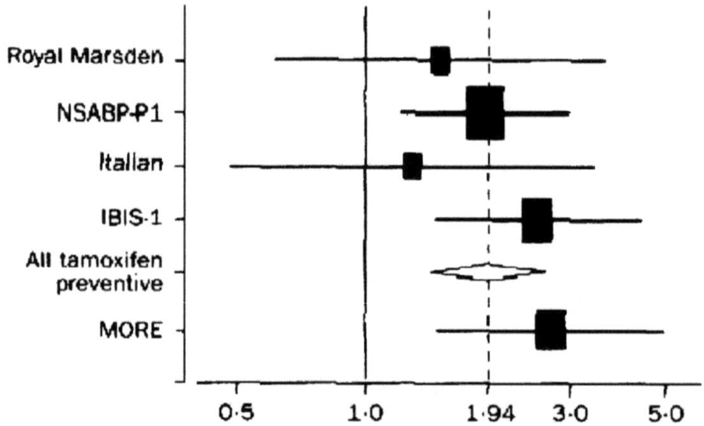

Fig. 10.9. Hazard ratio of presenting a venous thomboembolic event as the consequence of treatment with tamoxifen or raloxifene (MORE study). Reproduced with permission from Cuzick et al. (2003)

The Italian study subanalysis identifies as independent predictors of VTE: age > 60 years, height > 165 cm, and diastolic blood pressure > 90 mm. Also relevant is the association between high global cardiovascular risk scores and VTE incidence. This means that there is a correlation between arterial and venous risks, and consequently prevention of arterial complications will also mean lower venous risk (Decensi et al. 2005; Goldhaber 2005) (Fig. 10.9).

Considering the information presented, tamoxifen does not appear to be suitable for breast cancer prevention. Further studies are needed to reduce risks and increase efficiency either by reducing the dose or identifying those women likely to gain the highest benefit (Powles and Chang 1997). Meanwhile, new agents emerge as alternatives with similar or higher protective effects and fewer or different side effects (Fabian and Kimler 2005; Cuzick 2005).

10.6 Raloxifene and Breast Cancer

Raloxifene is a SERM devoid of stimulating effects on the uterus as is known from the initial studies (Delmas et al. 1997). Eliminating one of the major concerns raised by the experience gained with tamoxifen studies, both in prevention and adjuvant treatments, puts raloxifene in a place of privilege to be a rational alternative agent. At the same time it improves bone density, prevents osteoporosis and vertebral fracture, and reduces cardiovascular events in a subset of high-risk patients (Silverman et al. 2004). The evidences on the effects of raloxifene on the uterus are explained in detail in Chap. 10 of this book.

Experimental studies showed antitumoral effects of raloxifene in different in vitro preparations and animal models. Raloxifene has been able to inhibit the mitogenic effect induced by estrogens on ZR-75-1 cells, an estrogen responsive human breast cancer cell line (Poulin et al. 1989). In a well-accepted rat model of breast cancer induced by nitroso-methyl urea (NMU) raloxifene significantly suppressed the development of breast tumors and acted synergistically with 9 cis-retinoic acid (Anzano et al. 1996).

10.6.1 Clinical Studies

The strongest clinical information on the effects of raloxifen on breast cancer risks emerges from the MORE study. As a reminder, this study included 7705 osteoporotic women randomized either to placebo (2576) or raloxifene (5129), either 60 or 120 mg. Mammographic evaluation was optative during the first year but mandatory at the second, third, and fourth years. At the six-month followup controls the patients were asked about any mammary event, and in the case of surgery or biopsy the mammograms, pathological reports, specimens, and ER special staining slides were reviewed by an independent board for adjudication. There were no differences in family history between the placebo and the treated group, and no specific evaluation of breast cancer risk factors has been made.

From the first evaluations a positive effect of raloxifene tratment on the incidence of breast cancer was detected (Cummings et al. 1999). During the 4 years of treatment 79 breast cancer cases were detected and 77 of them were confirmed by the review board. In the placebo group 44 cases were identified, of which 39 were invasive, whereas in the raloxifene-treated group 33 cases were detected and 22 were invasive. The differences between both groups appeared progressively and tended to increase over time. This means a relative risk of 0.38 (IC: 95% 0.24–0.58) or, in other words, a reduction in the incidence of breast cancer of 68%.

Absolute risks can better reflect the clinical importance of the protective effect. In the placebo group the incidence was 5.3 cases per 1000 woman-years, while in the treated group only 1.9 cases per 1000 woman-year were diagnosed. If we only take into account invasive cancers, the figures would be 4.7 and 1.3, respectively, meaning a relative risk of 0.28 or a decrease of 72% (Cauley et al. 2001).

These encouraging results, similar to those observed with tamoxifen in the BP-1 study, lead to the design of CORE (Continuing Outcomes Relevant to Evista) with the primary objective of investigating the effect of four additional years of raloxifene treatment on the incidence of invasive breast cancer. In fact, the study was the continuation of MORE in a slightly reduced subset with a change in the primary endpoint. A final group of 4011 participants of MORE agreed to continue in CORE. They continued with the same assignment, raloxifene or placebo. Consequently, 1286 received placebo and 2725 raloxifene. The active treatment was 60 mg/d raloxifene because it is the dose approved for the prevention and treatment of osteoporosis and because the two dosage groups in MORE (60 and 120 mg/d) had similar reductions in the incidence of breast cancer. All participants had a bilateral mammogram within the year of enrollement and 2 and 4 years thereafter. The process of adjudication by an independent review board was similar to that implemented for MORE.

During the 4 years of the trial 61 cases of breast cancer were reported and confirmed. Of these, 30 were in the placebo group (28 invasive) and 31 were in the raloxifene group (24 invasive). This means a 59% reduction in the incidence of invasive breast cancer in the raloxifene group as compared with women receiving placebo (2.1 vs. 5.2 cases per 1000 woman-years; HR = 0.41, CI = 0.24 to 0.71). Only nine intraductal, noninvasive breast cancers were detected, seven in the raloxifene group and two in the placebo group. The treatment with raloxifene reduced the overall incidence of breast cancer by 50%. The results obtained in this second treatment period are very similar to those observed in MORE.

Considering all 7705 MORE participants from the moment of the initial randomization to the end of their participation in either MORE or CORE, a total number of 121 breast cancers were adjudicated, 56 cancers in the raloxifene group and 65 in the placebo group. Of these 58 in the placebo group (4.2 cases per 100 woman-years) and 40 in the raloxifene group (1.4 cases per 1000 woman-years) were invasive. Consequently, raloxifene induced a 66% reduction in the incidence of invasive breast cancer compared with the placebo group (HR = 0.34, 95% CI = 0.22–0.50) (Martino et al. 2004b) (Fig. 10.10).

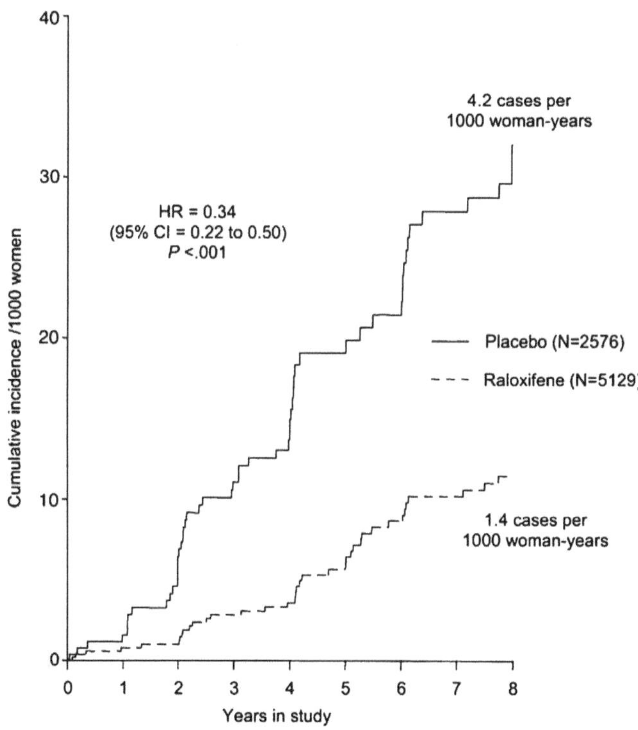

Fig. 10.10. Cumulative incidence of invasive breast cancers during 8 years of treatment either with raloxifene (*dotted line*) or placebo (*solid line*) Reproduced with permission from Martino et al. (2004)

10.6.2 Estrogen Receptor Status

It is also important to note that, as happened with tamoxifen, this decrease in risk concentrated exclusively in ER(+) tumors. ER status was determined for 88 cases, and 75% of these were considered positive. The decrease in risk induced by raloxifene administration during the total 8 years of MORE plus CORE reached 76% of the invasive ER(+) cases, compared with the placebo group (0.8 vs. 3.2 cases per 1000 woman-years; HR = 0.24; 95% CI = 0.15 to 0.40). There was no influence of the raloxifene treatment on the incidence of ER(−) invasive tumors (0.53 versus 0.51 cases per 1000 woman-years; HR = 1.06; 95% CI = 0.43 to 2.59). This confirms the hypothesis that raloxifene exerts its protective effect through its binding to breast cell ERs, avoiding the proliferative effect of estrogens to take place. Consequently ER(−) tumors cannot be influenced by the presence of raloxifene in the blood, and no difference in its incidence should be expected between placebo and treated groups (Cauley et al. 2001) (Fig. 10.11).

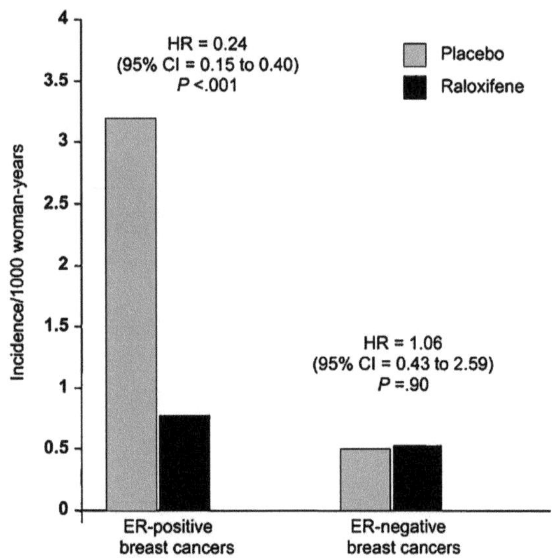

Fig. 10.11. Annual incidence rate per 1000 woman-years of followup for invasive breast cancers over the 8 years of CORE according to ER status. Reproduced with permission from Martino et al. (2004a)

10.6.3 Estrogen Circulating Levels and Raloxifene Protection

The hypothesis of protection based on the competition of raloxifene with estrogens for the occupation of ERs implies the need for circulating estrogens to compete with. For the same reason the higher the concentrations of estrogens circulating, the higher the expected risk of presenting an ER(+) breast cancer and, consequently, the higher the protection offered by the administration of a SERM. The validity of this hypothesis has been tested both in MORE and CORE.

Lippman et al. (2001) determined the basal serum estradiol levels of 7290 women participating in MORE at the moment of enrollement. The samples were analyzed in a central laboratory with a low-sensitivity radioinmuno analysis (RIA) allowing for discrimination only between samples containing more or less than 12 pmol/L. The incidence of invasive breast cancer was clearly higher among women in the placebo group, with values higher than 12 pmol/L. The number of cancers was similar in the treatment group irrespective of the estradiol concentrations. Thus the effect of raloxifene treatment was also more evident in the group of women with the higher estrogen levels.

Using a more sensitive RIA, but studying the same population, Cummings et al. (2002b) were able to discriminate between undetectable concentrations and those lower than 5, 6 to 10, and more than 10 pmol/L. In the placebo group the incidence of invasive breast cancer increased according to increases in the concentrations of circulating estradiol detected. As expected, the raloxifene-treated group presented the same incidence of breast cancer, irrespective of circulating levels of estradiol at recruitment, reflecting the ability of raloxifene to compete with any postmenopausal level of circulating estradiol. Since the incidence was higher in the high estrogen group, the degree of protection was also more important in these patients.

Finally, Martino et al. (2004a) analyzed the cases from MORE and CORE together using the basal data analyzed by Cummings et al. (2002). Participants were divided into three groups: those with baseline levels of < 5 pmol/L (N = 3655), 5–10 pmol/L (N = 983), or > 10 pmol/L (N = 2652). The incidence of invasive breast cancer cases was significantly reduced by 75% (HR = 0.25, 95% CI = 0.14–0.47; ARR = 46 cases per 10,000 woman-years) in the raloxifene group compared to placebo in women with serum estradiol > 10 pmol/L.

In those with serum estradiol concentrations of 5–10 pmol/L, invasive breast cancer incidence was reduced by 67% (HR = 0.33, 95% CI = 0.13–0.84; ARR = 40 cases per 10,000 woman-years) in the raloxifene group compared to those receiving placebo. In women with serum estradiol levels < 5 pmol/L, the 48% reduction in invasive breast cancer incidence for the raloxifene group compared to placebo was not significant (HR = 0.52, 95% CI = 0.26–1.06; ARR = 11 cases per 10,000 woman-years). However, the interaction test showed that the magnitude of reduction in breast cancer incidence with raloxifene was independent of estradiol level (interaction $p = 0.317$).

These figures lend support to the hypothesis that raloxifene prevents the progression of breast cancer by blocking the binding of estrogens to spe-

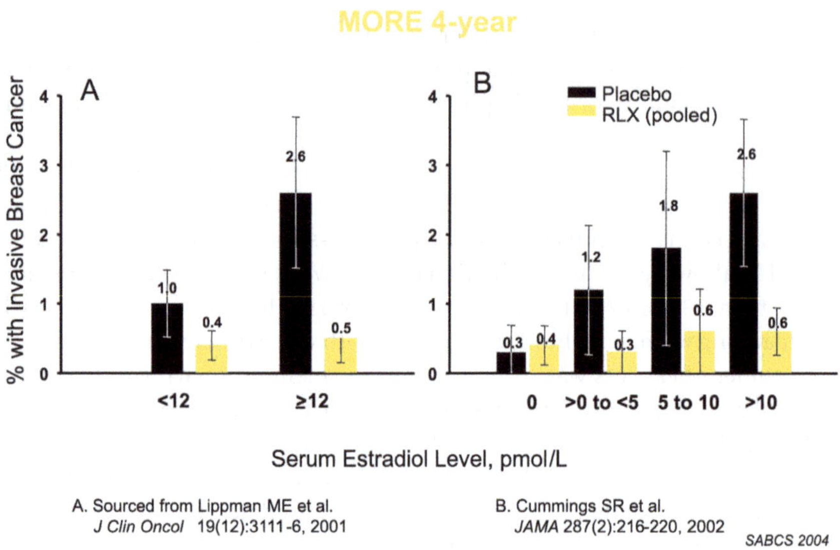

Fig. 10.12. Effect of raloxifene on the risk of invasive breast cancer at different serum estradiol levels evaluated in two different studies. Elaborated from Lippman et al. (2001) and Cummings et al. (2002a)

cific intracellular receptors and allows for the suggestion that the detection of relatively high estrogen concentrations can be a criterion for selecting women in which a pharmacological intervention would be cost-effective. This is not an easy task since the usual clinical RIA systems are not sensitive enough to discriminate among the very low estradiol levels circulating in postmenopausal women (Stanczyk 2002). However, this is technically feasible, and specific RIAs could be set up if such a selection system were shown, by prospective randomized studies, to be clinically useful (Cummings 2002b) (Fig. 10.12).

10.6.4 Bone Density and Effect of Raloxifene on the Breast

All women included in MORE met criteria for osteoporosis defined as a lumbar spine or femoral neck bone mineral density (BMD) T score equal to or less than 2.5 or as the presence of a radiographic vertebral fracture. These women are considered to be at lower risk for breast cancer than women with normal BMD since this parameter could partially reflect a woman's lifetime exposure to estrogens (Zhang et al. 1997). After the start of MORE, NHANES III criteria standardizing total hip BMD measurements became available allowing part of the MORE population to be recategorized as having osteopenia and the rest as being osteoporotic.

Delmas and coworkers (2005) have analyzed the impact of raloxifene treatment on breast cancer incidence over the 8 years of MORE plus CORE depending on the classification of the participants as osteopoenic or osteoporotic. For women assigned to placebo, more cases of invasive and ER(+) invasive breast cancers were reported in the osteopenic than in the osteoporotic group.

In postmenopausal women with osteopenia, 8 years of raloxifene, compared with placebo, was associated with a 65% lower incidence of invasive breast cancer and 78% lower incidence of ER(+) invasive breast cancer. In postmenopausal women with osteoporosis, 8 years of raloxifene, compared with placebo, was associated with a 69% lower incidence of invasive breast cancer and a 71% lower incidence of ER(+) invasive breast cancer. As mentioned previously, raloxifene performed better in protecting from ER(+) cancers, and consequently this effect was more evident in the osteopenic group, expected, according to the hypothesis, to have a higher estrogenic priming along reproductive life. Even if this reanalysis has the limitation of being based on a post hoc classification, according to new conventional criteria, it gives indications of the correlation between bone density and breast cancer risks and suggests that what is true for osteoporotic patients could also apply to women with normal BMD (Fig. 10.13).

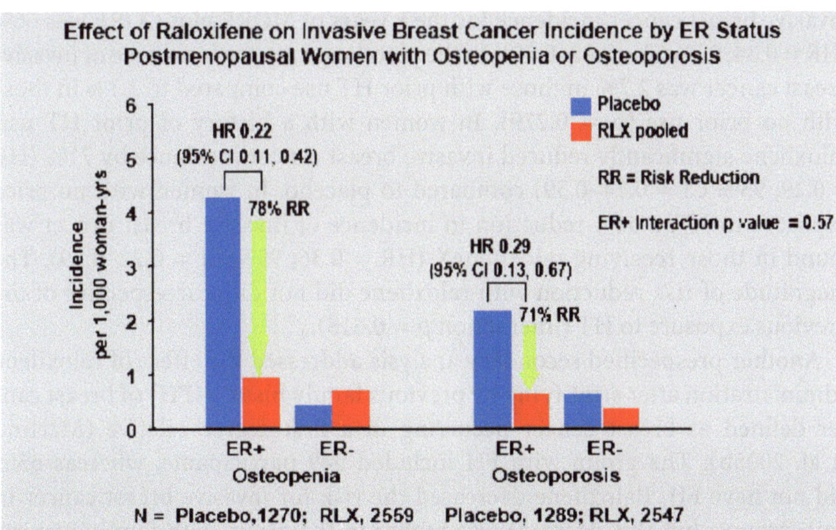

Fig. 10.13. Effect of raloxifene on invasive breast cancer incidence by ER status in postmenopausal women with osteopenia or osteoporosis. Reproduced with permission from Delmas et al. (2005)

10.6.5 Other Conditions Related to Raloxifene Protection

Several secondary analyses have evaluated the effect of raloxifene as compared to placebo after stratifying for different factors known to be related to invasive breast cancer incidence as age, family history, Gail score, or previous exposure to hormone treatment for menopausal symptoms. Martino et al. (2005a) stratified MORE + CORE participants according to age (< 65 and ≥ 65 years). The participants older than 65 had a 77% increase in the risk of presenting an invasive breast cancer vs. those < 65 years (hazard ratio 1.77, 95% CI = 1.01, 3.12). The invasive breast cancer rates were 29.6 and 51.0 per 10,000 woman-years in the age categories < 65 and ≥ 65 years, respectively. The absolute risk reduction (ARR) was 17.1 cases per 10,000 woman-years for the group younger than 65 years and 35.6 cases per 10,000 woman-years for those older than 65 years. Therapy by age group interaction was not significant ($p = 0.43$), and consequently raloxifene risk reduction was independent of age group.

As previously mentioned, HT is considered to increase risk for invasive breast cancer. The ability of raloxifene to reduce breast cancer risk was evaluted after MORE (Lippman 2001; Johnell et al. 2004) and has been evaluated recently with a consideration of all the breast cancer cases diagnosed after MORE + CORE (Purdie et al. 2004). Previous HT use was reported by 2235 women and no previous HT use by 5447 women. In these women, the overall reduction in invasive breast cancer incidence for the 8 years of MORE plus CORE was 66% (HR = 0.34; 95% CI = 0.22–0.50). In the placebo group the incidence of invasive breast cancer was 2.7% in those with prior HT use compared to 2.1% in those with no prior use ($p = 0.279$). In women with a history of prior HT use, raloxifene significantly reduced invasive breast cancer incidence by 71% (HR = 0.29; 95% CI = 0.14–0.59) compared to placebo. In women with no prior exposure to HT, a 64% reduction in incidence of invasive breast cancer was found in those receiving raloxifeneX (HR = 0.36; 95% CI = 0.22–0.59). The magnitude of risk reduction with raloxifene did not differ irrespective of the previous exposure to HT (interaction $p = 0.618$).

Another prespecified secondary analysis addressed the effect of raloxifene administration after stratifying by previous family history (FH) of breast cancer defined as breast cancer occurring in a first-degree relative (Martino et al. 2005b). The group with FH included 949 participants, whereas 6569 did not have FH. Raloxifene decreased the risk for invasive breast cancer in both groups, but this decrease was higher in the group with family history: HR = 0.11; (95% CI = 0.03–0.38) vs. HR = 0.42 (0.27–0.66) for the group without FH. Expressed in terms of absolute risk reduction (ARR), raloxifene avoided 72 cases per 10,000 woman-years in the FH group vs. 21 cases in the group with no FH ($p = 0.04$). Thus, compared with placebo, raloxifene significantly reduced the incidence of invasive breast cancer both in those postmenopausal osteoporotic women with and those without a FH of breast cancer, but this reduction was significantly greater in women with a FH.

As discussed in the preceding section, osteoporotic women are known to be at lower risk for invasive breast cancer. However, the incidence detected in the study was not lower than that expected for a similar general population. The breast cancer incidence rate for the placebo group in the CORE trial was 5.4 cases per 1000 woman-years, slightly higher than the 4.4–4.5 observed for a similar age group population as reported by the National Cancer Institute's Surveillance, Epidemiology and End Results Program (Kikuchi et al. 1997). Thus the CORE participants were not at lower risk for breast cancer despite having osteoporosis. To explain this situation Cauley and coworkers (2004) analyzed the basal risk for breast cancer as evaluated according to Gail's score (Gail et al. 1989).

Of the 5213 MORE participants included in the CORE primary analysis, 3996 had a Gail risk assessment; 2718 received 60 mg/d raloxifene and 1278 received placebo during CORE. The mean 5-year breast cancer risk for all women in CORE was 1.94, and 54% met the Gail criteria for breast cancer high risk (Gail's score > 1.67%). In the placebo group, the rate of invasive breast cancer was 2.7 times higher in the high-risk group than the low-risk group ($p = 0.034$). In the total cohort, there were 45 adjudicated cases of invasive breast cancer: 21 (0.8%) in the raloxifene group vs. 24 (1.9%) among those receiving placebo (HR = 0.42, 95% CI = 0.23, 0.75; $p = 0.002$ vs. placebo). In the high-risk group there were 31 cases of invasive breast cancer, 13 in the group receiving

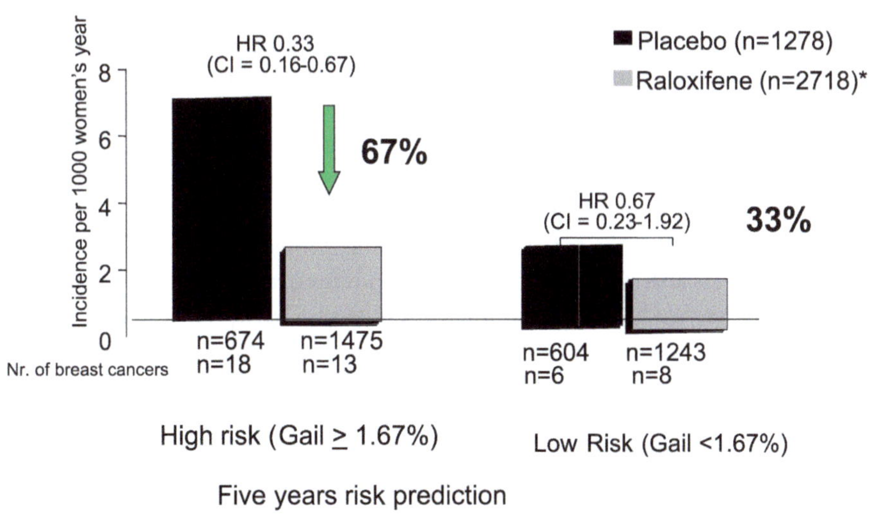

Fig. 10.14. Effect of raloxifene on incidence of invasive breast cancer after stratifying for risk evaluated with Gail's score. Redrawn from Cauley et al. (2004)

raloxifene (0.9%) and 18 (2.7%) in the pacebo group (HR = 0.33, 95% CI = 0.16, 0.67). Even if the protective effect was three times higher in the high-risk group, there was no significant difference in the effect of raloxifene between those patients at low and those at high risk of breast cancer based on the Gail model (interaction $p = 0.28$) (Fig. 10.14).

10.6.6 Raloxifen as a Breast Cancer Preventive Agent

In 1999 the American Society of Clinical Oncology working group on breast cancer risk reduction strategies concluded that "it was premature to recommend raloxifene use to lower the risk of developing breast cancer outside of a clinical trial setting" (Chlebowski et al. 1999). Five years later the amount and quality of information has increased significantly. The results obtained in the CORE study prove that what was true for a 5-year treatment with tamoxifen in BP1 can persist for at least 8 years with raloxifene. The most relevant lesson learned from all tamoxifen prevention trials is that the degree of protection is closely related to the risk profile of the participants. Even in osteoporotic women, CORE included a significant amount of high-risk women irrespective of the evaluation system used (age, family history, Gail's score, or estrogen levels), which probably explains the high degree of protection offered by raloxifene. Even not reaching significance, raloxifene always performed better in these high-risk subgroups. Consequently, more refined and updated scores than Gail's, including biological data such as estradiol levels, would decrese the number of women to treat (NNT) to avoid a new case. Such an evaluation should be considered in future strategies for breast cancer prevention.

On the other hand, efforts have to be made to reduce the major side effect shared by both tamoxifen and raloxifene: thromboembolism (Cuzick et al. 2003). This could be achieved through a careful selection of women at risk (Goldhaber 2005) and concomitant administration of preventive treatments like low-dose aspirin. At the present time tamoxifen is not the answer (Powles and Chang 1997) since for apparently similar protective effects it has similar venous effects and significant increase in endometrial cancer risk as compared to raloxifene. We have to wait for the results of STAR (Wickerham 2003), an ongoing breast cancer study comparing the ability of tamoxifen and raloxifene to reduce the incidence of breast cancer in postmenopausal women at high risk, and RUTH (Mosca 2001), a prospective, double-blind, randomized study comparing raloxifene an placebo in both secondary prevention of cardivascular disease and risk reduction of breast cancer in postmenopausal women. In the meantime we have to keep in mind that, for menopausal women with osteoporosis and increased breast cancer risk, raloxifene is a reasonable choice to treat osteoporosis and also reduce the risk of breast cancer (Kalidas et al. 2004).

10.7 New Perspectives

At the present time SERMs are the only alternative for pharmacological primary prevention of ER(+) breast cancer. Only a small percentage of the eligible women agree to enter into such a process, the most important reason being the uncertainty about the risk/benefit ratio. Consequently, new research aims to find substances or strategies maintaining the preventive ability at the level of the breast and bone and without the negative impact on venous thrombosis or uterine cancer (Fabian and Kimler 2005).

There are evidences showing that lower daily doses of tamoxifen, between 1 and 5 mg, can obtain antiproliferative effects on in situ or small invasive cancers similar to those observed with the usual dose of 20 mg (Decensi et al. 2003). If that proves to be true with respect to the protective effect in primary prevention, it would probably allow skipping the negative effects on endometrium and coagulation, both dose related.

New SERMS are in different development stages. Lasofoxifene has been shown to have positive effects on bone and lipid metabolism without negative impact on uterine growth (Ke et al. 1998). There is a large-sample, prospective, randomized clinical trial in progress in which breast cancer, together with fracture prevention, is one of the main outcomes.

Bazedoxifene has also demonstrated in experimental studies its ability to inhibit the growth of ER(+) tumors in mice and rats in the absence of uterotrophic effects (Greenberger et al. 2001). At the present time bazedoxifene's ability to counteract the estrogenic effects of CEE at the levels of both breast and endometrium is being tested in a multicentric study comparing calcium + vitamin D to bazedoxifene with and without a low dose of CEE in mild symptomatic postmenopausal women.

Arzoxifene, a third-generation SERM, has demonstrated in experimental, preclinical, and presurgical studies its ability to inhibit tumoral proliferation and prevent bone loss. A randomized trial of arzoxifene vs. placebo has been initiated in late postmenopausal women to evaluate its preventive effect on breast cancer and vertebral fractures.

All these new SERMs will be challenged by the emerging alternative in prevention: aromatase inhibitors (Santen et al. 2001; Cuzick 2005). Data from adjuvant trials suggest that these substances could be more efficient than tamoxifen in preventing new ER(+) cancers without the drawbacks of endometrial cancer and thromboembolic risks. However, they increase bone turnover and induce bone mineral loss leading to the need for coadministering an antiresortive agent. Two large studies, IBIS II and MAP3, are now in the recruitment period to evaluate the preventive effect of anastrazole and exemestane, respectively. IBIS II will also consider the coadministration of a bisphosphonate in case of initial low bone mass, and MAP3 will associate colecoxib to exemestane during the first 3 years in a subgroup of 5100 high-risk postmenopausal women.

When the results of these studies and STAR are made available, the choice between the two alternatives will likely be very complex. Decisions will be influenced by the profile of the women, the importance of the different (bone and breast) risks, and additional risk factors. With quality evidences available, wise clinical judgment will be made on a case-by-case basis.

References

1. Abe O, Abe R, Enomoto K et al. and the Early Breast Cancer Collaborative Group (1998) Tamoxifen for early breast cancer: an overview of the randomized trials. Lancet 351:1451–1467
2. Ames BN, Gold LS (1990) Too many rodent carcinogens: mitogenesis increases mutagenesis. Science 249:970–971
3. Anderson GL, Limacher M, Assaf AR et al. (2004) Effects of conjugated equine estrogens in postmenopausal women with hysterectomy. J Am Med Assoc 291:1701–1712
4. Anzano MA, Peer CW, Smith JM et al. (1996) Chemoprevention of mammary carcinogenesis in the rat: Combined use of Raloxifene an cis-retinoic acid. J Natl Cancer Inst 88:123–125
5. Black DM (1994) The genetics of breast cancer. Eur J Cancer 30a:1957–1961
6. Brinton LA, Devesa SS (1996) Etiology and pathogenesis of breast cancer. Epidemiologic factors. Incidence, demographics and environmental factors. In: Harris JR, Lippman ME, Morrow M, Hellman S (eds) Diseases of the breast. Lippincott-Raven, Philadelphia, pp 159–168
7. Buchanan RB, Blamey RW, Durrant KR et al. (1986) A randomized comparison of tamoxifen with surgical oophorectomy in premenopausal patients with advanced breast cancer. J Clin Oncol 4:1326–1330
8. Cauley JA, Norton L, Lippman ME et al. (2001) Continued breast cancer risk reduction in postmenopausal women treated with raloxifene: 4-year results from the MORE trial. Breast Cancer Res Treat 65[2],125–134
9. Cauley JA, Martino S, Barrett-Connor E et al. (2004) Effect of raloxifene on invasive breast cancer incidence in postmenopausal women stratified by Gail risk assessment: results of the Continuing Outcomes Relevant to Evista (CORE) trial. Abstract 1018. American Society of Clinical Oncology
10. Chlebowski RT, Collyar DE, Somerfield MR et al. (1999) American Society of Clinical Oncology technology assessment on breast cancer risk reduction strategies: tamoxifen and raloxifene. J Clin Oncol 17:1939–1955
11. Chlebowski RT, Col N, Winer EP et al. (2002) American Society of Clinical Oncology Technology assessment of pharmacologic interventions for breast cancer risk reduction including tamoxifen, raloxifene, and aromatase inhibition. J Clin Oncol 20(15):3328–3343
12. Chlebowski RT, Hendrix SL, Langer RD et al. (2003) Influence of estrogen plus progestin on breast cancer and mammography in healthy postmenopausal women. J Am Med Assoc 289:3243–3253
13. Colditz GA, Hankinson SE, Hunter DJ et al. (1995) The use of estrogens and progestins and the risk of breast cancer in postmenopausal women. N Eng J Med 332:1589–1593

14. Collaborative Group on Hormonal Factors in Breast Cancer (1997) Breast cancer and hormone replacement therapy: collaborative reanalysis of data from 51 epidemiological studies of 52,705 women with breast cancer and 108,411 women without breast cancer. Lancet 350:1047–1059
15. Colletti RB, Roberts JD, Devlin JT et al. (1989) Effect of tamoxifen on plasma insulin-like growth factor I in patients with breast cancer. Cancer Res 49:1882–1884
16. Cummings SR, Eckert S, Krueger KA et al. (1999) The effect of raloxifene on risk of breast cancer in postmenopausal women: Results from the MORE randomized trial. J Am Med Assoc 281(23):2189–2197
17. Cummings SR, Duong T, Kenyon E et al. (2002a) Serum estradiol level and risk of breast cancer during treatment with raloxifene. J Am Med Assoc 287:216–220
18. Cummings SR (2002b) Measurement of serum estradiol levels in postmenopausal women. J Am Med Assoc 288:451
19. Cuzick J (2005) Aromatase inhibitors for breast cancer prevention. J Clin Oncol 23:1636–1643
20. Cuzick J, Baum M (1985) Tamoxifen and contralateral breast cancer. Lancet ii:282
21. Cuzick J, Powles T, Veronesi U et al. (2003) Overview of the main outcomes in breast-cancer prevention trials. Lancet 361(9354):296–300
22. Decensi A, Robertson C, Viale G et al. (2003) A randomized trial of low dose tamoxifen on breast cancer proliferation and blood estrogenic biomarkers. J Natl Cancer Inst 95:779–790
23. Decensi A, Maisonneuve P, Rotmenz N et al. (2005) Effect of Tamoxifen on venous thromboembolic events in a breast cancer prevention trial. Circulation 111:650–656
24. Delmas P, Cauley JA, Burshell AL et al. (2005) Breast cancer risk reduction over 8 years in postmenopausal women with osteopenia or osteoporosis receiving raloxifene. Bone 36:S436–7
25. Dijkhuizen FPHLJ, Brölmann HAM, Oddens BJJ et al. (1996) Transvaginal ultrasonography and endometrial changes in postmenopausal breast cancer patients receiving tamoxifen. Maturitas 24:45–50
26. Early Breast Cancer Collaborative Group (1998) Tamoxifen for early breast cancer: an overview of the randomized trials. Lancet 351:1451–1467
27. Endogenous Hormones and Breast Cancer Collaborative Group (2003) Body mass index, serum sex hormones and breast cancer risk in post menopausal women. J Natl Cancer Inst 95:1218–1226
28. Fabian CJ, Kimler BF (2005) Selective estrogen receptor modulators for primary prevention of breast cancer. J Clin Oncol 23:1644–1655
29. Fisher B, Constantino JP, Wickerham DL et al. and other National Surgical Adjuvant Breast and Bowel Project Investigators (1998) Tamoxifen for prevention of breast cancer: report of the National Surgical Adjuvant Breast and Bowel Project P-1 study. J Natl Cancer Inst 90:1371–1388
30. Freiss G, Rochefort H, Vignon F (1990) Mechanisms of 4-hydroxytamoxifen antigrowth factor activity in breast cancer cells: alterations of growth factor receptor binding sites and tyroxine kinase activity. Biochem Biophys Res Commun 919–926
31. Gail MH, Brinton LA, Byar DP et al. (1989) Projecting individualized probabilities of developing breast cancer for white females who are being examined annually. J Natl Cancer Inst 81:1879–1986
32. Goldhaber SZ (2005) Tamoxifen, preventing breast cancer and placing the risk of deep vein thrombosis in perspective. Circulation 111:539–541
33. Grady D, Herrington D, Bittner V et al. for the HERS research group (2002) Cardiovascular disease outcomes during 6.8 years of hormone therapy: Heart and

Estrogen/progestin Replacement Study follow-up (HERS II). J Am Med Assoc 28:49–57
34. Holli K, Isola J, Cuzick J (1997) Hormone replacement therapy and biological aggressiveness of breast cancer. Lancet 350:1704–1705
35. Huff KK, Knabe C, Linsey R (1988) Multihormonal regulation of insulin-like growth factor-1-related protein in MCF-7 cells. Mol Endocrinol 2:200–208
36. Hulley S, Furberg C, Barret-Connor E et al. (2002) Noncardiovascular disease outcomes during 6.8 years of hormone therapy. J Am Med Assoc 288:58–66
37. IBIS (2002) First results from the international Breast Cancer Intervention Study (IBIS-I): a randomised prevention trial. Lancet 360:817–824
38. Ingle JN, Krook JE, Green SJ et al. (1986) Randomized trial of bilateral oophorectomy versus tamoxifen in premenopausal women with metastasic breast cancer. J Clin Oncol 4:178–185
39. Johnell O, Cauley JA, Kulkarni PM et al. (2004) Raloxifene reduces risk of vertebral fractures and breast cancer in postmenopausal women regardless of prior hormone therapy. J Fam Pract 53:789–796
40. Jordan CV (1994) Molecular mechanisms of antiestrogen action in breast cancer. Breast Cancer Res Treat 31:41–52
41. Kalidas M, Hilsenbeck S, Brown P (2004) Defining the role of raloxifene for the prevention of breast cancer. J Natl Cancer Inst 96(23):1731–1733
42. Ke HZ, Paralkar VM, Grasser WA et al. (1998) Effects of CP-336,156, a new, nonsteroidal estrogen agonist/antagonist, on bone, serum cholesterol, uterus, and body composition in rat models. Endocrinology 139:2068–2076
43. Kinsinger LS, Harris S (2002) Chemoprevention of breast cancer: a promising idea with an uncertain future. Lancet 360:813–814
44. Kleinman D, Karas M, Danilenko M (1996) Stimulation of endometrial cancer cell growth by tamoxifen is associated with increased insulin-like growth factor (IGF)-I induced tyrosine phosphorylation and reduction of IGF binding proteins. Endocrinology 137:1089–1095
45. Lee AV, Yee D (1995) Insulin-like growth factors and breast cancer. Biomed Pharmacother 49:415–421
46. Lippman ME, Krueger KA, Eckert S et al. (2001) Indicators of lifetime estrogen exposure: effect on breast cancer incidence and interaction with Raloxifene therapy in the multiple outcomes of Raloxifene evaluation study participants. J Clin Oncol 19(12):3111–3116
47. Love RR, Mazess RB, Barden HS et al. (1992) Effects of tamoxifen in bone mineral density in post menopausal women with breast cancer. N Engl J Med 326:852–856
48. Manier J, Johansson R, Lenner P (2004) Smoking is associated wtith post menopausal breast cancer in women with high levels of estrogens. Int J Cancer 112:324–328
49. Marchbanks PA, Mc Donald JA, Wilson HG et al. (2002) Oral contraceptives and the risk of breast cancer. N Engl J Med 27(346):2025–2032
50. Martino S, Cauley JA, Barrett-Connor E et al. (2004a) Continuing outcomes relevant to Evista: Breast cancer incidence in postmenopausal osteoporotic women in a randomized trial of raloxifene. J Natl Cancer Inst 96(23):1751–1761
51. Martino S, Powles T, Cauley JA et al. (2004b) Effect of raloxifene on incidence of invasive breast cancer in postmenopausal women stratified by baseline serum estradiol: results of the Continuing Outcomes Relevant to Evista (CORE) trial. San Antonio Breast Cancer Symposium

52. Martino S, Disch D, Dowsett S, Mershon J (2005a) Effect of raloxifene on invasive breast cancer incidence in postmenopausal women stratified by age (< 65 and > 65 years) Abstract: ASCO Annual Meeting
53. Martino S, Disch D, Dowsett S, Mershon J (2005b) Raloxifene and Breast Cancer Risk Reduction based on Breast Cancer Family History. Abstract. ASCO, San Francisco
54. McPherson K, Steel CM, Dixon JM (2000) ABC of breast cancer: Epidemiology, risk factors and genetics. Br Med J 321:624–628
55. McTiernan A, Rajan KB, Tworoger S et al. (2003) Adiposity and sex hormones in post menopausal breast cancer survivors. J Clin Oncol 21:1961–1966
56. McTiernan A, Rajan KB, Ulrich CM et al. (2004) Effect of exercise on serum estrogens in postmenopausal women: a 12-month randomized clinical trial. Cancer Res 64:2923–2928
57. Mosca L, Barrett-Connor E, Wenger NK et al. (2001) Design and methods of the Raloxifene Use for the Heart (RUTH) study. Am J Cardiol 88:392–395
58. Kikuchi Y, Hirata J, Kita T, Imaizumi E et al. (1997) SEER cancer statistics review. National Cancer Institute Bethesda, MD
59. Nolvadex Adjuvant Trial Organization (1983) Controlled trial of tamoxifen as adjuvant agent in management of early breast cancer; interim analysis at four years by Nolvadex Adjuvant Trial Organization. Lancet i:257–261
60. Pike MC, Krailo MD, Henderson BE (1983) "Hormonal" risk factors, "breast tissue age" and the age incidence of breast cancer. Nature 303:767–769
61. Poulin R, Merand Y, Poirier D et al. (1989) Antiestrogenic properties of keoxifene, trans-4-hydroxytamoxifen, and ICI 164384, a new steroidal antiestrogen, in ZR-75-1 human breast cancer cells. Breast cancer Res Treat 14:65–76
62. Powles TJ, Chang J (1997) Chemoprevention of breast cancer: why is tamoxifen not the answer? Endocrine-related cancer 4:135–139
63. Powles T, Eeles R, Ashley S (1998) Interim analysis of the incidence of breast cancer in the Royal Marsden Hospital tamoxifen randomizˌsed chemoprevention trial. Lancet 352:98–101
64. Purdie D, Cauley J, Disch D et al. (2004) Effect of raloxifene on incidence of invasive breast cancer in postmenopausal women having a history of prior hormone therapy use: results of the CORE trial Abstract. European Society of Medical Oncology (ESMO), Vienna
65. Russo J, Rivera R, Russo IH (1992) Influence of age and parity on the development of the human breast. Breast Cancer Res Treat 23:211–218
66. Russo J, Russo IH (1997) Role of differentiation in the pathogenesis and prevention of breast cancer. Endocrine-Rel Cancer 4:7–21
67. Rossouw JE, Anderson GL, Prentice RL et al. (2002) Risks and benefits of estrogen plus progestin in healthy postmenopausal women: principal results from the Women's Health Initiative
68. Santner SJ, Pauley RJ, Tait L (1997) Aromatase activity and expression in breast cancer and benign breast tissue stromal cells. J Clin Endocrinol Metab 82:200–208
69. Santen RJ (2002) To block estrogen's synthesis or action: That is the question. J Clin Endocrinol Metab 87(7):3007–3012
70. Santen RJ, Pinkerton J, McCartney C (2001) Clinical review 121: Risk of breast cancer with progestins in combination with estrogen as hormone replacement therapy. J Clin Endocrinol Metab 86(1):16–23
71. Silverman SL, Delmas PD, Kulkarni PM (2004) Comparison of fracture, cardiovascular event, and breast cancer rates at 3 years in postmenopausal women with osteoporosis. J Am Geriatr Soc 52(9):1543–1548

72. Stanczyk FZ (2002) Measurement of serum estradiol levels in postmenopausal women. J Am Med Assoc 288:450–451
73. Toniolo PG, Levitz M, Zeleniuch-Jacquotte N (1995) A prospective study of endogenous estrogens and breast cancer in postmenopausal women. J Natl Cancer Inst 87:190–197
74. Veronesi U, Maisonneuve P, Costa A (1998) Prevention of breast cancer with tamoxifen: preliminary findings from the Italian randomised trial among hysterectomised women. Italian Tamoxifen Prevention Study. Lancet 352:93–97
75. Veronesi U, Maisonneuve P, Sacchini V et al. (2002a) Tamoxifen for breast cancer among hysterectomised women. Lancet 359:1122–1124
76. Veronesi U, Maisonneuve P, Rotmenz N et al. (2002b) Italian randomised trial among women with hysterectomy: tamoxifen and hormone dependent breast cancer in high-risk women. J Natl Cancer Inst 94:160–165
77. Wellings SR, Jensen HM, Marcum RG (1975) An atlas of subgross pathology of 16 human breasts with special reference to possible precancerous lesions. J Natl Cancer Inst 55:231–275
78. Wickerham DL (2003) Tamoxifen's impact as a preventive agent in clinical practice and an update of the STAR trial. Recent Results Cancer Res 163:87–95
79. Wolman SR, Heppner GH, Wolman E (1997) New directions in breast cancer research. FASEB J 11:535–543
80. Young RL (1999) Selective estrogens and breast tissue. Am J Managed Care 5(Suppl 3):S180–S189
81. Zhang Y, Kiel DP, Kreger BE et al. (1997) Bone mass and the risk of breast cancer among postmenopausal women. N Engl J Med 336:611–617

CHAPTER 11

Endometrial Effects of SERMs

SANTIAGO PALACIOS

11.1
Introduction

SERMs (Selective Estrogen Receptor Modulators) are compounds with a molecular structure different from that of steroids. They share with steroids their selective binding to estrogen receptors (ERs), which is followed by an agonistic or antagonistic effect, depending on the target cell and the hormonal environment. Initially known as antiestrogens, and developed for treatment of breast cancer, the two better known SERMs tamoxifen and raloxifene are being used currently in the prevention and treatment of breast cancer and osteoporosis, respectively. A recently published review of a total of 37,000 women in 55 trials confirmed that, when used as an additional treatment, tamoxifen significantly improved 10-year survival in women with breast cancer positive for ER (Early Breast Cancer Trialists' Collaborative Group 1998). Nevertheless, the incidence of endometrial cancer appeared to double after 1 to 2 years of treatment, and nearly quadrupled when treatment lasted for 5 years (Early Breast Cancer Trialists' Collaborative Group 1998).

These clinical observations demonstrate that the effect of tamoxifen and other SERMs on the endometrium needs to be studied in depth in order to offer objective evidence-based information on these compounds to our patients. This chapter provides a summary of the information available on the mechanism of action and on the clinical data of SERMs on the endometrium.

11.2
Mechanism of Action in the Endometrium

As has been widely commented in previous chapters, the agonist/antagonist profile of a given SERM is determined by the type of compound and the particular target tissue.

Members of the different SERM families bind to the ligand-binding domain (LBD) of the ER, whose particular crystal structure has been revealed for estradiol and for raloxifene (Brzozowski et al. 1997). Once inserted into the binding cavity, estradiol makes direct hydrogen bonds bewteen its A-ring and the carboxylate of Glu 353, the guanidinium group of Arg 394, and between a water molecule, and between its D-ring and His 524 (Brzozowski et al. 1997). As a consequence of the estradiol insertion within the LBD, the large helix 12 of the ER folds over and traps the steroid, thus exposing three specific amino acids, 540, 543, and 547, critical within the activating function-2 (AF-2) region for binding coactivators (Tzukerman et al. 1994).

Raloxifene is also anchored to the same three amino acids as estradiol by direct hydrogen bonds, but it also interacts with Asp 351. The final orientation of raloxifene within the binding pocket determines that its side chain displaces helix 12. Then, helix 12 becomes reoriented and cannot seal the pocket containing the ligand (MacGregor et al. 1998). The repositioned AF-2 region impairs the formation of transcription complex by coactivators, and the signal transduction is blocked.

11.2.1 Tamoxifen

Together with other members of the triphenylethylene family, tamoxifen has been shown to act as an AF-2 antagonist, a trait shared with raloxifene. However, tamoxifen and other triphenylethylene derivatives act as partial agonists in the uterus, an effect that seems opposite to that of raloxifene. It may, therefore, be postulated that at the endometrial level (where both tamoxifen and raloxifene share the same tissue and promoter context), the contrasting action of those compounds may be due to particular details of the conformational change induced on the ligand–receptor complex, at either the AF-2 or other domain. Recent results obtained in mice further support the notion that tamoxifen acts in the endometrium as a classical impeded estrogen and that the AF-1 domain regulates its effects (Zhang et al. 2005).

The proliferative effects of tamoxifen on the endometrium have been supported by molecular data. The expression of both ER and progesterone receptors (PRs) was found to be consistently positive in endometria from women treated with tamoxifen for 1 month (Cano et al. 2000). That positivity has been reported to be even higher than that found in a control group of premenopausal women (Kommoss et al. 1998). Tamoxifen also mimicked estradiol treatment in up-regulating ERs, c-fos, and glyceraldehyde phosphate dehydrogenase mRNAs, together with other estrogen-induced genes (Rivera-Gonzalez et al. 1998; Robertson et al. 1998). The bromo-deoxyuridine index, an indicator of cell mitogenesis, has been shown to increase in endometrial cells from tamoxifen-treated uteri (Karlsson et al. 1998; Carthew et al. 1999). In this connection, the expression of markers of proliferation, e.g., Ki67, was potentiated by tamoxifen in human endometrium (Elkas et al.

1998). More recently, tamoxifen increased Ki67 expression in the human endometrial adenocarcinoma Ishikawa cell line (Koda et al. 2004). An increased susceptibility to genetic lesions associated with carcinogenesis linked to tamoxifen was suggested by a study on endometrium of surgically postmenopausal cynomolgus macaques, where the drug induced p53 positivity, although at a lower level than conjugated equine estrogens (CEE) (Isaksson et al. 1999).

The available experimental information is still of little help in clarifying whether tamoxifen is genotoxic and oncogenetic in human endometrium. There is, nonetheless, a great deal of debate about the actual relevance of minor concentrations of adducts (as detected by high-perfomance liquid chromatography and other modern technology), compared with the high concentrations induced in rat hepatic tumors, or the equally elevated concentrations formed in human DNA as a result of enviromental sources (Swenberg et al. 1997). Accordingly, if tamoxifen is an endometrial carcinogen, as classified by the International Agency for Research on Cancer (IARC), its mechanism of action is possibly different from that reported in rat liver.

An alternative oncogenetic mode of action of tamoxifen on human endometrium may derive from its proliferative activity. It is possible that the increase in the rate of mitoses in a given tissue entails an augmented risk of mutation, the first step toward malignancy (Ames et al. 1990). Therefore, it is possible that the oncogenetic attributes of estrogens in tissues where they induce a proliferative effect (e.g., breast or endometrium) might be influenced by the mutagenic potential derived from a higher mitotic activity. This might also be the main pathway for the oncogenetic action of tamoxifen in the uterus, where one study showed that an increase in uterine weight by tamoxifen was accompanied by a doubled uterine expression of insulinlike growth factor-I (IGF-I), whereas the opposite occurred when the pure antiestrogen ICI 182780 was used instead of tamoxifen (Huynh et al. 1993). In a subsequent study, the same investigators showed that the expression of insulinlike growth factor-binding protein (IGFBP)-3, the principal quantitative binder of IGF-I, was similarly suppressed by estradiol and tamoxifen (Huynh et al. 1994).

The dysregulation of transforming growth factor-β (TGFβ) has also been suggested as an additional epigenetic (nongenotoxic) mechanism of tamoxifen carcinogenicity (Carmichael et al. 1998). It has been postulated that the tamoxifen-induced dysregulation of the TGFβ signalling pathway may create an environment that selects for the cells with genetic alterations in the signal system (Carmichael et al. 1998). Cells with mutations in this pathway become refractory to mitosis inhibitory signals, thus developing into end-stage tumors.

11.2.2 Raloxifene

Crystallographic studies have confirmed that a critical difference in the antiestrogenic action of raloxifene lies in the interaction of the alkylaminoethoxy side chain with the amino acid aspartate at position 351. The peculiar orientation of this side chain of the raloxifene molecule, an essential determinant of the antiestrogenic properties of the drug, is believed to account for its lack of endometrial activity (Clark et al. 1976; Grese et al. 1997; Bryant et al. 1998).

Biochemical data support the lack of agonistic activity of raloxifene on uterine tissue (Somjen et al. 1996). Raloxifene has exhibited little uterothropic activity in rodents (Black and Goode 1980, 1981; Black et al. 1983) and has not resulted in increases in uterine weight or in stimulation of epithelial cell height and eosinophilic infiltration (Bryant et al. 1998). In other experiments on ovariectomized rats, raloxifene was similar to the no-treatement controls with regard to uterine epithelial cell height myometrial thickness and stromal expansion (Black et al. 1994; Sato et al. 1996). There are, however, discrepant data showing increases in uterine weight and uterine epithelial thickness in ovariectomized (Sato et al. 1996) or immature (Ashby et al. 1997) rats. Interestingly, raloxifene has been shown to block the stimulating endometrial effects of estrogen and tamoxifen (Bryant et al. 1998; Black et al. 1994; Sato et al. 1996; Palacios et al. 2000), an effect confirmed on an endometrial carcinoma cell line grown in athymic mice (Kleinman et al. 1996).

Table 11.1. Actions of SERMs on uterus. Preclinical data (Gottardis et al. 1990)

- In ovariectomized rats
  - Tamoxifen produces a trophic effect:
    - ↑ weight of uterus
    - ↑ thickness of endometrium
    - ↑ thickness of myometrium
- Raloxifene produces a minimum effect on:
  - Weight of uterus
  - Endometrium
  - Myometrium
- Ovariectomized rats treated with estrogens
  - Tamoxifen produces a partial blockade of the estrogenic effect (partial agonistic effect)
  - Raloxifene blocks the estrogenic effect (antagonist)
- Intact rats

  Mature:
  - Tamoxifen ↓↓ the weight of the uterus
  - Raloxifene ↓↓ the weight of the uterus

A summary of preclinical data on the uterus is given in Table 11.1 (Gottardis et al. 1990).

11.3 Tamoxifen and Endometrium: Clinical Consideration

Descriptive as well as case-control and cohort studies have shown that tamoxifen may cause alterations, including cancer, in human endometrium. The findings have been observed in studies using ultrasound technology or histology data.

11.3.1 Ultrasonographic Findings

Studies carried out with transvaginal ultrasound (TVU) in postmenopausal women with breast cancer have shown that the endometrium is thickened more frequently in women receiving tamoxifen than in those not treated with the drug. For example, in a transversal study Cohen et al. observed that 94.6% of women treated with tamoxifen and nonsymptomatic from a gynecological point of view had an endometrial thickness $\geq$ 5 mm, an observation that was present in only 40% of women who did not receive this treatment (Cohen et al. 1994).

Further, postmenopausal women taking tamoxifen for secondary prevention of breast cancer for an average of 24 months seemed to have a uterus significantly larger and with a greater volume than those who did not take the drug. Their endometrium was also significantly thicker (average of 9.1 vs. 4.8 mm, respectively). Yet, although the normal appearance of the endometrium was more frequent in the untreated group, this difference was not significant. However, the image of thickened cystic endometrium was significantly more frequent in the tamoxifen group (Kedar et al. 1994).

11.3.2 Hystological Findings

The presence of an enlarged endometrium ($\geq$ 5 mm) may be associated with endometrial abnormalities, principally polyps, hyperplasia, or even adenocarcinoma of the endometrium, in the postmenopausal woman (Dijkhuizen et al. 1996; Granberg et al. 1991; Holbert 1997). It seems that treatment with tamoxifen in postmenopausal women sustains this association. Thus, in the previously mentioned study by Cohen et al. (1994), the only endometrial abnormalities were found in those women whose endometrium had a thickness

$\geq$ 5 mm. The endometrial pathology was seen more frequently in tamoxifen-treated women (35.5% vs. 20%). The histology of the endometrial biopsies obtained in women on tamoxifen was reported as proliferative endometrium (24.74%), polyps (5.38%), cancer of the endometrium (3.2%), and hyperplasia (2.15%). In the case of women not on tamoxifen, no material was obtained from biopsy in 80% of cases, and in the rest the diagnosis was proliferative endometrium. Although a clear relationship between length of treatment and the presence of pathological endometrium could not be demonstrated, all tamoxifen-treated women with abnormal endometrium had received treatment for approximately 1 year (Cohen et al. 1994). Healthy postmenopausal women were also associated with histological alterations of the endometrium when treated with tamoxifen.

A randomized placebo-controlled trial found that 39% of the tamoxifen-treated women had an endometrial abnormality, a percentage that was reduced to 10% of women on placebo ($p < 0.0001$) (Kedar et al. 1994), though no cases of endometrial cancer were diagnosed in this study. The histological abnormalities found in the tamoxifen group were atypical hyperplasia (16%), proliferative endometrium (13%), polyps (8%), or presence of mitosis (2%). The authors concluded that the predicative value of an endometrium thickness $\geq$ 8 mm was 100% for the presence of atypical hyperplasia or endometrial polyps. No correlation could be found between the presence of endometrial pathology and the length of treatment with tamoxifen (Kedar et al. 1994).

In contrast to the data from that study, other authors have suggested that the increased endometrial thickness found in postmenopausal women treated with tamoxifen is less frequently associated with endometrial abnormalities, even in the presence of a marked thickening and cystic appearance (Achiron et al. 1996; McGonigle et al. 1998). Those ultrasonographic findings often represent subendometrial processes such as cysts or stromal edema (Bese et al. 1996; Bornstein et al. 1994; Achiron et al. 1995).

In this respect McGonigle et al. (1998) have observed that after an average of 2.4 years the endometrial abnormalities associated with tamoxifen in a group of postmenopausal women were polyps (66%), found more frequently in women with vaginal bleeding previous to surgery, cysts covered with an atrophic endometrium, or cystic endometrial atrophy (29%). Although one of the polyps proved to be a leiomyoma, no cases of atypical hyperplasia or adenocarcinoma were found among the women studied, thus supporting the idea that endometrial thickening does not seem to reflect serious endometrial pathology in most cases. The authors suggest that the presence of cystic endometrial atrophy could explain the endometrial abnormalities detected by TVU and that do not correspond with polyps, hyperplasia, or adenocarcinoma. Given that TVU cannot differentiate between polyps, hyperplasia, and cysts, the authors recommended the use of sonohysterography in those cases where a taximofen-treated woman has a thickened endometrium and a benign histology after an endometrial biopsy. If sonohysterography does not reveal the presence of polyps, it is very possible that the patient will have a cystic endometrial atrophy (McGonigle et al. 1998).

An important criticism to most of the available information on tamoxifen-induced changes in endometrium has been that the initial status of the endometrium has not been assessed (Berlière et al. 1998). To establish a link between tamoxifen and endometrial changes, it has been said, the endometrium needs to be evaluated before and during treatment.

Three prospective studies have initially assessed the endometrium (Berlière et al. 1998; Neven et al. 2000; Gal et al. 1991). In two of them (Neven et al. 1990; Gal et al. 1991), the low number of women studied, 16 and 12, could be responsible for the lack of endometrial alterations detected prior to treatment and for their low incidence as a result of treatment. The third study (Berlière et al. 1998), however, which included 264 nonsymptomatic postmenopausal women with breast cancer, detected a high prevalence of endometrial abnormalities prior to treatment, 17.4%, polyps being the most frequent (77%). Note that one case of endometrial adenocarcinoma and another of atypical hyperplasia were detected in the pretreatment evaluation. Women with and without lesions were followed separately and, after 3 years of treatment (20 mg/d), the incidence of lesions with/without atypias was significantly greater in the group with lesions prior to treatment. The incidence of benign lesions was similar in both groups (9.8 vs. 11.1%), but atypic endometrial hyperplasia, and adenocarcinoma, had a significantly higher incidence in women with endometrial lesions before treatment with tamoxifen.

Interestingly, the authors observed that the severity of the lesions seemed to increase with the length of exposure to tamoxifen. Women with previous alterations would be, they suggested, more sensitive to the carcinogenetic effects of tamoxifen, an indication favoring the concept that lesions would represent a risk factor (Berlière et al. 1998). However, contrary to what was observed by other researchers (Sasco et al. 1995; Magriples et al. 1993), the adenocarcinomas diagnosed during the study were well differentiated (Berlière et al. 1998). It was then postulated that, as observed for endometrial tumors associated with estrogen replacement therapy, tamoxifen would induce a high proportion of highly differentiated tumors with a better prognosis. Nevertheless, this hypothesis still lacks conclusive data.

11.3.3 Tamoxifen and Risk of Endometrial Cancer

The partial agonistic effect of tamoxifen on the uterus has caused concern not only regarding an increased incidence of endometrial pathology but also regarding a potential increase in endometrial cancer. The probability that a woman will develop endometrial cancer is low, varying from 12 cases per 100,000 women at 40 years to 84 cases per 100,000 women at 60 years (Rose 1996). Tamoxifen has been found to increase the risk for endometrial cancer in the majority of studies. The relative risks (RRs) seem to vary between 1,3 (van Leeuwen et al. 1994) and 6.4 (Early Breast Cancer Trialist's Collaborative Group; Fornander et al. 1989; Andersson et al. 1991, 1992; Fisher et al. 1998) for dosages of 20–40 mg/d. However, some studies did not detect any increase in risk (Fisher et al. 1989; Stewart et al. 1989; Nayfield et al. 1991; Cook et al. 1995).

In a case-control study (van Leeuwen et al. 1994) in which 98 cases of invasive endometrial carcinoma were diagnosed at least 3 months after diagnosis of primary breast cancer, it was observed that the use of tamoxifen was associated with a RR of 1.3. The risk appeared to have a tendency to increase during treatment, from 0.6 for less than a year to 3.0 for more than 5 years of treatment. It should be noted that the accumulated dose of tamoxifen was significantly associated with risk of endometrial cancer. However, the average daily dose used (20–40 mg/d) did not seem to influence risk. Other authors have also observed that the increase in risk is only detected when a determined accumulated dose is attained (van Leeuwen et al. 1994; De Muylder et al. 1991).

The observation that women with breast cancer receiving tamoxifen had a reduced incidence of contralateral cancer was the basis for the NSABP-PI study, a randomized, double-blind, placebo-controlled trial that began in 1992. The main objective was to ascertain whether tamoxifen might effectively reduce the risk for breast cancer in women with a high risk of developing this disease. A total of 13,388 women $\geq$ 35 years old were randomized to either tamoxifen (20 mg/d) or placebo for 5 years. In 1998, the trial was prematurely interrupted as the hypothesis of the study was confirmed (Fisher et al. 1998). However, the reduction in breast cancer risk with tamoxifen was accompanied by an increase in the incidence of invasive endometrial cancer (mean RR = 2.53). The increased risk was seen principally among women $\geq$ 50 years old with a RR of 4.01, while among women $\leq$ 49 years old the RR was 1.21.

During the 66 months of the study the accumulated incidence of endometrial cancer was 5.4/1000 women in the placebo group and 13.0/1000 women in the treatment group. Fourteen out of the 15 cancers in the placebo group were diagnosed in stage 1 of the FIGO classification, and one cancer was diagnosed in stage IV. The 36 invasive endometrial tumors diagnosed in the tamoxifen-treated women were in stage I. Three out of the 4 cases of carcinomas in situ were detected in the placebo group. The only death due to endometrial cancer occurred in the placebo group. In light of these results, the authors commented that the concern about the excess of risk of endometrial cancer associated with tamoxifen could be somewhat exaggerated, in agreement with their and other studies (Fisher 1996; Fisher et al. 1994), the endometrial tumors associated with tamoxifen did not seem to be either more aggressive or to have a worse prognosis or mortality than those arising in women untreated or on estrogen therapy.

In a recent British case-control study, treatment information on 813 patients who had endometrial cancer after being diagnosed with breast cancer was compared to 1067 control patients with breast cancer but no subsequent endometrial cancer. The use of tamoxifen was associated with an increased risk of endometrial cancer (odds ratio = 2.4). Based on the concluding information, the majority of researchers recommended that women taking tamoxifen should be carefully evaluated from an endometrial point of view, both before starting treatment and periodically during its use, and that a physician be consulted in the case of abnormal vaginal bleeding. This risk should be considered for both premenopausal and postmenopausal women for at least 5 years after the last treatment (Swerdlow et al. 2005).

11.4 Raloxifene

None of the clinical trials carried out to evaluate the effects of raloxifene, extending from 8 weeks to 4 years, detected stimulating effects of the drug on endometrium. Consequently, an antiestrogenic, or neutral, profile of raloxifene on endometrium has been vindicated.

11.4.1 Data Obtained from Biopsy

The clarification of whether raloxifene has any potential agonistic effect on the endometrium has been investigated through quantification of the ratio of estrogenicity. This effect has been assessed by studying endometrial tissue samples obtained though biopsy. In one clinical trial by Draper et al. (1996) on 251 healthy postmenopausal women, the treatment with raloxifene at a dose of 200 or 600 mg/d for 8 weeks did not produce changes in the degree of estrogenicity of the endometria when compared with biopsies taken before initiating treatment. In contrast, a group of women randomly assigned to CEE (0.625 mg/d) in the same study exhibited a significant increase in the aforementioned ratio after 8 weeks of treatment. Even the placebo-treated women had a estrogenicity significantly superior to that of women receiving raloxifene (Draper et al. 1996).

In a subsequent study, Boss et al. (1997) confirmed that raloxifene (200 or 600 mg/d) did not produce significant morphological changes in the glandular epithelium or in the stroma when compared with placebo. As expected, treatment with CEE (0.625 mg/d) induced changes clearly proliferative. Curiously, treatment with raloxifene produced, similarly to estrogens, an improved quality in the sample obtained from biopsy, that is to say, the percentage of samples obtained with intact glands and with stromal tissue increased with respect to samples obtained prior to treatment. The authors suggested that raloxifene could produce a lighter edematous endometrium, which in turn would enlarge the cervical orifice, facilitating its entrance and increasing the surface of the sample (Boss et al. 1997).

11.4.2 Ultrasonographic Data and Symptomatology

Delmas et al. (1997) carried out a clinical trial on 601 healthy postmenopausal women to evaluate the antiosteoporotic effect of 2 years of raloxifene treatment at a dose of 30, 60, or 150 mg/d vs. placebo. In this study TVU was used to evaluate the effect of raloxifene on the thickness of the endometrium. No change was observed in endometrial thickness in the 4 groups during the whole study. Vaginal bleeding was observed in 3.0% of women on 60 mg/d raloxifene, which was not significantly different from the 2.2% observed in the control group. Endometrial thickness in these women who bled was in all cases $\leq$ 5 mm, an indication favoring the hypothesis that the bleeding came from atrophic endometrium.

Another clinical trial on women treated with raloxifene at dosages of 60 or 120 mg/d for 6 months confirmed a low incidence in vaginal bleeding, 5 and 3%, respectively. This incidence was similar to that observed in the placebo group (5%) and significantly less than in the group on hormonal treatment (0.625 mg/d of CEE + 2.5 mg/d of MPA), where bleeding attained 45%. No dropouts were produced as a result of bleeding in either of the raloxifene-treated groups or in the placebo group, whereas 9% of women treated with hormones dropped out of the study for this reason (Walsh et al. 1998).

Cohen et al. (2000) presented integrated data from two identically designed, randomized, double-blind, placebo-controlled trials, including 969 healthy women less than 60 years old who were followed for a period of 3 years. Dosages of 30, 60, and 150 mg of raloxifene were used. Endometrial thickness was measured by TVU at the initial stage and then regularly at 6-month intervals for 2 years and again at 3 years. There was no statistical difference between the groups in terms of the endometrial thickness at the initial stage. None of the raloxifene dosages increased vaginal bleeding, affected endometrial thickness, or was associated with uterine pathologies. These findings were confirmed in studies comparing raloxifene with hormone therapy (Christodoulacos et al. 2002; Neven et al. 2000) (Fig. 11.1).

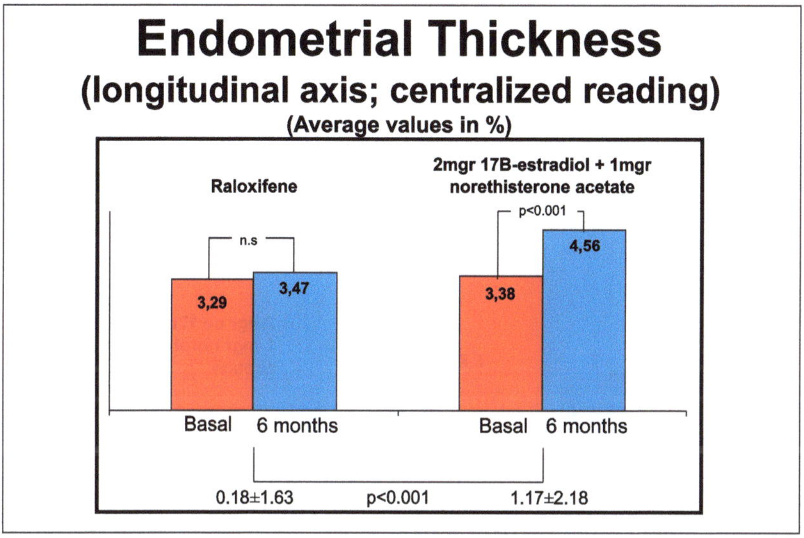

Fig. 11.1. Effects of raloxifene on endometrial thickness compared to combined continuous Hormones: 2 mgr of 17 B-estradiol and 1 mgr of noretisterone acetate for 6 months. (Palacios et al. 2000)

As concluded from the above-mentioned data, the presence of bleeding or spotting is rare during treatment with raloxifene, the incidence being similar to that of placebo. In another study (Christodoulacos et al. 2002), only 7.7% of patients who took raloxifene presented sporadic spotting during the first 6 months of treatment. The incidence of bleeding–spotting was similar in the placebo group and significantly lower than in a group receiving a continuous combined hormonal formulation (estradiol plus norethisterone acetate [NETA]). These results are similar to those of the Euralox study (Neven et al. 2000) and those of Fugere et al. (2000), who reported an incidence of 6.8 and 9%, respectively. All these results further reinforce the notion that raloxifene does not stimulate the endometrium.

Recently Neven et al. (2003) published data of the Euralox study in which the use of raloxifene was not associated with an increase in vaginal bleeding or spotting or in uterine volume after 6 and 12 months of treatment (Fig. 11.2). In this trial, where raloxifene was compared with a formulation containing continuous combined estrogen plus progestin therapy, women using hormones had a higher incidence of benign endometrial pathology, which required more frequent protocol-specific gynecological assessment and followup (Table 11.2) (Neven et al. 2004).

In another study where raloxifene (60 mg/d) was compared with placebo in postmenopausal women for up to 5 years, a similar incidence of vaginal

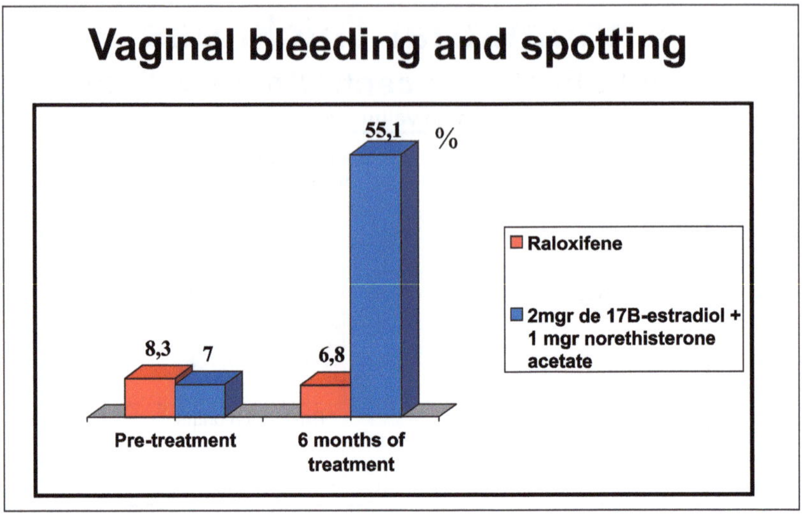

Fig. 11.2. Percentage of women who referred to vaginal bleeding or spotting previous to treatment and after 6 months of treatment with Raloxifene or continuous combined therapy with 2 mgr of 17B-estradiol and 1 mgr of noretisterone acetate (Neven et al. 2003)

bleeding or a mean endometrial thickness of more than 5 mm was found. No diagnosis of endometrial hyperplasia or endometrial cancer was made in either group (Jolly et al. 2003).

Additionally it has been observed that raloxifene reduces the risk of breast cancer by 58–66%, without producing an increased risk of endometrial cancer in postmenopausal women (Cummings et al. 1999; Jordan et al. 1998). The Multiple Outcomes of Raloxifene Evaluation (MORE) clinical trial is particularly eloquent in this regard (Cummings et al. 1999). A total of 7704 postmenopausal women (average age 66.5 years) with osteoporosis and without history of breast or endometrial cancer were included. The trial, which was randomized and double-blind, used two doses of raloxifene (60 or 120 mg/d) or placebo to as-

Table 11.2. Uterine effects of estrogen plus progestin therapy and raloxifene (Euralox study) (Neven et al. 2004)

	Estrogen/progestin therapy vs. raloxifene Average values in %	
Benign endometrial proliferation	8.8 vs. 1.2	$p < 0.001$
Endometrial polyps	4.3 vs. 2	$p = 0.048$
Cystic atrophy	5.5 vs. 1.2	$p < 0.001$

sess whether raloxifene reduced the number of fractures more effectively than placebo. Apart from the successful effect against fractures, raloxifene significantly reduced the risk of breast cancer (RR = 0.26) with respect to placebo after an average of 28.9 months of followup. Moreover, raloxifene did not significantly change the incidence of endometrial cancer (Cummings et al. 1999). This neutral effect was subsequently confirmed after 48-month followup in the MORE study (Cauley et al. 2001).

11.5 Others SERMs

11.5.1 Arzoxifene

Arzoxifene is an orally active third-generation selective ER modulator. Arzoxifene has been shown to induce apoptosis in an ER-positive cell line through a mechanism that includes induction of TGFβ (Colletta et al. 1990). The capacity to induce TGF-β expression may contribute to the potential antiproliferative effects of arzoxifene in hormonally responsive uterine.

In preclinical models, arzoxifene exerts an estrogen agonistic effect on bone and on the lipid profile and an estrogen antagonistic effect in breast and endometrium (Sato et al. 1998; Russo et al. 1990; Ma et al. 1998). Thus, in both the ovariectomized rat and the ovary-intact rat arzoxifene did not stimulate uterine weight gain (Russo et al. 1990).

Clinical phase I and II data reveal arzoxifene to be safe, well tolerated, and efficacious. Two multi-institutional phase II trials including 100 women with metastatic or recurrent endometrial cancer have demonstrated significant activity of arzoxifene at 20 mg/d in patients with metastatic or recurrent endometrial cancer. The observed clinical response rates were 25 and 31%, with a mean response duration of 19.3 and 13.9 months, respectively. Progression of the disease was stabilised in a substantial number of women. Toxicity was mild, except for two cases of pulmonary embolism that might have been drug related (Burke et al. 2003).

Phase III trials on treatment and prevention of postmenopausal osteoporosis are in progress.

11.5.2 Bazedoxifene Acetate

Bazedoxifene acetate is a third-generation SERM. In in vitro studies bazedoxifene competitively inhibited 17β-estradiol binding to both ERα (Ki = 0.1 nM) and ERβ (Ki = 0.03 nM). Bazedoxifene's ability to competitively bind to ERs while exhibiting estrogenlike activity in a promoter and cell-type selective manner is the hallmark of SERM-type action and a prominent characteristic of this drug (Miller et al. 2002).

Bazedoxifene's primary indication is the treatment and prevention of postmenopausal osteoporosis (Miller et al. 2002). In animal models bazedoxifene displays estrogenlike agonistic activity on bone loss and significantly reduces total cholesterol levels with doses as low as 0.1 mg/kg (Miller et al. 2002). Also in these models, there is no evidence of an estrogenic stimulatory effect on the endometrial epithelial cell (Miller et al. 2001).

Clinical phase I and II data reveal bazedoxifene to be safe, very well tolerated, and efficacious. Phase III trials are currently in progress.

11.5.3 Lasofoxifene

This is a third-generation SERM. It binds with high affinity to human estrogen receptors and acts as a tissue-selective estrogen antagonist or agonist.

In preclinical models of postmenopausal osteoporosis, lasofoxifene inhibited bone turnover and prevented bone loss throughout the skeleton (Maeda et al. 2004). The primary indication of lasofoxifene is the treatment and prevention of postmenopausal osteoporosis. In preclinical models, lasofoxifene inhibited breast tumor formation and reduced serum cholesterol (Maeda et al. 2004). Lasofoxifene-treated animals did not differ from ovariectomized controls with respect to endometrial thickness and superficial and basal endometrial gladular epithelial luminal area (Maeda et al. 2004; Ke et al. 2004).

The clinical phase I and II trials correlate well with the preclinical pharmacology. Phase III trials are currently in progress.

11.5.4 Ospemifene

Ospemifene is a novel third-generation SERM that in animal models has been shown to have agonistic effects on bone and the cardiovascular system and antagonistic effects in uterus and breast.

In a double-blind, placebo-controlled phase I study, ospemifene exerted a very weak estrogenic effect on endometrial histology, and no clinically significant changes were seen in endometrial thickness at any dose level (Voipio et al. 2002). In another double-blind study, ospemifene at daily doses of 30 to 90 mg did not stimulate growth of endometrial thickness (Rutanen et al. 2003).

11.6 Conclusions

The preclinical data indicate that SERMs exert a specific action depending not only on the tissue on which they act but also on the hormonal enviroment. Tamoxifen, through its partial estrogenic agonism on the uterus, seems to produce a trophic effect in the endometrium and myometrium in ovariectomized rats. Raloxifene behaves as an estrogenic antagonist at this level, producing a minimum effect on the uterus. However, both raloxifene and tamoxifen produced a decrease in the weight of the uterus in intact rats, although to a lesser degree than that produced by surgical castration.

According to results from clinical trials, the agonistic effects of tamoxifen detected in animals were also observed in the human uterus as it produces a trophic effect and an increase in the incidence of endometrial pathology, which is related to endometrial thickening ($\geq$ 4 mm). Its use seems to be associated with an increase in endometrial cancer, which is related to the length of treatment and the accumulated dose of tamoxifen. Nevertheless, these tumors do not seem to be more aggressive or to have a worse prognosis than those found in women who do not follow this treatment or who receive hormone therapy.

Clinical evidence indicates that the use of tamoxifen increases survival up to 10 years in women with breast cancer. Tamoxifen also seems to diminish the incidence of breast cancer in healthy women with a high risk of suffering from the tumor. Its use as a therapy in breast cancer should be accompanied by careful periodic vigilance of the endometrium. In healthy women, a careful evaluation of the risk/benefit for each and every woman should be imposed.

Unlike tamoxifen, raloxifene seems to have a minimum effect on the uterus in postmenopausal women. It does not seem to produce any estrogenic effect on the endometrium or the myometrium from a histological or ultrasonographic point of view. The low incidence of vaginal bleeding is similar to that observed in untreated women, and these data should be taken into consideration as they will facilitate adherence to treatment. An important strength of raloxifene is its efficacy in the prevention and treatment of osteoporosis without increasing the risk of endometrial cancer, at least during 4 years of treatment.

References

1. Achiron R, Lipitz S, Sivan E, Goldenberg M, Mashiach S (1995) Sonohysterography for ultrasonographic evaluation of tamoxifen-associated cystic thickened endometrium. J Ultrasound Med 14:685–688
2. Achiron R, Grisaru D, Golan-Porat, Lipitz S (1996) Tamoxifen and the uterus: an old drug tested by new modalities. Ultrasound Obstet Gynecol 7:374–378

3. Ames BN, Gold LS (1990) Too many rodent carcinogens: mitogenesis increases mutagenesis. Science 249(4972):970–971
4. Andersson M, Storm HH, Mouridsen HT (1991) Incidence of new primary cancers after adjuvant tamoxifen therapy and radiotherapy for early breast cancer. J Natl Cancer Inst 83:1013–1017
5. Andersson M, Storm HH, Mouridsen HT (1992) Carcinogenic effects of adjuvant tamoxifen treatment and radiotherapy for early breast cancer. Acta Oncol 31:259–263
6. Ashby J, Odum J, Foster JR (1997) Activity of raloxifene in immature and ovariectomized rat uterotrophic assays. Regul Toxicol Pharmacol 25(3):226–231
7. Berlière M, Charles A, Galant C, Donnez J (1998) Uterine side effects of tamoxifen: a need for systematic pretreatment screening. Obstet Gynecol 91:40–44
8. Bese T, Kösebay D, Demirkiran F, Arvas M, Bese N, Mandel N (1996) Ultrasonographic appearence of endometrium in postmenopausal breast cancer patients receiving tamoxifen. Eur J Obstet Gynecol Reprod Biol 67:157–162
9. Black LJ, Goode RL (1980) Uterine bioassay of tamoxifen, trioxifene and a new estrogen antagonist (LY117018) in rats and mice. Life Sci 26(17):1453–1458
10. Black LJ, Goode RL (1981) Evidence for biological action of the antiestrogens LY117018 and tamoxifen by different mechanisms. Endocrinology 109(3):987–989
11. Black LJ, Jones CD, Falcone JF (1983) Antagonism of estrogen action with a new benzothiophene derived antiestrogen. Life Sci 32(9):1031–1036
12. Black LJ, Sato M, Rowley ER, Magee DE, Bekele A, Williams DC, Cullinan GJ, Bendele R, Kauffman RF, Bensch WR, et al. (1994) Raloxifene (LY139481 HCI) prevents bone loss and reduces serum cholesterol without causing uterine hypertrophy in ovariectomized rats. J Clin Invest 93(1):63–69
13. Bornstein J, Auslender R, Pascal B, Gutterman E, Isakov D, Abramovici H (1994) Diagnostic pitfalls of ultrasonographic uterine screening in women treated with tamoxifen. J Reprod Med 39:674–678
14. Boss SM, Huster WJ, Neild JA, Glant MD, Eisenhut CC, Draper MW (1997) Effects of raloxifene hydrochloride on the endometrium of postmenopausal women. Am J Obstet Gynecol 177:1458–1464
15. Bryant HU, Dere WH (1998) Selective estrogen receptor modulators: an alternative to hormone replacement therapy. Proc Soc Exp Biol Med 217(1):45–52
16. Brzozowski AM, Pike AC, Dauter Z, Hubbard RE, Bonn T, Engstrom O, Ohman L, Greene GL, Gustafsson JA, Carlquist M (1997) Molecular basis of agonism and antagonism in the oestrogen receptor. Nature 389(6652):753–758
17. Burke TW, Walker CL (2003) Arzoxifene as therapy for endometrial cancer. Gynecol Oncol 90(2 Pt 2):S40–46
18. Cano A, Hermenegildo C (2000) The endometrial effects of SERMs. Hum Reprod Update 6(3):244–254
19. Carmichael PL, Mills JJ, Neven P (1998) An epigenetic mechanism for tamoxifen-associated uterine carcinogenesis? Eur J Cancer 34(Suppl 4):S10–S11
20. Carthew P, Edwards RE, Nolan BM (1999) Uterotrophic effects of tamoxifen, toremifene, and raloxifene do not predict endometrial cell proliferation in the ovariectomized CD1 mouse. Toxicol Appl Pharmacol 158(1):24–32
21. Cauley JA, Norton L Lippman ME, Eckert S, Krueger KA, Purdie DW, et al. (2001) Continued breast cancer risk reduction in postmenopasusal women treated with raloxifene: 4 year results from the MORE trial. Breast Cancer Res Treatment 65:125–134
22. Christodoulacos G, Panoulis C, Botsis D, Rizoz D, Kassanos D, Creatsas G (2002) Transvaginal sonographic monitoring of the uterine effects of raloxifene and a continuous combined replacement therapy in postmenopausal women. Maturitas 42:77–84

23. Clark ER, Jordan VC (1976) Oestrogenic, anti-oestrogenic and fertility effects of some triphenylethanes and triphenylethylenes related to ethamoxytriphetol (MER 25). Br J Pharmacol 57(4):487–493
24. Cohen I, Rosen DJ, Shapira J, Cordoba M, Gilboa S, Altaras MM, et al. (1994) Endometrial changes with tamoxifen: comparison between tamoxifen-treated and nontreated asymptomatic, postmenopausal breast cancer patients. Gynecol Oncol 52:185–190
25. Cohen FJ, Watts S, Shah A, Akers S, Plouffe L (2000) Uterine effects of 3-years raloxifene therapy in postmenopausal women younger than age 60. Obstet Gynecol 95(1):104–111
26. Colletta AA, Wakefield LM, Howell FV, van Roozendaal KE, Danielpour D, Ebbs SR, Sporn MB, Baum M (1990) Anti-oestrogens induce the secretion of active transforming growth factor beta from human fetal fibroblasts. Br J Cancer 62(3):405–409
27. Cook LS, Weiss NS, Schwartz SM, White E, McKnight B, Moore DE, et al. (1995) Population-based study of tamoxifen therapy and subsequent ovarian, endometrial, and breast cancers. J Natl Cancer Inst 87:1359–1364
28. Cummings SR, Eckert S, Krueger KA, Grady D, Powles TJ, Cauley JA, et al. (1999) The effect of raloxzifene on risk of breast cancer in postmenopausal women:results from MORE randomized trial. Multiple Outcomes of Raloxifene Evaluation. J Am Med Assoc 281:2189–2197
29. Delmas PD, Bjarnason NH, Mitlak BH, Ravoux AC, Shah AS, Huster WJ, et al. (1997) Effects of raloxifene on bone mineral density, serum cholesterol concentrations, and uterine endometrium in postmenopausal women. N Engl J Med 337:1641–1647
30. De Muylder X, Neven P, De Somer M, Van Belle Y, Vanderick G, De Muylder E (1991) Endometrial lesions in patients undergoing tamoxifen therapy. Int J Gynaecol Obstet 36:127–130
31. Dijkhuizen FP, Brölmann HA, Potters AE, Bongers MY, Heintz AP (1996) The accuracy of transvaginal ultrasonography in the diagnosis of endometrial abnormalities. Obstet Gynecol 87:345–349
32. Draper MW, Flowers DE, Huster WJ, Neild JA, Harper KD, Arnaud C (1996) A controlled trial of raloxifene (LY139481) HCl: impact on bone turnover and serum lipid profile in healthy postmenopausal women. J Bone Miner Res 11:835–842
33. Early Breast Cancer Trialists' Collaborative Group (1998) Tamoxifen for early breast cancer: an overview of the randomised trials. Lancet 351(9114):1451–1467
34. Elkas J, Gray K, Howard L, Petit N, Pohl J, Armstrong A (1998) The effects of tamoxifen on endometrial insulin-like growth factor-1 expression. Obstet Gynecol 91(1):45–50
35. Fisher B (1996) A commentary on endometrial cancer deaths in tamoxifen-treated breast cancer patients. J Clin Oncol 14:1027–1039
36. Fisher B, Costantino J, Redmond C, Poisson R, Bowman D, Couture J, et al. (1989) A randomized clinical trial evaluating tamoxifen in the treatment of patients with node-negative breast cancer who have estrogen-receptor-positive tumors. N Engl J Med 320(8):479–484
37. Fisher B, Costantino JP, Redmond CK, Fisher ER, Wickerham DL, Cronin WM (1994) Endometrial cancer in tamoxifen-treated breast cancer patients: findings from the National Surgical Adjuvant Breast and Bowel Project (NSABP) B-14). J Natl Cancer Inst 86:527–537
38. Fisher B, Costantino JP, Wickerham L, Redmond CK, Kavanah M, Cronin WM, et al. (1998) Tamoxifen for prevention of brest cancer: report of the National Surgical Adjuvant Breast and Bowel Project P-1 Study. J Natl Cancer Inst 90:1371–1388
39. Fornander T, Rutqvist LE, Cedermark B, Glas U, Mattsson A, Silfversward C, et al. (1989) Adjuvant tamoxifen in early breast cancer: occurrence of new primary cancers. Lancet 1(8630):117–120

40. Fugere P, Scheele WH, Shah A, et al. (2000) Uterine effects of raloxifene in comparison with continuous-combined hormone replacement therapy in postmenopausal women. Am J Obstet Gynecol 182:568–574
41. Gal D, Kopel S, Basheukin M, Lebowicz J, Lev R, Tancer L (1991) Oncogenic potential of tamoxifen on endometria of postmenopausal women with breast cancer. Preliminary report. Gynecol Oncol 42:120–123
42. Gottardis MM, Ricchio ME, Satyaswaroop PG, Jordan VC (1990) Effect of steroidal and nonsteroidal antiestrogens on the growth of a tamoxifen-stimulated human endometrial carcinoma (EnCa101) in athymic mice. Cancer Res 50(11):3189–3192
43. Granberg S, Wikland M, Karlsson B, Norström A, Friberg L (1991) Endometrial thickness as measured by endovaginal ultrasonography for identifying endometrial abnormality. Am J Obstet Gynecol 164:47–52
44. Grese TA, Sluka JP, Bryant HU, Cullinan GJ, Glasebrook AL, Jones CD, Matsumoto K, Palkowitz AD, Sato M, Termine JD, Winter MA, Yang NN, Dodge JA (1997) Molecular determinants of tissue selectivity in estrogen receptor modulators. Proc Natl Acad Sci USA 94(25):14105–14110
45. Holbert TR (1997) Transvaginal ultrasonographic measurement of endometrial thickness in postmenopausal women receiving estrogen replacement therapy. Am J Obstet Gynecol 176:1334–1339
46. Huynh HT, Pollak M (1993) Insulin-like growth factor I gene expression in the uterus is stimulated by tamoxifen and inhibited by the pure antiestrogen ICI 182780. Cancer Res 53(23):5585–5588
47. Huynh H, Pollak M (1994) Uterotrophic actions of estradiol and tamoxifen are associated with inhibition of uterine insulin-like growth factor binding protein 3 gene expression. Cancer Res 54(12):3115–3119
48. Isaksson E, Cline JM, Skoog L, Soderqvist G, Wilking N, von Schoultz E, von Schoultz B (1999) p53 expression in breast and endometrium during estrogen and tamoxifen treatment of surgically postmenopausal cynomolgus macaques. Breast Cancer Res Treat 53(1):61–67
49. Jolly EE, Bjarnason NH, Neven P, Plouffe L Jr, Johnston CC Jr, Watts SD, Arnaud CD, Mason TM, Crans G, Akers R, Draper MW (2003) Prevention of osteoporosis and uterine effects in postmenopausal women taking raloxifene for 5 years. Menopause 10(4):337–344
50. Jordan VC, Glusman JE, Eckert S, Lippman M, Powles T, Costa A, et al. (1998) Incident primary breast cancer are reduced by raloxifen: integrated data from multicenter, double-blind, randomized trial in ~ 12,000 postmenopausal women. Proc Am Soc Clin Oncol 17:122a (abstract)
51. Karlsson S, Iatropoulos MJ, Williams GM, Kangas L, Nieminen L (1998) The proliferation in uterine compartments of intact rats of two different strains exposed to high doses of tamoxifen or toremifene. Toxicol Pathol 26(6):759–768
52. Ke HZ, Foley GL, Simmons HA, Shen V, Thompson DD (2004) Long-term treatment of lasofoxifene preserves bone mass and bone strength and does not adversely affect the uterus in ovariectomized rats. Endocrinology 145(4):1996–2005
53. Kedar RP, Bourne TH, Powles TJ, Collins WP, Ashley SE, Cosgrove DO, et al. (1994) Effects of tamoxifen on uterus and ovaries of postmenopausal women in a randomised breast cancer prevention trial. Lancet 343:1318–1321
54. Kleinman D, Karas M, Danilenko M, Arbell A, Roberts CT, LeRoith D, Levy J, Sharoni Y (1996) Stimulation of endometrial cancer cell growth by tamoxifen is associated with increased insulin-like growth factor (IGF)-I induced tyrosine phosphorylation and reduction in IGF binding proteins. Endocrinology 137(3):1089–1095

55. Koda M, Jarzabek K, Haczynski J, Knapp P, Sulkowski S, Wolczynski S (2004) Differential effects of raloxifene and tamoxifen on the expression of estrogen receptors and antigen Ki-67 in human endometrial adenocarcinoma cell line. Oncol Rep 12(3):517–521
56. Kommoss F, Karck U, Prompeler H, Pfisterer J, Kirkpatrick CJ (1998) Steroid receptor expression in endometria from women treated with tamoxifen. Gynecol Oncol 70(2):188–191
57. Ma L, Palkowitz A, Bryant HU, Rowley E, Adian MD, Cole HW, Shetler P, Smith S, Turner CH, Yao W, et al. (1998) Long-term dosing of LY353381HC1 preserves bone quality, reduces turnover and lowers cholesterol levels in ovariectomized rats. Bone 23(Suppl 5):S609
58. MacGregor JI, Jordan VC (1998) Basic guide to the mechanisms of antiestrogen action. Pharmacol Rev 50(2):151–196
59. Maeda T, Ke HZ, Simmons H, Thompson D (2004) Lasofoxifene, a next generation estrogen receptor modulator: preclinical studies. Clin Calcium 14(10):85–93
60. Magriples U, Naftolin F, Schartz PC, Carcangiu ML (1993) High-grade endometrial carcinoma in tamoxifen-treated breast cancer patients. J Clin Oncol 11:485–490
61. McGonigle KF, Shaw SL, Vasilev SA, Odom-Maryon T, Roy S, Simpson JF (1998) Abnormalities detected on transvaginal ultrasonography in tamoxifen-treated postmenopausal breast cancer patients may represent endometrial cystic atrophy. Am J Obstet Gynecol 178:1145–1150
62. Miller CP, Collini MD, Tran BD (2001) Design, synthesis, and preclinical characterization of novel, highly selective indole estrogens. J Med Chem. 44:1654–1657
63. Miller CP, Harris HA, Konmin BS (2002) Bezedoxifene Acetate. Drugs Future 27(2):117–121
64. Nayfield SG, Karp JE, Ford LG, Dorr FA, Kramer BS (1991) Potential role of tamoxifen in prevention of breast cancer. J Natl Cancer Inst 83:1450–1459
65. Neven P, De Muylder X, Van Belle Y, Vanderick G, De Muylder E (1990) Hysteroscopic follow-up during tamoxifen treatment. Eur J Obstet Gynecol Reprod Biol 35:235–238
66. Neven P, Lunde T, Benedetti-Panicini P, et al. (2000) A multicentre randomized trial to compare the uterine effects of raloxifene(evista) with a continuous combined hormone replacement therapy (kliogest); results from Euralox I. Gynecol Endocrinol 14(2):77
67. Neven P, Lunde T, Benedetti-Panici P, Tiitinen A, Marinescu B, Villiers T, Hillard T, Cano A, Peer E, Quail D, Nickelsen T (2003) A multicentre randomised trial to compare uterine safety of raloxifene with a continuous combined hormone replacement therapy containing oestradiol and norethisterone acetate. Br J Obstet Gynaecol 110:157–167
68. Neven P, Quail D, Levrier M, Aguas F, The HS, De Geyter C, Glant MD, Beck H, Bosio-LeGoux B, Schmitt H, Hottgenroth A, Nickelsen T (2004) Uterine effects of estrogen plus progestin therapy and raloxifene: adjudicated results from the EURALOX study. Obstet Gynecol 103(5 Pt 1):881–891
69. Palacios S, Cifuentes I, Menendez C, von Helde S (2000) Los SERMs y el utero. In: Cano A, Calaf J (eds) Moduladores selectivos de los receptores de estrogenos (SERM). Ediciones Doyma, Barcelona
70. Rivera-Gonzalez R, Petersen DN, Tkalcevic G, Thompson DD, Brown TA (1998) Estrogen-induced genes in the uterus of ovariectomized rats and their regulation by droloxifene and tamoxifen. J Steroid Biochem Mol Biol 64(1–2):13–24
71. Robertson JA, Bhattacharyya S, Ing NH (1998) Tamoxifen up-regulates oestrogen receptor-alpha, c-fos and glyceraldehyde 3-phosphate-dehydrogenase mRNAs in ovine endometrium. J Steroid Biochem Mol Biol 67(4):285–292
72. Rose PG (1996) Endometrial carcinoma. N Engl J Med 335:640–649

73. Russo J, Gusterson BA, Rogers AE, Russo IH, Wellings SR, van Zwieten MJ (1990) Comparative study of human and rat mammary tumorigenesis. Lab Invest 62(3):244–278
74. Rutanen EM, Heikkinen J, Halonen K, Komi J, Lammintausta R, Ylikorkala O (2003) Effects of ospemifene, a novel SERM, on hormones, genital tract, climacteric symptoms, and quality of life in postmenopausal women: a double-blind, randomized trial. Menopause 10(5):433–439
75. Sasco AJ, Raffi F, Satge D, Goburdhun J, Fallou HB, Leduc B (1995) Endometrial müllerian carcinosarcoma after cessation of tamoxifen therapy for breast cancer. Int J Gynaecol Obstet 48:307–310
76. Sato M, Rippy MK, Bryant HU (1996) Raloxifene, tamoxifen, nafoxidine, or estrogen effects on reproductive and nonreproductive tissues in ovariectomized rats. FASEB J 10(8):905–912
77. Sato M, Zeng GQ, Rowley E, Turner CH (1998) LY353381 × HCl: an improved benzothiophene analog with bone efficacy complementary to parathyroid hormone-(1–34). Endocrinology 139(11):4642–4651
78. Somjen D, Waisman A, Kaye AM (1996) Tissue selective action of tamoxifen methiodide, raloxifene and tamoxifen on creatine kinase B activity in vitro and in vivo. J Steroid Biochem Mol Biol 59(5–6):389–396
79. Stewart HJ, Knigth GM (1989) Tamoxifen and the uterus and endometrium. Lancet 1:375–376
80. Swenberg JA (1997) Clinical relevance of laboratory and animal data on tamoxifen. Oncology (Huntingt) 11(2 Suppl 1):39–44
81. Swerdlow AJ, Jones ME, British Tamoxifen Second Cancer Study Group (2005) Tamoxifen treatment for breast cancer and risk of endometrial cancer: a case-control study. J Natl Cancer Inst 97(5):375–384
82. Tzukerman MT, Esty A, Santiso-Mere D, Danielian P, Parker MG, Stein RB, Pike JW, McDonnell DP (1994) Human estrogen receptor transactivational capacity is determined by both cellular and promoter context and mediated by two functionally distinct intramolecular regions. Mol Endocrinol 8(1):21–30
83. van Leeuwen FE, Benraadt J, Coebergh JW, Kiemeney LA, Gimbrère CH, Otter R, et al. (1994) Risk of endometrial cancer after tamoxifen treatment of breast cancer. Lancet 343:448–452
84. Voipio SK, Komi J, Kangas L, Halonen K, DeGregorio MW, Erkkola RU (2002) Effects of ospemifene (FC-1271a) on uterine endometrium, vaginal maturation index, and hormonal status in healthy postmenopausal women. Maturitas 43(3):207–214
85. Walsh BW, Kuller LH, Wild RA, Paul S, Farmer M, Lawrence JB, et al. (1998) Effects of raloxifene on serum lipids and coagulation factors in healthy postmenopausal women. J Am Med Assoc 279:1445–1451
86. Zhang H, McElrath T, Tong W, Pollard JW (2005) The molecular basis of tamoxifen induction of mouse uterine epithelial cell proliferation. J Endocrinol 184(1):129–140

Chapter 12

Benign Gynecological Diseases and SERMs

Stefano Palomba · Fulvio Zullo

12.1
Introduction

The most common benign gynecological diseases, for prevalence and related economic costs, are probably uterine leiomyomas and endometriosis (Stewart 2001; Missmer et al. 2003). Notwithstanding the fact that both conditions are characterized by a sex-hormone-related development and by the possibility of a medical treatment consisting of hormonal manipulation, at present the main approach to these conditions is surgical excision (Palomba et al. 2006a; Olive et al. 2001).

The present chapter describes current knowledge regarding the effects of selective estrogen receptor modulators (SERMs) on these two gynecological conditions.

First we shall describe the effects of tamoxifen, a first-generation SERM used as adjuvant treatment in women with breast cancer, on uterine leiomyomas and endometriosis. Considerable space will be devoted to raloxifene, a second-generation SERM administered for the prevention and treatment of postmenopausal women recently tested for the treatment of these two sex-hormone-related diseases. Unfortunately, at present no or very little data are available on the new third-generation SERMs such as lasofoxifene, idroxifene, droloxifene, ospemifene, azomifene, fulvestrant, and MDL 103.323.

12.2
Uterine Leiomyomas

Uterine leiomyomas are the most frequent benign disease of the female reproductive apparatus. At least 20–25% of women of fertile age and 50% of women studied in postmortem have uterine leiomyomas (Stewart 2001; Palomba et al. 2005a). In between 20 and 50% of cases, the uterine leiomyomas cause a clinically relevant symptomatology (such as menorrhagia, infertility, recurrent abortion, pelvic pain, and so on) and treatment is required (Stewart 2001; Palomba et al. 2006a). Thus, this disease is one of the main causes of health expense in the field of gynecology (Stewart 2001; Palomba et al. 2006a). In fact, symptomatic uterine leiomyomatosis is the surgical indication for about 2/3 of hysterectomies, and these data are all the more relevant considering the fact that hysterectomy is the most frequent intervention of major surgery (Stewart 2001; Palomba et al. 2006a).

Despite the fact that the pathogenesis of uterine leiomyomas is still poorly defined, it has been demonstrated that uterine leiomyomas are estrogen-dependent monoclonal tumors (Chegini et al. 1996; Englund et al. 1998; Higashijima et al. 1996). The primum movens is probably a genetic mutation and thus an alteration of the intratumoral estrogenic metabolism (Pasqualini et al. 1990; Yamamoto et al. 1984; Bulun et al. 1994; Benassayag et al. 1999). The transcription and expressivity of the estrogen receptor (ER), in fact, is increased in myoma tissue when compared to healthy myometrium (Yamamoto et al. 1984; Bulun et al. 1994). A specific distribution of ER subtypes has been demonstrated (Benassayag et al. 1999). The simple action of estrogens does not seem, moreover, to be the only pathogenic cause. Progesterone could play a pivotal role in the transformation of the normal myometrial cell to a myomatous cell (Rein et al. 1995; Tiltman 1985). High progesterone levels, such as those detected in the luteal phase of the menstrual cycle or in the administration of medroxyprogesterone acetate, are related to an increase in mitotic activity of the myoma cells (Kawaguchi et al. 1989; Rein 2000). Finally, in myomatous tissue, as in ERs, there is an overexpression of the progesterone receptor (Englund et al. 1998).

12.2.1 Treatments of Uterine Leiomyomas

To date, the standard treatment for uterine leiomyomas is their laparotomic/laparoscopic excision in women who want to preserve their fertility, whereas the use of a more extensive surgery, such as the hysterectomy, is reserved for disseminating uterine leiomyomatosis, generally in the perimenopausal period (Stewart 2001; Palomba et al. 2006a).

Moreover, given the pathogenesis of uterine leiomyomas (see below), it is clear that future treatments of fibroids will be essentially medical and consist of hormonal therapies. In recent years, in fact, several medical therapies have been proposed for the treatment of this benign disease (Table 12.1). In clinical practice it is very common to administer oral contraceptives in patients affected by uterine leiomyomas. Even if few data are available regarding the effects of estroprogestin associations on uterine leiomyomas (Friedman et al. 1995; Marshall et al. 1998), in clinical practice is very common to administer oral contraceptives in patients affected by uterine leiomyomas. They should be administered to regularize menstrual bleeding so as to decrease the duration of bleedings and the severity of menorrhagia (Friedman et al. 1995). Moreover, some studies have also determined that oral contraceptives can cause tumoral growth (Barbieri 1997; Marshall et al. 1998). The use of mifepristone (RU486), a drug with a weak antiprogestin action, at a dosage of 10 mg/d, induces the reduction of progesterone receptors and leiomyoma dimensions (Murphy et al. 1993; Kertel et al. 1994). Also, the use of gestrinone at doses of 2.5 or 5 mg two to three times a week has been proposed as treatment for uterine leiomyomas (Coutinho et al. 1989; Coutinho 1989, 1990). Danazol is also effective for treating patients with uterine leiomyomas (De Leo et al. 1999). In particular, it has been demonstrated that 400 mg daily of danazol for 4 months leads to a decrease of about 25% in the size of leiomyomas due to the actions of hypoestrogenism and antiprogestin (De Leo et al. 1999). Moreover, in both therapeutic regimens the treatment has several side effects related to the androgenic action of the drugs such as weight gain, seborrhea, acne, and hirsutism (Palomba et al. 2006a).

Virtually the only medical therapeutic approach that is currently used in clinical practice is the administration of GnRH agonists (GnRH-a) (Palomba et al. 2006a). GnRH-a, a group of drugs with an agonist action on the GnRH receptor, induces, after a rapid and initial synthesis and secretion of gonadotropins

Table 12.1. Medical therapies for uterine leiomyomas (Palomba et al. 2000a)

Treatment	Efficacy	Side effects	Main form of administration	Duration of therapy	Cost
Progestins	No	Possible increase in tumor size	Os	Long term	Low
Oral contraceptive	Poor	Possible increase in tumor size	Os	Long term	Low
Danazol	Good	Weight gain, mild hyperandrogenism	Os	Long term	Not expensive
Gestrinone	Good	Weight gain, mild hyperandrogenism	Os	Long term	Low
Mifepristone	Good	Mild hot flashes	Os	Long term	Low
GnRH agonist	Very good	Climacteric-like symptoms, metabolic syndrome, bone loss	IM	Short term	Very expensive
GnRH agonist plus add-back therapy	Very good	Very long-term data unknown	IM, os	Long term	Very expensive
GnRH antagonist	Unknown	Unknown	IM	Short term	Very expensive
Raloxifene	No	Leg cramps	Os	No data	Expensive

(the "flare up" effect), a profound down-regulation of the pituitary followed by postreceptor message blockage of the gonadotropin synthesis and secretion with inhibition of follicular development, anovulation, and a reversible hypogonadotropic hypogonadism state (Palomba et al. 2005a). GnRH-a induce a significant reduction in the size of leiomyomas within only 8–10 weeks, achieving the highest reduction after the 14th week of treatment. After this period, the volume reduction achieves a steady state. Even if some evidences seem to show a direct action of the GnRH-a on leiomyoma tissue (Palomba et al. 2005a), after treatment withdrawal, estrogen levels will return to their normal range within about 1 month and the leiomyomas will resume their pretreatment sizes within about 3 months (Palomba et al. 2005a). The disease will again be symptomatic in relation to the regrowth of the leiomyomas.

The hypoestrogenism induced by GnRH-a causes several climacteric-like symptoms such as hot flashes, vaginal dryness, reduction in libido, metabolic alterations, cognitive deficit, and, above all, bone loss, which varies from 0.8% to 7% after 12 months of GnRH-a administration (Palomba et al. 2005a). Notwithstanding the metabolic alterations, which have been studied recently in women treated with GnRH-a (Palomba et al. 2004b), at present there is no clear evidence regarding the cardiovascular risk related to GnRH-a treatment (Palomba et al. 2005a).

For GnRH-a administration beyond 6 months, it has been postulated that the addition of low doses of steroids ("add-back therapy") may avoid the adverse effects of prolonged hypoestrogenism without reducing the efficacy of the analog alone (Pickersgill 1998; Palomba et al. 1998; Palomba et al. 1999). Furthermore, with respect to the high costs of treatment, the use of GnRH-a plus add-back therapy has little clinical impact (Palomba et al. 2005a).

Finally, new hypotheses of treatment were recently published (Minakuchi et al. 1999; De Leo et al. 2001; Palomba et al. 2002b; Shozu et al. 2003; Gainer et al. 2005; Spitz 2003). At present, only SERMs, i.e., raloxifene, seem to hold any real promise in terms of future development.

12.2.2 SERMs and Uterine Leiomyomas

12.2.2.1 *Tamoxifen*

Tamoxifen, a first-generation SERM, is a nonsteroidal triphenylethylene derivate routinely used in clinical practice for the treatment and prevention of breast cancer in high-risk populations (Robertson 2004). This drug produces an estrogen antagonist effect on the breast and an estrogen agonist effect on the reproductive organs, e.g., uterus, ovary, and endometrium (Robertson 2004).

The first data on the effects of tamoxifen on uterine leiomyomas were obtained in a rat model. They showed that tamoxifen increased tumor latency and decreased tumor size (Howe et al. 1995). These findings were confirmed more recently by Walker et al. (2000). In the same period, moreover, several case reports were published showing an increase in uterine leiomyoma dimensions following tamoxifen administration (Dilts et al. 1992; Leo et al. 1994; Ugwumadu et al. 1994).

The scientific data on the effects of tamoxifen on uterine leiomyomas are generally extrapolated from safety data on the use of tamoxifen in women with breast cancer, and for this reason the studies available are essentially clinical studies on human models.

In premenopausal women with uterine leiomyomas, Lumsden et al. (1989a) showed that 20 mg/d tamoxifen prolongs the luteal phase, increasing the secretion of gonadotropins by antagonizing the effects of estradiol at the central level, but it has no effect on the dimensions of uterine tumors. On the contrary, when tamoxifen was administered in women treated with GnRH-a, despite the profound pituitary–ovarian suppression, no significant changes in uterine and leiomyoma volume were observed during combined therapy, suggesting that tamoxifen acts as an estrogen agonist in hypoestrogenic women (Lumsden et al. 1989b).

The effects of tamoxifen on uterine leiomyomas have been studied also in postmenopausal patients with breast cancer (Schwartz et al. 1998). After an average treatment of about 1 year, uterine and leiomyoma volumes increased significantly, confirming an agonistic effect of tamoxifen on the uterus. No significant difference in agonist effect on the uterus has been detected between tamoxifen and toremifene (Tomas et al. 1995).

Notwithstanding these somewhat discouraging data, a clinical trial has been designed to study the efficacy of tamoxifen in women affected by uterine fibroids (Sadan et al. 2001). In this, the most recent, study, Sadan et al. demonstrated that 20 mg/d tamoxifen confers no benefit in premenopausal women with symptomatic leiomyomas.

12.2.2.2
Raloxifene

Raloxifene hydrochloride is a synthetic nonsteroidal drug derived from the benzothiophene and afferent to SERMs. It is known that raloxifene acts on metabolism, the skeleton, and the cardiovascular system as an estrogenic agonist (Khovidhunkit et al. 1999; Ettinger et al. 1999; Walsh et al. 1998), whereas it shows an estrogenic antagonist effect on reproductive organs such as the breast and the uterus (Cummings et al. 1999; Goldstein et al. 2000; Cohen et al. 2000). Data on the central nervous system are still unclear (Lacreuse et al. 2002; Yaffe et al. 2001).

Raloxifene is a SERM with desirable mixed agonist/antagonist effects. In fact, unlike tamoxifen, it does not cause uterine stimulation, and it seems to have no effect on the reproductive system.

Preclinical Studies

Black et al. (1994) first reported that raloxifene was effective in terms of bone loss prevention and lipid pattern without any stimulatory effect on the uterus. Specifically, the histological examination of uteri from ovariectomized rats treated with raloxifene alone shows poor effects on myometrial thickness and a uterine weight slightly higher than untreated ovariectomized rats (Black et al. 1994).

Later, Fuchs-Young et al. (1996) demonstrated that raloxifene inhibited proliferation of rat leiomyoma cells in culture. In the same year, in one of the first reviews of the pharmacology of raloxifene, Bryant et al. (1996) showed that raloxifene exerted on animal models a dose-related capacity for blocking estrogen-induced stimulation of uterine weight gain.

More recently, it has been demonstrated that raloxifene induces a fast regression of abdominal-wall estrogen-induced leiomyomas in guinea pigs (Porter et al. 1998). Finally, Walker et al. (2000) have confirmed that treatment with tamoxifen or with a raloxifene analog reduces the size of leiomyomas and their incidence by 40–60% in the rat.

Clinical Studies

The first clinical data on the humans were published by Palomba et al. (2001). Based on previous experimental studies (Black et al. 1994; Fuchs-Young et al. 1996; Bryant et al. 1996; Porter et al. 1998), the effect of raloxifene administration on uterine leiomyomas was tested in postmenopausal women. These data (Palomba et al. 2001) confirmed that raloxifene was effective in reducing leiomyoma dimensions. In particular, after six cycles of raloxifene administration, a significant reduction in mean uterine and uterine leiomyoma size was observed (Fig. 12.1). This reduction was not observed in subjects treated with placebo. During raloxifene administration, a high rate of amenorrhea with a low number of spotting episodes was observed. No significant differences were observed in the length and severity of abnormal uterine bleedings among women treated with raloxifene in comparison with those treated with placebo tablets (Palomba et al. 2001).

A relevant finding of this study was the selective action of raloxifene on leiomyoma tissue highlighted by a significant increase in the difference be-

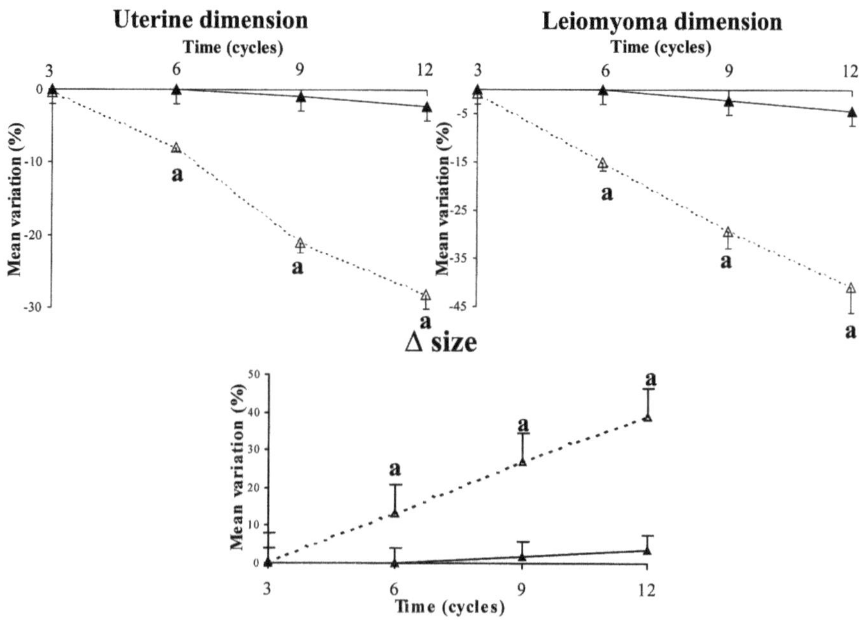

Fig. 12.1. Variation (%) from baseline in uterine and leiomyoma sizes and in Δ size after 3, 6, 9, and 12 cycles of treatment. Values are reported as mean ± SD. [a] $p < 0.05$ vs. baseline. △ = group A; ▲ = group B (Palomba et al. 2001). Permission to publish from Elsevier

tween uterine and leiomyoma sizes (nonleiomyoma tissue size) (Fig. 12.1) (Palomba et al. 2001). In particular, in postmenopausal women raloxifene seems to induce a significant reduction in leiomyoma size, without any significant action on a normal myometrium. The reduction in uterine size, in fact, is due essentially to a reduction in leiomyoma dimensions. An explanation for these data may be the selective action of raloxifene on leiomyoma tissue. The selective action of raloxifene on leiomyoma tissue, just as on other target tissues, is probably due to the varying distribution of ER subtypes. In fact, as was already specified in previous chapters, at least two ERs exist in humans, encoded by two independent ER genes (Paech et al. 1997; Kuiper et al. 1997). ERα binds estrogens with high affinity and low capacity, while ERβ binds estrogens with low affinity and high capacity (Paech et al. 1997; Kuiper et al. 1997). The estradiol activation of the two different ERs gives two different regulatory signals inducing, respectively, activation and inhibition of transcription (Paech et al. 1997; Kuiper et al. 1997). Furthermore, to date no clear consensus exists about the presence of sex hormone receptors in leiomyomas (Palomba et al. 2005a).

An excellent experimental work (Benassayag et al. 1999) showed an overexpression of the genes regulated by sex hormones in leiomyoma tissue, such as in pregnant compared with nonpregnant myometrium. In leiomyoma tissue, like the pregnant myometrium, higher levels of ERα and ERβ mRNA were detected (Benassayag et al. 1999). Notwithstanding the high level of ERα mRNA present in leiomyoma tissue, high concentrations of ERα for estradiol have not been shown (Benassayag et al. 1999). This result may be explained by the presence of ERα variants lacking estradiol binding sites for posttranscriptional modification or a faulty translation of ERα mRNA. In contrast, the concentrations of ERβ were two- to threefold higher in leiomyoma in comparison with non-pregnant myometrium (Benassayag et al. 1999). The differential expression of these two ER genes could play a pivotal role in the normal or abnormal growth of the myometrium.

To date, experimental data regarding the cellular mechanisms by which raloxifene acts on uterine and leiomyoma tissue are provided by only two papers (Walker et al. 2000; Palomba et al. 2005b). In the first study (Walker et al. 2000) it was shown in a rat model that the effect of raloxifene analog LY 326315 in reducing leiomyoma incidence and size is mediated exclusively by a decrease in cell proliferation without any action on the apoptotic index. In contrast, in the second study (Palomba et al. 2005b) a significant effect of raloxifene on both cell indexes was observed. In particular, a 3-month course of 180 mg/d raloxifene induced a significant decrease in proliferating cell nuclear antigen (PCNA)/total cells (TC) and in Bcl-2/Bax ratios in comparison with placebo showing that raloxifene acts on uterine leiomyomas, reducing cell proliferation and enhancing cell apoptosis (Palomba et al. 2005b). In addition, the raloxifene effect on the apoptotic index seems to be specific to leiomyoma tissue. In fact, no difference in the apoptotic index was observed in the myometrium of subjects treated with raloxifene when compared to control samples (Palomba et al. 2005b).

The discrepancy between these two studies (Walker et al. 2000; Palomba et al. 2005c) are probably due to the different models used. This suggestion is supported by the absence of a correspondence between beneficial effects of tamoxifen on uterine leiomyomas in the rat (Walker et al. 2000) and findings obtained in clinical studies in humans (Leo et al. 1994; Ugwumadu et al. 1994; Lumsden et al. 1989a,b; Schwartz et al. 1998; Tomas et al. 1995; Sadan et al. 2001). In fact, it has been clearly shown, as detailed earlier, that tamoxifen in women with breast cancer exerts a proliferative estrogenlike effect on uterine leiomyomas (Leo et al. 1994; Ugwumadu et al. 1994; Lumsden et al. 1989a,b; Schwartz et al. 1998; Tomas et al. 1995; Sadan et al. 2001).

Raloxifene has been shown also to exert a more mild but significant effect on normal myometrium in terms of cell proliferation inhibition, as suggested by a PCNA/TC ratio that is lower in raloxifene than in placebo groups (Palomba et al. 2005b). This finding could explain the observation of a reduced incidence in new tumors observed in premenopausal women treated with 180 mg/d raloxifene (Palomba et al. 2002a). To define the relationship, if any, between proliferation and apoptotic indexes and raloxifene's effect on uterine and leiomyoma dimensions, a linear correlation between PCNA/TC and Bcl-2/Bax ratios and the percent change in uterine and leiomyomas sizes was performed (Palomba et al. 2005c). Proliferation and apoptotic indexes resulted significantly related to the percent change in the dimension of leiomyomas alone, whereas no significant relationship was observed with a percent change in uterine size (Palomba et al. 2005c).

At present, no explanation of these data is available. A possible hypothesis could be that raloxifene acts on cell proliferation and apoptosis, decreasing the intratumoral insulin growth factor (IGF)-1 concentrations with an antagonist effect on ERs (Gao et al. 2001). In fact, several data suggest that IGF-1 may be involved in the regulation of leiomyoma growth as a local mediator of the growth-promoting actions of sex hormones (Gao et al. 2001). The altered expression of different ER subtypes in leiomyomas could play a role (Benassayag et al. 1999; Brandon et al. 1995).

To test the real efficacy in clinical practice of raloxifene in the treatment of uterine leiomyomas, a randomized, placebo-controlled study was performed in premenopausal women with asymptomatic uterine leiomyomas using conventional (60 mg/d) and high (180 mg/d) doses of raloxifene (Palomba et al. 2002a). No significant effect on uterine and leiomyoma sizes was observed after six cycles of raloxifene administration at either dose (Palomba et al. 2002a). However, our results should not be considered completely negative (Table 12.2). In fact, after six cycles of raloxifene treatment at the high dosage, in only two women was an increase in tumor size detected, whereas in a high percentage of cases the leiomyoma size was unmodified. Indeed, it seems that the use of 180 mg/d raloxifene acts more to prevent tumoral growth than to reduce leiomyoma size. A higher incidence of new leiomyomas has been observed in the groups treated with 60 mg/d raloxifene or with placebo, suggesting a dose-related response of raloxifene treatment (Table 12.2) (Palomba et al. 2002a). Unfortunately, it was not possible to perform an appropriate statistical analysis to evaluate the raloxifene effect on the prevention of leiomyomas for the small group of women and the short treatment period.

A possible explanation for these results may be twofold. First, the raloxifene doses were too low to reduce or reverse the proliferative effect of serum estradiol in normal ovulatory women. In fact, in postmenopausal women serum estradiol levels are about tenfold lower in comparison with normally cycled premenopausal women. Second, it is possible that in postmenopausal women ERs have a different intratumoral pattern in terms of concentration, expression, and affinity in comparison with premenopausal women.

No significant effect was observed on endometrial thickness or on the length and severity of uterine bleedings after raloxifene treatment at doses of 60 and 180 mg/d in premenopausal women (Palomba et al. 2002a). Unfortunately,

Table 12.2. Number and percentage of women with unmodified, decreased, and increased uterine and leiomyoma sizes after 3 and 6 cycles of 60 mg/d raloxifene (group A), 180 mg/d raloxifene (group B), and placebo (group C) (Palomba et al. 2002a)

	Unmodified (%)	Decreased (%)	Increased (%)
Group A (*n* = 29)			
3rd cycle	27 (93.1)	– (0)	2 (6.9)
6th cycle	22 (75.9)	1 (3.4)	6 (20.7)
Group B (*n* = 30)			
3rd cycle	27 (90.0)	1 (3.3)	2 (6.7)
6th cycle	26 (86.7)	2 (6.7)	2 (6.7)
Group C (*n* = 29)			
3rd cycle	25 (86.2)	1 (3.4)	3 (10.3)
6th cycle	21 (72.4)	1 (3.4)	7 (24.1)

during the different phases of the menstrual cycle, only the plasma FSH, estradiol, and progesterone levels were studied. In contrast, in the study of Baker et al. (1998) the endocrine effects of raloxifene in premenopausal women were studied extensively. No alteration in LH surge, FSH, progesterone, and estradiol levels was detected while raloxifene was being administered at doses of 400 mg/d for 5 d during the follicular, periovulatory, and luteal phases and at doses of 100 or 200 mg/d for 28 d/month in healthy premenopausal women (Baker et al. 1998). Indeed, all women ovulated regularly, and only in some cases was an increase of estradiol and FSH levels observed (Baker et al. 1998).

More recently, in a randomized, open-label, controlled clinical trial Janseng et al. (Jerecek et al. 2004) demonstrated that high doses (180 mg/d) of raloxifene inhibited leiomyoma growth in premenopausal women. However, several criticisms have been made of this study (Palomba et al. 2004a). In perimenopausal women with low sex hormone levels, high doses of raloxifene could probably only inhibit leiomyoma growth and not have any clinical effect on uterine and leiomyoma dimensions (Palomba et al. 2004a).

Based on these findings, our team has studied the efficacy of raloxifene as an "add-back therapy" in women with uterine leiomyomas treated with GnRH-a (Palomba et al. 2002b; Palomba et al. 2002c). In this study's protocol, we compared, in a randomized, single-blind, placebo-controlled fashion, the administration of GnRH-a plus raloxifene vs. GnRH-a alone (Palomba et al. 2002b; Palomba et al. 2002c). A significant decrease in uterine, leiomyoma, and nonleiomyoma sizes was detected in both treatment groups in comparison with the baseline (Fig. 12.2) (Palomba et al. 2002b). Significantly lower leiomyoma sizes were observed in the GnRH-a plus raloxifene group than in the GnRH-a alone group, but no difference was observed in leiomyoma-related symptoms between groups throughout the study period (Fig. 12.2) (Palomba et al. 2002b).

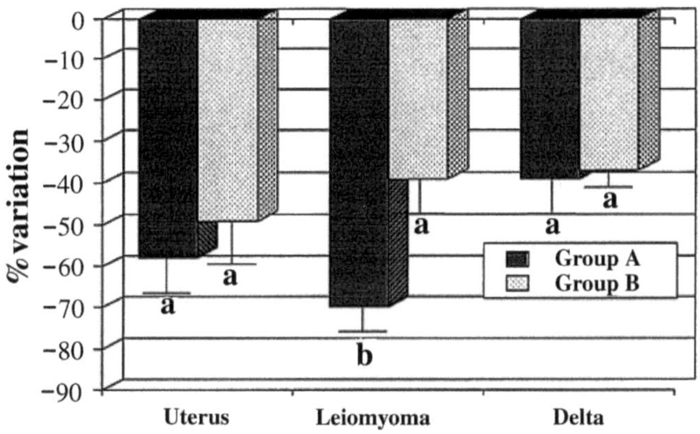

Fig. 12.2. Variation (%) from baseline in uterine and leiomyoma sizes and in Δ size after 6 cycles of treatment in groups A (GnRH analog plus raloxifene) and B (GnRH analog plus placebo). Values are reported as mean ± SD. [a] $p < 0.05$ vs. baseline; [b] $p < 0.05$ vs. baseline and group A (Palomba et al. 2002b). Permission to publish from Oxford University Press

In this view, the effectiveness of raloxifene on leiomyoma reduction in postmenopausal women and in premenopausal women treated with GnRH-a could explain partially the ineffectivess of raloxifene in normally cycled women. Specifically, it seems, as supposed, that raloxifene achieves a clinical result only in patients with low serum estrogen levels.

In this sample of women treated with GnRH-a, raloxifene proved to be efficacious also in the prevention of GnRH-a-related bone loss (Palomba et al. 2002c). In fact, no significant variation in bone metabolism and mineral density was detected during treatment with GnRH-a plus raloxifene (Palomba et al. 2002c). The safety and effectiveness of GnRH-a plus raloxifene treatment were also tested following a long-term study (Palomba et al. 2004c) that showed improvements in mood and quality of life (Palomba et al. 2004d). Unfortunately, raloxifene did not reduce GnRH-a-related vasomotor symptoms.

In a subanalysis of the study (Palomba et al. 2004b), it was observed that GnRH-a altered serum lipoprotein and homocycsteine levels and increased insulin resistance. In contrast, when raloxifene was added to GnRH-a, these acute metabolic changes were prevented or reduced (Palomba et al. 2004b). However, raloxifene did not reduce the cognitive deficits observed during GnRH analog administration (Palomba et al. 2004d).

Finally, raloxifene has been successfully used in a symptomatic premenopausal woman with benign metastasizing leiomyomas (Rivera et al. 2004). In particular, 60 mg/d raloxifene, in coadministration with anastrozole 1 mg/d, induced a regression of the symptoms within few days, but a worsening of the symptomatology was observed when the woman stopped the treatment (Rivera et al. 2004). Raloxifene (120 mg/d) plus anastrozole (2 mg/d) was again administered inducing a regression of symptoms. After a 2-year followup, the woman remained clinically well (Rivera et al. 2004).

12.2.2.3 *Other New-Generation SERMs*

Lasofoxifene is a new potent nonsteroidal SERM that binds with high affinity to ERs acting as a tissue-selective estrogen antagonist or agonist (Maeda et al. 2004).

In preclinical studies designed to evaluate the effects of lasofoxifene on the uterus, a slight increase in wet uterine weight was observed in immature and aged female rats, but this difference was not observed in dry uterine weight, suggesting that the increased uterine weight was due to increased water content in the tissue (Maeda et al. 2004). When lasofoxifene was administered in combination with estrogens, it blocked the hypertrophic effects of estrogen specifically in the uterus. In immature and aged female rats, lasofoxifene did not affect uterine weight or uterine histology (Maeda et al. 2004).

12.3 Endometriosis

Endometriosis is an estrogen-dependent disorder mostly occurring in reproductive-age women characterized by a growth of the endometrium outside the uterine cavity (Oral et al. 1997; Child et al. 2001). Explanations of how the tissue stains this abnormal placement are controversial, although the predominant theory is that retrograde menstruation is the cause (Oral et al. 1997; Child et al. 2001). Additional factors that may be pivotal in the disease's pathogenesis include immunologic abnormalities, endometrial disorders, and peritoneal dysfunction (Oral et al. 1997; Child et al. 2001).

The main manifestations and symptoms of endometriosis are infertility/subfertility and pelvic pain (Missmer et al. 2003; Olive et al. 2001). Retrospective data have, in fact, shown that women with subfertility are at a high risk of having endometriosis, and prospective studies have demonstrated that endometriosis is related to a low relative risk for pregnancy (D'Hooghe et al. 2003; Akande et al. 2004).

In addition, about 15% of cases of pelvic pain are due to endometriosis, and most primary care physicians consider pelvic pain to be a common clinical problem that accounts for as much as 25% of routine gynecologic office visits (Hurd 1998). Endometriosis is frequently associated with several types of pelvic pain such as dysmenorrhea, chronic pelvic pain, deep dyspareunia, and, occasionally, painful defecation (Hurd 1998). Specifically, endometriosis was found in 37 to 74% of women undergoing laparoscopy for chronic pelvic pain (Demco 1998; Porpora et al. 1997).

The severity of pelvic pain and the incidence of infertility are not related to the localization of the lesions or to the stage of the disease (Gruppo Italiano per lo Studio dell'Endometriosi 2001), as categorized according to the revised American Fertility Society (r-AFS) guidelines (American Fertility Society 1985). In fact, the r-AFS classification system is inadequate to express the severity of the symptomatology because it does not reflect the disease in terms of cellular mass or activity.

12.3.1 Treatments of Endometriosis

The treatment of endometriosis is strongly related to its clinical manifestations. In women with infertility, the surgical treatment is probably the main therapeutic approach (Olive et al. 2001). In particular, if the endometriosis is of sufficient severity to cause distortion of the pelvis, the anatomic alteration could probably be treated by surgery (Olive et al. 2001). More controversial is the situation in women with early-stage endometriosis (Check 2003a,b,c). In fact, the effect of surgery is probably significant but too small to be acceptable (Marcoux et al. 1997; Parazzini 1999; Jacobson et al. 2004). In these cases a medical approach to infertility, such as induction of ovulation plus intrauterine insemination or assisted reproductive techniques, could be more appropriate (Olive et al. 2001).

When pelvic pain is the characterizing symptom of the disease, medical treatment could have a significant role. Several medical treatments have been proposed to treat secondary chronic pelvic pain due to endometriosis (Stones et al. 2004). Moreover, few data are available regarding the effectiveness of the treatments for endometriosis on the quality of life of these patients that seems to be deeply impaired (Carter 1998).

Medical treatment of endometriosis has focused on the hormonal alteration of the menstrual cycle in an attempt to produce a pseudopregnancy, pseudomenopause, or chronic anovulation (Olive et al. 2001).

Like the medical treatment of uterine leiomyomas, danazol, gestrinone, mifepristone, and GnRH-a, with or without add-back therapy, have been proposed for the treatment of endometriosis as well (Olive et al. 2001; Stones et al. 2004), but unlike leiomyomas, oral contraceptive pills, in cyclic or continuous administration, and medroxyprogesterone acetate also seem to be effective (Olive et al. 2001; Stones et al. 2004). A significant benefit in terms of pelvic pain relief also is obtained with the use of nonsteroidal anti-inflammatory drugs (Olive et al. 2001; Stones et al. 2004).

Furthermore, about 20% of women with chronic pelvic pain due to endometriosis are not responsive to medical treatment, and in these cases surgery represents the final diagnostic and therapeutic option (Olive et al. 2001; Stones et al. 2004). Several procedures have been described to treat medically untreatable pelvic pain (Carter 1998). Nonconservative procedures, such as hysterectomy (Rannestad et al. 2001; Lefebvre et al. 2002), are effective in terms of pain relief, but they can be associated to the decrease in the quality of life (MacDonald et al. 1999), and considered unacceptable to women who wish to preserve intact their reproductive apparatus.

The goal of conservative surgery is to remove all apparent endometriosis from the abdomen and pelvis and restore normal anatomical relations. Several data show that the conservative surgical treatment of endometriosis is effective, in terms of pain relief and quality of life in women with secondary pelvic pain (Sutton et al. 1994; Palomba et al. 2006b). In addition, other surgical procedures can be used as a first course of action or added to surgical endometriosis treatment (Palomba et al. 2006b). These procedures, known as pelvic denervations, consist essentially in the interruption of a majority of cervical and uterine sensory nerve fibers (Palomba et al. 2006b).

Recently, several other medical treatments of endometriosis have been proposed (Olive 2002; D'Hooghe 2003; Chwalisz et al. 2002; Saito et al. 2003). However, their use is currently only potential.

12.3.2 SERMs and Endometriosis

The estrogen agonist effects of tamoxifen on eutopic endometrium have been widely described (Riggs et al. 2003; Fotiou et al. 1998). Several data have confirmed that tamoxifen acts also on ectopic endometrium as an estrogen agonist (Cohen et al. 1997; Parrott et al. 2001; Rose et al. 2000; Abad de Velasco et al. 2003; Chang et al. 2003; Bese et al. 2003).

A high incidence of histologically diagnosed adenomyosis has been detected in postmenopausal women with breast cancer taking tamoxifen when compared with those not taking tamoxifen (53.6% vs. 18.2%) (Cohen et al. 1997). Toremifene seems to exert the same effect as tamoxifen in the induction of adenomyotic foci in the rat (Parrott et al. 2001). In addition, in hypoestrogenic premenopausal women with breast cancer, tamoxifen has been shown to stimulate massively and rapidly an ectopic endometrium (Rose et al. 2000; Abad de Velasco et al. 2003; Chang et al. 2003; Bese et al. 2003), inducing a rapid condition requiring surgical treatment. Tamoxifen-induced endometriosis can be severe, making necessary a demolitive surgery (Bese et al. 2003).

Based on these considerations, a history of endometriosis should be considered a contraindication for treatment with tamoxifen, and considerable attention should be paid to the widespread use of tamoxifen as prophylactic treatment for the prevention of breast cancer in premenopausal women.

Raloxifene seems to have pharmacological proprieties that make its administration useful in women with endometriosis. Raloxifene, in fact, has been investigated in animal models with good results. Furthermore, just as with the other novel therapies for endometriosis, original articles on the effect of raloxifene on this condition are still lacking.

Recently, a Japanese research group published preclinical safety and efficacy data of an oral antiestrogen (TZE-5323) (Saito et al. 2003). This drug has been shown to have a strong affinity for human ERα and ERβ and a dose-dependent capacity to inhibit estradiol-stimulated transcriptional activation (Saito et al. 2003). In the experimental endometriosis model in rats, TZE-5323 dose-dependently reduced the volume of the endometrial implant with an effectiveness similar to that of danazol and leuprorelin acetate without causing significant changes in bone mineral density and in serum estradiol levels (Saito et al. 2003).

12.4 Conclusions

At present, the only SERMs routinely used in clinical practice are tamoxifen and raloxifene. Tamoxifen is used essentially as adjuvant treatment in women with breast cancer. Its use is related to estrogenic effects on the uterus. Specifically, tamoxifen can be associated with an increase not only in endometrial hyperplasia and cancer risk but also in uterine leiomyoma dimensions and in a risk of developing active endometriotic lesions.

Raloxifene is actually used for the treatment and prevention of postmenopausal osteoporosis. Also, if raloxifene has been shown to have any effect on uterine leiomyomas in vitro and in animal models, to date no concrete efficacy has been demonstrated in normally cycled premenopausal women. Moreover, the addition of raloxifene to GnRH-a administration can be useful for limiting GnRH-a-related side effects and increasing the rate of reduction in tumor size.

Regarding the use of SERMs in women with endometriosis, the efficacy of raloxifene or other compounds is only potential. Experimental studies to determine if SERMs have a greater potency against uterine leiomyomas and endometriosis are currently in progress.

References

1. Abad de Velasco L, Cano A (2003) Acute abdomen due to endometriosis in a premenopausal woman taking tamoxifen. Eur J Obstet Gynecol Reprod Biol 109:234–235
2. Akande VA, Hunt LP, Cahill DJ, Jenkins JM (2004) Differences in time to natural conception between women with unexplained infertility and infertile women with minor endometriosis. Hum Reprod 19:96–103
3. American Fertility Society (1985) Revised American Fertility Society classification of endometriosis: 1985. Fertil Steril 43:351–355
4. Baker VL, Draper M, Paul S, Allerheiligen S, Glant M, Shifren J, Jaffe RB (1998) Reproductive endocrine and endometrial hydrochloride, a selective estrogen receptor modulator, in women with regular menstrual cycles. J Clin Endocrinol Metab 83: 6–13
5. Barbieri RL (1997) Reduction in the size of a uterine leiomyoma following discontinuation of an estrogen-progestin contraceptive. Gynecol Obstet Invest 43:276–277
6. Benassayag C, Leroy MJ, Rigourd V, Robert B, Honore JC, Mignot TM (1999) Estrogen receptors (ERalpha/ERbeta) in normal and pathological growth of the human myometrium: pregnancy and leiomyoma. Am J Physiol 276:1112–1118
7. Bese T, Simsek Y, Bese N, Ilvan S, Arvas M (2003) Extensive pelvic endometriosis with malignant change in tamoxifen-treated postmenopausal women. Int J Gynecol Cancer 13:376–380
8. Black LJ, Sato M, Rowley ER, Magee DE, Bekele A, Williams DC (1994) Raloxifene (LY139481 HCL) prevents bone loss and reduces serum cholesterol without causing uterine hypertrophy in ovriectomized rats. J Clin Invest 93:63–69
9. Brandon DD, Erickson TE, Keenan EJ, Strawn EY, Novy MJ, Burry KA (1995) Estrogen receptor gene expression in human uterine leiomyomata. J Clin Endocrinol Metab 80:1876–1881
10. Bryant HU, Glasebrook AL, Yang NN, Sato M (1996) A pharmacological review of raloxifene. J Bone Miner Metab 14:1–9
11. Bulun SE, Simpson ER, Word RA (1994) Expression of the CYP19 gene and its product aromatase cytochrome P450 in human uterine leiomyoma tissue and cells in culture. J Clin Endocrinol Metab 78:736–743
12. Carter JE (1998) Surgical treatment for chronic pelvic pain. J Soc Laparoendoscop Surgeons 2:129–133
13. Chang CK, Chen P, Leu FJ, Lou SM (2003) Florid polypoid endometriosis exacerbated by tamoxifen therapy in breast cancer. Obstet Gynecol 102:1127–1130
14. Check JH (2003a) The association of minimal and mild endometriosis without adhesions and infertility with therapeutic strategies. Clin Exp Obstet Gynecol 30:13–18
15. Check JH (2003b) The association of minimal and mild endometriosis without adhesions and infertility with therapeutic strategies. Clin Exp Obstet Gynecol 30:19–34
16. Check JH (2003c) The association of minimal and mild endometriosis without adhesions and infertility with therapeutic strategies. Clin Exp Obstet Gynecol 30:35–39
17. Chegini N, Rong H, Dou Q, Kipersztok S, Williams RS (1996) Gonadotropin-releasing hormone (GnRH) and GnRH receptor gene expression in human myometrium and leiomyomata and the direct action of GnRH analogs on myometrial smooth muscle cells and interaction with ovarian steroids in vitro. J Clin Endocrinol Metab 81:3215–3221
18. Child TJ, Tan SL (2001) Endometriosis: aetiology, pathogenesis and treatment. Drugs 61:1735–1750

19. Chwalisz K, Garg R, Brenner RM, Schubert G, Elger W (2002) Selective progesterone receptor modulators (SPRMs): a novel therapeutic concept in endometriosis. Ann NY Acad Sci 955:373–388
20. Cohen FJ, Watts S, Shah A, Akers R, Plouffe L (2000) Uterine effects of 3-year raloxifene therapy in postmenopausal women younger than age 60. Obstet Gynecol 95:104–110
21. Cohen I, Beyth Y, Shapira J, Tepper R, Fishman A, Cordoba M, Bernheim J, Yigael D, Altaras MM (1997) High frequency of adenomyosis in postmenopausal breast cancer patients treated with tamoxifen. Gynecol Obstet Invest 44:200–205
22. Coutinho EM (1989) Gestrinone in the treatment of myomas. Acta Obstet Gynecol Scand 150:39–46
23. Coutinho EM (1990) Treatment of large fibroids with high doses of getrinone. Gynecol Obstet Invest 30:44–47
24. Coutinho EM, Goncalves MT (1989) Long-term treatment of leiomyomas with gestrinone. Fertil Steril 51:939–946
25. Cummings SR, Eckert S, Krueger KA, Grady D, Powles TJ, Cauley JA, Norton L, Nickelsen T, Bjarnason NH, Morrow M, Lippman ME, Black D, Glusman JE, Costa A, Jordan VC (1999) Effects of raloxifene on breast cancer risk in postmenopausal women. J Am Med Assoc 281:2189–2197
26. De Leo V, La Marca A, Morgante G (1999) Short-term treatment of uterine fibromyomas with danazol. Gynecol Obstet Invest 47:258–262
27. De Leo V, La Marca A, Morgante G, Severi FM, Petraglia F (2001) Administration of somatostatin analogue reduces uterine and myoma volume in women with uterine leiomyomata. Obstet Gynecol 75:632–633
28. Demco L (1998) Mapping the source and character of pain due to endometriosis by patient-assisted laparoscopy. J Am Assoc Gynecol Laparosc 5:241–245
29. D'Hooghe TM (2003) Immunomodulators and aromatase inhibitors: are they the next generation of treatment for endometriosis? Curr Opin Obstet Gynecol 15: 243–249
30. D'Hooghe TM, Debrock S, Hill JA, Meuleman C (2003) Endometriosis and subfertility: is the relationship resolved? Semin Reprod Med 21:243–254
31. Dilts PV Jr, Hopkins MP, Chang AE, Cody RL (1992) Rapid growth of leiomyoma in patient receiving tamoxifen. Am J Obstet Gynecol 166:167–168
32. Englund K, Blanck A, Gustavsson I, Lundkvist U, Sjoblom P (1998) Sex steroids receptors in human myometrium and fibroids: changes during the menstrual cycle and gonadotropin-releasing hormone treatment. J Clin Endocrinol Metab 83:92–96
33. Ettinger B, Black DM, Mitlak BH, Knickerbocker RH, Nickelsen T, Genant NK (1999) Reduction of vertebral fracture risk in postmenopausal women with osteoporosis treated with raloxifene. J Am Med Assoc 282:637–645
34. Fotiou S, Tserkezoglou A, Hadjieleftheriou G, Apostolikas N, Karydas I, Stravolemos K (1998) Tamoxifen associated uterine pathology in breast cancer patients with abnormal bleeding. Anticancer Res 18:625–629
35. Friedman AJ, Thomas PP (1995) Does low-dose combination oral contraceptive use affect uterine size or menstrual flow in premenopausal with leiomyomas? Obstet Gynecol 85:631–635
36. Fuchs-Young R, Howe S, Hale L, Miles R, Walker C (1996) Inhibition of estrogen stimulated growth of uterine leiomyomas by selective estrogen receptor modulators. Mol Carcinog 17:151–159
37. Gainer EE, Ulmann A (2003) Pharmacologic properties of CDB(VA)-2914. Steroids 68:1005–1011

38. Gao Z, Matsuo H, Wang Y, Nakago S, Maruo T (2001) Up-regulation by IGF-I of proliferating cell nuclear antigen and Bcl-2 protein expression in human uterine leiomyoma cells. J Clin Endocrinol Metab 86:5593–5599
39. Goldstein SR, Scheele WH, Rajagopalan SK, Wilkie JL, Walsh BW, Parsons AK (2000) A 12-month comparative study of raloxifene, estrogen, and placebo on the postmenopausal endometrium. Obstet Gynecol 95:95–103
40. Gruppo Italiano per lo Studio dell'Endometriosi (2001) Relationship between stage, site and morphological characteristics of pelvis endometriosis and pain. Hum Reprod 16:2668–2671
41. Higashijima T, Kataoka A, Nishida T, Yakushiji M (1996) Gonadotropin-releasing hormone agonist therapy induces apoptosis in uterine leiomyoma. Eur J Obstet Gynecol Reprod Biol 68:169–173
42. Howe SR, Gottardis MM, Everitt JI, Walker C (1995) Estrogen stimulation and tamoxifen inhibition of leiomyoma cell growth in vitro and in vivo. Endocrinology 136:4996–5003
43. Hurd WW (1998) Criteria that indicate endometriosis is the cause of chronic pelvic pain. Obstet Gynecol 92:1029–1032
44. Jacobson TZ, Barlow DH, Koninckx PR, Olive D, Farquhar C (2004) Laparoscopic surgery for subfertility associated with endometriosis. Cochrane Library, Issue 4. Update Software, Oxford
45. Jirecek S, Lee A, Pavo I, Crans G, Eppel W, Wenzl R (2004) Raloxifene prevents the growth of uterine leiomyomas in premenopausal women. Fertil Steril 81:132–136
46. Kawaguchi K, Fujii S, Konishi I, Nanbu Y, Nonogaki H, Mori T (1989) Mitotic activity in uterine leiomyomas during the menstrual cycle. Am J Obstet Gynecol 160:637–641
47. Kertel LM, Murphy AA, Morales AJ, Yen SS (1994) Clinical efficacy of antiprogesterone RU 486 in the treatment of endometriosis and uterine fibroids. Hum Reprod 9:116–120
48. Khovidhunkit W, Shoback DM (1999) Clinical effects of raloxifene hydrocloride in women. Ann Intern Med 130:431–439
49. Kuiper GGJM, Carlsson B, Grandien K , Enmark E, Haggblad J, Nilsson S, Gustafsson JA (1997) Comparison of the ligand binding specificity and transcript tissue distribution of estrogen receptors α and β. Endocrinology 138:863–870
50. Lacreuse A, Wilson ME, Herndon JG (2002) Estradiol, but not raloxifene, improves aspects of spatial working memory in aged ovariectomized rhesus monkeys. Neurobiol Ag 23:589–600
51. Lefebvre G, Allaire C, Jeffrey J (2002) Clinical Practice Gynaecology Committee and Executive Committeee and Council, Society of Obstetricians and Gynaecologists of Canada. SOGC clinical guidelines. Hysterectomy. J Obstet Gynaecol Can 4:37–61
52. Leo L, Lanza A, Re A, Tessarolo M, Bellino R, Lauricella A, Wierdis T (1994) Leiomyomas in patients receiving tamoxifen. Clin Exp Obstet Gynecol 21:94–98
53. Lumsden MA, West CP, Baird DT (1989a) Tamoxifen prolongs luteal phase in premenopausal women but has no effect on the size of uterine fibroids. Clin Endocrinol 31:335–343
54. Lumsden MA, West CP, Hillier H, Baird DT (1989b) Estrogenic action of tamoxifen in women treated with luteinizing hormone-releasing hormone agonists (goserelin)-lack of shrinkage of uterine fibroids. Fertil Steril 52:924–929
55. MacDonald SR, Klock SC, Milad MP (1999) Long-term outcome of nonconservative surgery (hysterectomy) for endometriosis-associated pain in women < 30 years old. Am J Obstet Gynecol 180:1360–1363
56. Maeda T, Ke HZ, Simmons H, Thompson D (2004) Lasofoxifene, a next generation estrogen receptor modulator: preclinical studies. Clin Calcium 14:85–93

57. Marcoux S, Maheux R, Berube S (1997) Laparoscopy surgery in infertile woman with minimal or mild endometriosis. Canadian Collaborative Group on Endometriosis. N Engl J Med 337:217–222
58. Marshall LM, Spiegelman D, Goldman MB, Manson JE, Colditz G, Barbieri RL, Stampfer MJ, Hunter DJ (1998) A prospective study of reproductive factors and oral contraceptive use in relation to the risk of uterine leiomyomata. Fertil Steril 70:432–439
59. Minakuchi K, Kawamura N, Tsujimura A (1999) Remarkable and persistent shrinkage of uterine leiomyoma associated with interferon alfa treatment for hepatitis. Lancet 353:2127–2128
60. Missmer SA, Cramer DW (2003) The epidemiology of endometriosis. Obstet Gynecol Clin North Am 30:1–19
61. Murphy AA, Kettel LM, Morales AJ, Roberts VJ, Yen SSC (1993) Regression of uterine leiomyomata in response to the antiprogesterone RU 486. J Clin Endocrinol Metab 76:513–517
62. Olive DL (2002) Role of progesterone antagonists and new selective progesterone receptor modulators in reproductive health. Obstet Gynecol Surv 57:S55–63
63. Olive DL, Pritts EA (2001) Treatment of endometriosis. N Engl J Med 345:266–275
64. Oral E, Arici A (1997) Pathogenesis of endometriosis. Obstet Gynecol Clin North Am 24:219–233
65. Paech K, Webb P, Kuiper GGJM, Nilsson S, Gustafsson J, Kushner PJ, Scanlan TS (1997) Differential ligand activation of estrogen receptors ERα and ERβ at AP1 sites. Science 277:1508–1510
66. Palomba S, Zullo F (2006b) Pelvic denervations procedures as surgical management of pelvic pain due to endometriosis. In: Sutton C, Jones K, Adamdson GD (eds) Modern Management of Endometriosis. Taylor and Francis, London; 167–176; Palomba et al. 2006a
67. Palomba S, Affinito P, Tommaselli GA, Nappi C (1998) A clinical trial on the effects of tibolone association with gonadotropin-releasing hormone analogues for the treatment of uterine leiomyomata. Fertil Steril 70:111–118
68. Palomba S, Affinito P, Di Carlo C, Bifulco G, Nappi C (1999) Long term administration of tibolone plus gonadotropin-releasing hormone agonist for treatment of uterine leiomyomas: effectiveness and effects on vasomotor symptoms, bone mass, and lipid profile. Fertil Steril 72:889–895
69. Palomba S, Sammartino A, Di Carlo C, Affinito P, Zullo F, Nappi C (2001) Effects of raloxifene treatment on uterine leiomyomas in postmenopausal women. Fertil Steril 76:38–43
70. Palomba S, Orio F Jr, Morelli M, Russo T, Pellicano M, Zupi E, Lombardi G, Nappi C, Benedetti Panici PG, Zullo F (2002a) Raloxifene administration in premenopausal women with uterine leiomyomas: a pilot study. J Clin Endocrinol Metab 87:3303–3308
71. Palomba S, Russo T, Orio F jr, Tauchmananovà L, Zupi E, Benedetti Panici PG, Nappi C, Lombardi G, Colao A, Zullo F (2002b) Effectiveness of combined GnRH analogue plus raloxifene administration in the treatment of uterine leiomyomas: a prospective, randomized, single-blind, placebo-controlled clinical trial. Hum Reprod 17:3213–3219
72. Palomba S, Orio F Jr, Morelli M, Russo T, Pellicano M, Nappi C, Mastrantonio P, Lombardi G, Colao A, Zullo F (2002c) Raloxifene administration in women treated with gonadotropin releasing hormone agonist for uterine leiomyomas: effects on bone metabolism. J Clin Endocrinol Metab 87:4476–4481
73. Palomba S, Zullo F, Orio F Jr, Lombardi G (2004a) Does raloxifene inhibit the growth of uterine fibroids? Fertil Steril 81:1719–1720

74. Palomba S, Russo T, Orio F Jr, Sammartino A, Sbano FM, Nappi C, Colao A, Mastrantonio P, Lombardi G, Zullo F (2004b) Lipid, glucose, and homocysteine metabolism in women treated with a gonadotropin-releasing hormone agonist with or without raloxifene. Hum Reprod 19:415–421
75. Palomba S, Orio F Jr, Russo T, Falbo A, Cascella T, Doldo P, Nappi C, Lombardi G, Mastrantonio P, Zullo F (2004c) Long-term effectiveness and safety of GnRH agonist plus raloxifene administration in women with uterine leiomyomas. Hum Reprod 19:1308–1314
76. Palomba S, Orio F Jr, Falbo A, Russo T, Amati A, Zullo F (2005b) Gonadotropin-releasing hormone agonist with or without raloxifene: effects on cognition, mood, and quality of life. Fertil Steril 84:154–161
77. Palomba S, Falbo A, Russo T, Zullo F (2005a) Emerging drugs in uterine leiomyomas. Exp Opin Emerg Drugs (in press)
78. Palomba S, Falbo A, Russo T, Zullo F (2006a) GnRH analogs use for the treatment of symptomatic leiomyomas. Gynecol Surg 2:7–13
79. Palomba S, Orio F Jr, Russo T, Falbo A, Tolino A, Lombardi G, Cimini V, Zullo F (2005b) Anti-proliferative and pro-apoptotic effects of raloxifene on uterine leiomyomas in postmenopausal women. Fertil Steril (in press)
80. Parazzini F (1999) Ablation of lesions or no treatment in minimal-mild endometriosis in infertile women: a randomized trial. Gruppo Italiano per lo Studio dell'Endometriosi. Hum Reprod 14:1332–1334
81. Parrott E, Butterworth M, Green A, White INH, Greaves P (2001) Adenomyosis: a result of disordered stromal differentiation. Am J Pathol 159:623–630
82. Pasqualini JR, Cornier E, Grenier J, Vella C, Schatz B, Netter A (1990) Effect of decapeptyl, an agonost analog of gonadotropin-releasing hormone on estrogens, estrogen sulfates, and progesterone receptors in leiomyomata and myometrium. Fertil Steril 53:1012–1017
83. Pickersgill A (1998) GnRH agonists and add-back therapy: is there a perfect combination? Br J Obstet Gynaecol 105:475–485
84. Porpora MG, Gomel V (1997) The role of laparoscopy in the management of pelvic pain in women of reproductive age. Fertil Steril 68:765–769
85. Porter KB, Tsibris JC, Porter GW, Fuchs-Young R, Nicosia SV, O'Brien WF (1998) Effects of raloxifene in a guinea pig model for leiomyomas. Am J Obstet Gynecol 179:1283–1287
86. Rannestad T, Eikeland OJ, Helland H (2001) The quality of life in women suffering from gynecological disorders is improved by means of hysterectomy. Absolute and relative differences between pre- and postoperative measures. Acta Obstet Gynecol Scand 80:46–51
87. Rein MS (2000) Advanced in uterine leiomyoma research: the progesterone hypothesis. Environ Health Perspect 108:791–793
88. Rein MS, Barbieri RL, Friedman AJ (1995) Progesterone: a critical role in pathogenesis of uterine myomas. Am J Obstet Gynecol 172:14–18
89. Riggs BL, Hartmann LC (2003) Selective estrogen-receptor modulators: mechanisms of action and application to clinical practice. N Engl J Med 348:618–629
90. Rivera JA, Christopoulos S, Small D, Trifiro M (2004) Hormonal manipulation of benign metastasizing leiomyomas: report of two cases an review of the literature. J Clin Endocrinol Metab 89:3183–3188
91. Robertson JF (2004) Selective oestrogen receptor modulators/new antioestrogens: a clinical perspective. Cancer Treat Rev 30:695–706

92. Rose PG, Alvarez B, Maclennan GT (2000) Exacerbation of endometriosis as a result of premenopausal tamoxifen exposure. Am J Obstet Gynecol 183:507–508
93. Sadan O, Ginath S, Sofer D, Rotmensch S, Debby A, Glezerman M, Zakut H (2001) The role of tamoxifen in the treatment of symptomatic uterine leiomyomata: a pilot study. Eur J Obstet Gynecol Reprod Biol 96:183–186
94. Saito T, Yoshizawa M, Yamauchi Y, Kinoshita S, Fujii T, Mieda M, Sone H, Yamamoto Y, Koizumi N (2003) Effects of the novel orally active antiestrogen TZE-5323 on experimental endometriosis. Arzneimittelforschung 53:507–514
95. Schwartz LB, Rutkowski N, Horan C, Nachtigall LE, Snyder J, Goldstein SR (1998) Use of transvaginal ultrasonography to monitor the effects of tamoxifen on uterine leiomyoma size and ovarian cyst formation. J Ultrasound Med 17: 699–703
96. Shozu M, Murakami K, Segawa T, Kasai T, Inoue M (2003) Successful treatment of a symptomatic uterine leiomyoma in a perimenopausal woman with a nonsteroidal aromatase inhibitor. Fertil Steril 79:628–631
97. Spitz IM (2003) Progesterone antagonists and progesterone receptor modulators: an overview. Steroids 68:981–993
98. Steward EA (2001) Uterine fibroids. Lancet 357:293–298
99. Stones RW, Mountfield J (2004) Interventions for treating chronic pelvic pain in women. Cochrane Library, Issue 2. Update Software, Oxford
100. Sutton CJ, Ewen SP, Whitelaw N (1994) Prospective, randomized double-blind controlled trial of laser laparoscopy in the treatment of pelvic pain associated with minimal, mild and moderate endometriosis. Fertil Steril 62:696–700
101. Tiltman AJ (1985) The effect of progestins on the mitotic activity of uterine fibromyomas. Int J Gynecol Pathol 4:89–96
102. Tomas E, Kauppila A, Blanco G, Apaja-Sarkkinen M, Laatikainen T (1995) Comparison between the effects of tamoxifen and toremifene on the uterus in postmenopausal breast cancer patients. Gynecol Oncol 59:261–266
103. Ugwumadu AH, Harding K (1994) Uterine leiomyomata and endometrial proliferation in postmenopausal women treated with the anti-oestrogen tamoxifen. Eur J Obstet Gynecol Reprod Biol 54:153–156
104. Walker CL, Burroughs KD, Davis B, Sowell K, Everitt JI, Fuchs-Young R (2000) Preclinical evidence for therapeutic efficacy of selective estrogen receptor modulators for uterine leiomyoma. J Soc Gynecol Invest 7:249–256
105. Walsh BW, Kuller LH, Wild RA, Paul S, Farmer M, Lawrence JB, Shah AS, Anderson PW (1998) Effects of raloxifene on serum lipids and coagulation factors in healthy postmenopausal women. J Am Med Assoc 279:1445–1451
106. Yaffe K, Krueger K, Sarkar S, Grady D, Barrett-Connor E, Cox DA, et al. (2001) Cognitive function in postmenopausal women treated with raloxifene. N Engl J Med 344:1207–1213
107. Yamamoto T, Takamori K, Okada H (1984) Estrogen biosynthesis in leiomyomata and myometrium of the uterus. Horm Metab Res 16:678–679

[illegible]

Chapter 13

Other Clinical Effects of SERMs

P. Acién · F. Quereda · M.I. Acién

As shown in previous chapters, selective estrogen receptor modulators (SERMs) are drugs that bind to estrogen receptors (ERs); in some tissues they act like estrogen (agonists), while in other tissues they oppose the action of estrogen (antagonists). The SERM tamoxifen acts as an estrogen antagonist in the breast in that it prevents and treats breast cancer, but it acts as an estrogen agonist in the endometrium, where it can increase the risk of cancer. So the resulting estrogen agonistic or antagonistic activity of SERMs is tissue and organ dependent. The complexity of these interactions becomes even more confusing when one takes into consideration that different SERMs may act similarly in certain tissues, as in the case with tamoxifen and raloxifene in the breast, and dissimilarly in others, as seen with these same two in the endometrium. Therefore, each individual SERM may have, within itself, differing effects on different tissues and organs. This is what makes them so interesting. And since there are ERs in almost every tissue, SERMs are also likely to have some effect on nearly all the organs of the human body.

Descriptions exist of several SERMs: ethamoxytriphetol, cyclofenil, clomiphene, tamoxifen, raloxifene, arzoxifene, rolxifene, lasofoxifene, basodoxifene, levormeloxifene, ospemifene, tofupill/femarelle (DT56a) – a new phytoselective estrogen receptor modulatorlike substance – and fulvestrant, the first of a new class of drugs, an ER down regulator that may have advantages over tamoxifen in the treatment of estrogen-dependent diseases. But after several years of use of clomiphene citrate in the induction of ovulation, the first widely used SERM was tamoxifen in the treatment and prevention of breast cancer. Raloxifene is another SERM in clinical use, and it was developed to avoid some of the undesirable estrogen agonistic actions of other SERMs in order to improve the drug safety profile. It has been introduced for clinical use in the treatment and prevention of postmenopausal osteoporosis. All the other SERMs are still undergoing further research, a scrutiny that is even more necessary in those clinically introduced. This requirement is strengthened by the wide distribution of ERs in organs and systems distinct from the traditional targets, the genital apparatus and the breast. The actions of SERMs on those relevant systems, such as the cardiovascular tree, the bones, or the central nervous system, have been widely analyzed, together with several actions on the reproductive organs, in other chapters. Therefore, in this chapter we will review other clinical actions of SERMs that can be of clinical interest.

13.1 Urogenital Tract

13.1.1 Vaginal Trophism and Dyspareunia

In general, SERMs have an antiestrogenic or null estrogenic effect on the epithelium and on the vaginal trophism. Some, however, such as ospemifene have a significant estrogenic effect on the vaginal epithelium, as evidenced by an increase in intermediate and superficial cells in repeated Pap smears (Rutanen et al. 2003). Nevertheless, Morales et al. (2004) have recently studied the effects of tamoxifen and third-generation aromatase inhibitors on menopausal symptoms of breast cancer patients. Musculoskeletal pain and dyspareunia significantly increased with first-line nonsteroidal aromatase inhibitors, while patients using tamoxifen had a significant decrease in sexual interest. At a younger patient age, tamoxifen has been associated with hot flashes and vaginal dryness after 1 and 3 months of therapy. The relative incidence and correlation of subjective and psychosexual symptoms have also been studied during and after tamoxifen treatment by Mourits et al. (2002) in 98 breast cancer patients < 56 years of age in a randomized study comparing different doses of adjuvant chemotherapy, followed by radiotherapy and tamoxifen. During tamoxifen treatment there were complaints of vaginal dryness and/or dyspareunia in 47%, decreased sexual desire in 44%, and musculoskeletal symptoms in 43%. Decreased sexual interest correlated with vaginal dryness and/or dyspareunia. After discontinuation of tamoxifen, symptoms improved significantly. However, hot flashes, disturbed sleep, and vaginal dryness persisted more often in patients who remained postmenopausal after high doses of chemotherapy.

Likewise, raloxifene's effect on the postmenopausal vagina has been neutral in some studies, unlike estrogen's beneficial effect (Davies et al. 1999); in relation to placebo it does not increase the incidence of events related to vaginal atrophy. There are, however, few data on the effects of these drugs on urogenital atrophy (Robinson et al. 2003). In the paper by Modugno et al. (2003), raloxifene was not different from placebo with respect to comfort during sexual intercourse in postmenopausal women with osteoporosis, but the authors warn that no conclusion can be made about the effect of raloxifene on sexual function in premenopausal women, in younger postmenopausal women, or in women experiencing menopausal symptoms.

13.1.2 Pelvic Floor Function and Urinary Disorders

It has traditionally been considered that exogenous estrogens could improve incontinence and urinary control in postmenopausal women. In 2001, however, a large randomized blinded study compared oral daily estrogen plus progestin therapy vs. placebo in postmenopausal women with incontinence (Grady et al. 2001). Among the women who were assigned to hormonal treatment, incontinence was more likely to worsen and less likely to improve when compared with women who received placebo. The number of incontinent episodes per week increased an average of 0.7 in the hormone group and decreased by 0.1 in the placebo group ($p < 0.001$). It must be pointed out that the urethra and trigone of the bladder are covered by nonkeratinizing squamous epithelium of similar origin to the vagina and that these tissues have estrogen receptors and respond to estrogen (Bergman et al. 1990). The evidence of this randomized study, however, contradicted the traditional clinical teaching, which held that the administration of exogenous estrogen improves urinary control in postmenopausal women.

More recently, Robinson and Cardozo (2003) reviewed the role of estrogens in female lower urinary tract dysfunction and conclude that, although the role of estrogen replacement therapy (ERT) in the management of postmenopausal urinary incontinence (UI) remains controversial, its use in the treatment of women with urogenital atrophy is now well established. Estrogen therapy alone has little effect on the management of urodynamic stress UI, although in combination with an alpha-adrenergic agonist it may improve urinary leakage. Additionally, estrogen therapy may be of benefit for the irritative symptoms of urinary urgency and frequency and urge UI, although this effect may result from reversal of urogenital atrophy rather than a direct action on the lower urinary tract. Moreover, there is now some evidence that vaginal administration may be effective.

Concerning genital prolapse, the gynecological literature has traditionally favored the notion that postmenopausal atrophy of fascial and muscular support elements seems to be the important precipitating factor in older patients. It is unclear whether this is simply an aging phenomenon or is related to estrogen deprivation. Connective tissues may be weakened during the aging process as a result of decreases in collagen content (Affinito et al. 1999). Estrogen deprivation, which is associated generally with the postmenopausal state, has been considered to result in pelvic floor atrophy and the subsequent increased incidence of pelvic floor relaxation in older women (Rekers et al. 1992). Again, traditional teaching holds that ERT has positive effects on pelvic floor relaxation (Casper et al. 1998), although there have been no randomized trials to validate this.

Several clinical trials, however, demonstrated a neutral or antiestrogenic effect of raloxifene on the endometrium and uterus (Goldstein et al. 2000; Cohen et al. 2000), and, as previously mentioned, unlike estrogen's beneficial effect on the postmenopausal vagina, raloxifene's effect seems neutral (Davies et al. 1999). Thus, it becomes even more intriguing that, in an analysis of safety data of 3 raloxifene trials that included 6926 postmenopausal women, the relative risk of undergoing a surgical procedure for pelvic floor relaxation was 0.5 (95% CI, 0.31, 0.81) compared with the placebo control subjects (Goldstein et al. 2001). Therefore, raloxifene therapy was associated with a significantly reduced risk of pelvic floor surgery (1.51% vs. 0.75%) through 3 years of treatment (Fig. 13.1).

Hendrix and McNeely (2001) reviewed published and unplublished data on the effect of SERMs on reproductive tissues other than the endometrium. They identified the pharmaceutical companies developing or marketing SERMs, and the investigators at each company responsible for the conduct of investigational trials were contacted and queried about reports of adverse events in any ongoing or completed trials involving SERMs produced by their company. Levormeloxifene and idoxifene trials noted a higher proportion of surgery for pelvic organ prolapse in treated vs. untreated women. The development of these pharmaceutical agents was discontinued, primarily due to concerns over effects on the endometrium. Nevertheless, pelvic organ prolapse was reported to the FDA as an adverse event associated with both drugs. Study weaknesses preclude a definitive association between the agents and pelvic organ prolapse, since the treated groups were not necessarily similar due to confounding fac-

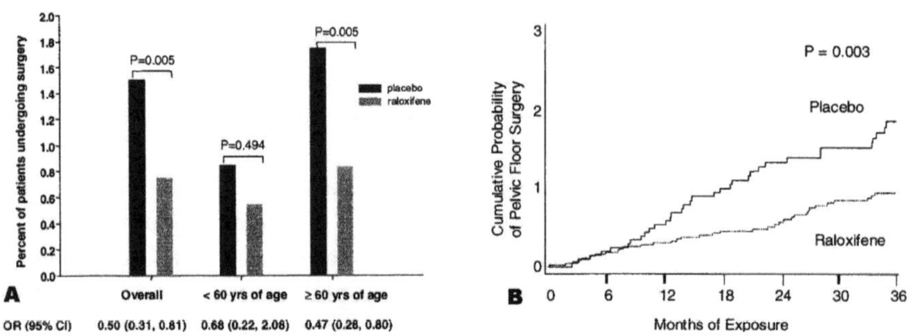

Fig. 13.1. **A** Incidence of surgery for pelvic floor relaxation in postmenopausal women followed for up to 3 years represented as a percentage of all randomized patients. Overall incidence and incidence in subgroups defined by age are shown. Statistical significance of the difference between placebo and raloxifene groups was assessed by a Cochran-Mantel-Haenszel test. **B** The cumulative probability of pelvic floor surgery for women in the placebo group as compared with those in the raloxifene group is represented as a percentage of women enrolled in the trial. Statistical significance of the difference between placebo and raloxifene groups was assessed by the log rank test (from Goldstein et al. 2001).

tors such as age, parity, obesity, cigarette smoking, and other risk factors for pelvic organ prolapse.

Later, Goldstein and Nanavati (2002) reported the adverse events associated with the SERM levormeloxifene in the aborted phase III osteoporosis treatment study. This study was stopped abruptly after 10 months because of the magnitude of adverse events compared to placebo. Thus, no bone mineral efficiency data were evaluated, nor was the comparability of the treatment groups at baseline analyzed statistically, though because it was a randomized study of > 2900 women, it is likely that the groups would be similar. Among the 2924 women who were studied, those who were treated with levormeloxifene had a marked increase compared with placebo in leukorrhea (30% vs. 3%), increased endometrial thickness on ultrasound scan (19% vs 1%), enlarged uterus (17% vs. 3%), uterovaginal prolapse (7% vs. 2%), urinary incontinence (17% vs. 4%), increased micturition frequency (9% vs. 4%), lower abdominal pain (17% vs. 6%), hot flashes (10% vs. 3%), and leg cramps (6% vs. 0.8%). All of these differences were highly statistically significant (Table 13.1). Therefore, the treatment group (with the SERM levormeloxifene 0.5 mg or 1.25 mg daily) had a > 3-fold increase in the risk of developing uterovaginal prolapse and an almost 5-fold increased risk of developing UI compared with placebo.

Subsequently, Goldstein (2002), in an update on nonuterine gynecological effects of raloxifene, insisted on the results formerly shown and that, unlike levormeloxifene, in the raloxifene-treated patients there was a decrease of

Table 13.1. Comparison of selected adverse event risk ratios during treatment (all patients who received levormeloxifene are combined vs. placebo) (from Goldstein and Nanavati 2002)

Body system (World Health Organization terminology)	Levormeloxifene total vs. placebo		
	P value	Risk ratio	95% CI
Reproductive disorders			
Endometrial disorder	0.0001	14.96	8.60–26.00
Leukorrhea	0.0001	14.30	9.60–21.51
Uterine disorder	0.0001	6.43	4.37–9.45
Uterovaginal prolapse	0.0001	3.44	2.13–5.56
Vaginal discomfort	0.0001	4.62	2.11–10.07
Urinary system disorders			
Micturition frequency	0.0001	2.40	1.70–3.39
Urinary incontinence	0.0001	4.99	3.55–7.00
Gastrointestinal disorders			
Abdominal pain	0.0001	2.85	2.16–3.75
Constipation	0.0001	1.70	1.34–2.16
Body as a whole (general disorders)			
Hot flashes	0.0001	3.84	2.55–5.79
Leg cramps	0.0001	7.12	3.47–4.6

50% in surgery for pelvic organ prolapse and/or UI. It should be noted, however, that these trials were not designed to assess the effect of raloxifene on the pelvic floor and that there was no systematic evaluation for pelvic organ relaxation.

Robinson and Cardozo (2003) concluded saying that the long-term effects of SERMs on the urogenital tract remain to be determined, and there are few data on the effects of these drugs on UI and urogenital atrophy.

13.2 Central nervous system

Animal studies have suggested that raloxifene may affect brain function, although the effects of SERMs on the human brain remain to be established (Nickelsen et al. 1999). Before mentioning them, it is worthwhile to review the actions of estrogens.

Evidence from randomized, controlled trials and from cross-sectional and longitudinal studies show that ERT preferentially protects against a decline in verbal memory in healthy postmenopausal women and decreases the risk of Alzheimer's disease (AD) (Sherwin 2002). Although results are not consistent across studies, they indicate that treatment with estrogen during the postmenopausal years might protect against cognitive aging in women during the latter part of their life. Experimental studies demonstrate a consistent beneficial effect on verbal memory, but these are short-term studies of the more acute effects of ERT. The observational studies suggest that there may be a long-lasting effect of continued ERT on cognitive functioning, and that with respect to the effects of ERT on AD, such therapy is associated with a decreased risk for dementia; however, there is little evidence for a positive effect on cognition in women with AD. Consequently, it is pointed out that definitive answers to questions about the long-term effects of ERT on cognitive aging and risk of developing AD should be provided by ongoing clinical trials (Zec et al. 2002).

The CNS is one of the main target tissues for sex steroid hormones, which act both through genomic mechanisms, modulating synthesis, release, and metabolism of many neuropeptides and neurotransmitters and through nongenomic mechanisms, influencing electrical excitability, synaptic function, and morphological features. The identification of the brain as a *de novo* source of neurosteroids modulating cerebral function suggests that the modifications in mood and cognitive performance occurring in postmenopausal women could also be related to a modification in the levels of neurosteroids, particularly allopregnanolone and DHEA, GABA-A agonist, and antagonist (Bernardi et al. 2003). Likewise, Shively and Bethea (2004) state that ovarian steroids have multiple effects on serotonin synthesis, reuptake, and degradation, on neural activity that drives serotonin release, and on receptor activation in primates. Moreover, as already mentioned, several studies have suggested that estrogen may improve cognitive function or prevent the development of dementia, but other studies have not shown benefits.

Certainly, to evaluate the effect of estrogen plus progestin on the incidence of dementia and mild cognitive impairment compared with placebo, the Women's Health Initiative Memory Study (WHIMS), a randomized, double-blind, placebo-controlled clinical trial, was designed, and it began enrolling participants from the Women's Health Initiative (WHI) estrogen plus progestin trial in May 1996. Of the 4894 eligible participants of the WHI study, 4532 (92.6%) postmenopausal women aged 65 years or older were free of probable dementia. Participants received either 1 daily tablet of 0.625 mg of conjugated equine estrogen plus 2.5 mg of medroxyprogesterone acetate (n = 2229) or a matching placebo (n = 2303). The incidence of probable dementia (primary outcome) and mild cognitive impairment (secondary outcome) were identified through a structured clinical assessment. The mean time between the date of randomization into WHI and the last Modified Mini-Mental State Examination for all WHIMS participants was 4.05 (1.19) years. Overall, 61 women were diagnosed with probable dementia, 40 (66%) in the estrogen plus progestin group and 21 (34%) in the placebo group. Therefore, the hazard ratio (HR) for probable dementia was 2.05 (95% CI, 1.21–3.48; 45 vs. 22 per 10,000 person-years; p = 0.01), and this increased risk would result in 23 additional cases of dementia per 10,000 women per year. Treatment effects on mild cognitive impairment did not differ between groups. So the conclusion of the authors (Shumaker et al. 2003) was that the estrogen plus progestin therapy increased the risk for probable dementia in postmenopausal women aged 65 years or older. In addition, estrogen plus progestin therapy did not prevent mild cognitive impairment in these women.

These results are not congruent, however, with all the previously published studies on the value of estrogens as neuroprotective agents with potential effects on the pathogenesis of AD. Conflicting findings may be due to differences in the types of hormone therapy given, specifically the addition of progestin. Moreover, some posterior studies, to be commented on later (Eberling et al. 2004), provide both physiological as well as anatomical evidence for the neuroprotective effects of estrogen.

With the recognition that SERMs have differential tissue-dependent effects on ER function, there has been recent interest in the effects of raloxifene, tamoxifen, and other SERMs on mood, sleep, cognitive function, and AD severity. What follows is an analysis of the effects of SERMs on several conditions.

13.2.1
Hot Flashes and Beta Endorphins

The most commonly observed side effect in patients taking raloxifene or tamoxifen was hot flashes (Agnusdei 1999; Muchmore 2000; Miller 2002). In the study by Mourits et al. (2002) in breast cancer patients < 56 years of age, the most frequent complaints during tamoxifen treatment were hot flashes (85%) and disturbed sleep (55%), whereas in the CORE study (Martino et al. 2004) hot flashes were observed in 12.5% of the raloxifene group vs. 6.9% in the placebo group.

Recently, Aldrighi et al. (2004) analyzed the predictors of hot flashes in postmenopausal women who received raloxifene therapy to assess the clinical usefulness of various therapeutic strategies for their reduction. In this randomized, double-blind, placebo-controlled study, 487 unselected postmenopausal women were assigned randomly to receive treatment for 8 months with raloxifene, which was administered either at a dose of 60 mg/d every other day for 2 months followed by 60 mg/d (slow-dose escalation) or 60 mg/d throughout (raloxifene), or placebo. Data on the number, duration, intensity, and severity of hot flashes and awakenings due to night sweats were collected, and logistic regression models were used to examine the predictive value of various demographic and menopausal factors on the development or worsening of hot flashes. At baseline, 40.4% of all randomly assigned patients did not have flashes, but the mean number of hot flashes (3–5 per week) was low. Fewer years postmenopause, surgical menopause, and previous estrogen or estrogen/progestin therapy were significant predictors of hot flashes at baseline but were not predictive of incident hot flashesduring treatment with raloxifene. Of the women who received raloxifene therapy who had preexisting hot flashes/during apart at baseline, 36% had none at the end point. Early postmenopause and surgical menopause were significant predictors of a biologically relevant increase in hot flashes ($\geq$ 14 flashes/week). Early postmenopause, previous estrogen/progestin therapy, high body mass index, and greater duration of hot flashes at baseline were significant predictors of the need for symptomatic treatment. After 2 months of treatment, women in early postmenopause had significantly more hot flashes with raloxifene therapy than with slow-dose escalation ($p = 0.042$), whereas there was no significant difference between raloxifene therapy and slow-dose escalation among women in later postmenopause. In the 50 patients who requested symptomatic treatment during the study, phytohormones or veralipride did not reduce the number of hot flashes markedly.

In conclusion, a shorter time since menopause and surgical menopause are important predictors of hot flashes not only before but also during treatment with raloxifene. Previous estrogen/progestin therapy also increases the risk of hot flashes at baseline. For women in early postmenopause, slow-dose escalation of raloxifene therapy may be a suitable therapeutic strategy for the reduction of the risk of hot flashes.

Finally, it should be noted that Neele et al. (2002) have observed that raloxifene treatment significantly increases plasma levels of beta endorphin in postmenopausal women but does not significantly affect climateric symptoms with the exception of worsening vasomotor symptoms, so that the increase of hot flashes with raloxifene could be related to the changes in the beta endorphins.

13.2.2 Mood, Sleep, Waking Episodes

Nickelsen et al. (1999) studied raloxifene effects on cognition and mood in postmenopausal women participating in a randomized, double-blind osteoporosis treatment trial. After 12 months of treatment there were no significant differences between the raloxifene groups and the placebo one, suggesting that raloxifene does not affect mood in postmenopausal women treated for 1 year. Natale et al. (2004) have also studied its effect on psychological functions in 49 women. This SERM does not appear to affect adversely any psychological function such as libido, mood, or memory. And though it may worsen attention, it reduces waking episodes, so it may improve sleep.

As for tamoxifen, in the aforementioned studies by Mourits et al. (2002) on breast cancer patients analyzing the effects on subjective and psychosexual well-being, disturbed sleep (55% of patients) correlated with hot flashes and concentration problems.

13.2.3 Cognitive Function, Alzheimer's Disease (AD)

As previously mentioned, Nickelsen et al. (1999) analyzed the safety assessment of raloxifene effects on cognitive function and mood in postmenopausal women participating in a randomized, double-blind osteoporosis treatment trial. The results did not suggest that raloxifene impaired cognition or affected mood in postmenopausal women treated for 1 year. Additionally, Lacreuse et al. (2002) examined the effects of ERT and raloxifene on cognitive function in a rhesus monkey model ovariectomized long term (10–16 years). Estradiol was able to enhance some aspects of spatial working memory in aged monkeys despite many years of estrogen deprivation, while raloxifene did not affect cognitive function after long-term ovarian hormone deprivation. Bernardi et al. (2003), however, state that raloxifene administration in postmenopausal women has an estrogenlike effect on circulating beta endorphin and allopregnanolone levels, and it restores the response of beta endorphin and allopregnanolone to neuroendocrine tests encouraging the positive effects of estrogens with fewer side effects. In one study by Yaffe et al. (2001) as well as in a more recent one by Natale et al. (2004), raloxifene treatment did not affect overall cognitive scores. Finally, the randomized clinical trial by Haskell and Richardson (2004) on 50 postmenopausal women receiving raloxifene 60 mg or placebo, for 8 weeks, drew identical conclusions, stating that the results showed no significant effect attributable to treatment with raloxifene on cognitive, psychological, or health variables.

As for tamoxifen, several studies have shown cognitive decline in women receiving it for the treatment of breast cancer, but the focus of those studies was on the effects of chemotherapy. For this reason Shilling et al. (2001) designed a pilot study to examine whether hormone therapy for breast cancer (with anatrozole, tamoxifen alone, or combined) affects cognition. The authors included not only the 94 patients but also another group of women without breast cancer ($n = 35$) who completed the battery of neuropsychological measures (Jenkins et al. 2004). The results showed specific impairments in processing speed and verbal memory in women receiving hormone therapy. The authors point out that verbal memory may be especially sensitive to changes in estrogen levels and that in view of the increased use of hormone therapies in an adjuvant and preventative setting, their impact on cognitive functioning should be investigated more thoroughly.

In this sense, then, the most recent and interesting material is the study by Eberling et al. (2004) on the estrogen- and tamoxifen-associated effects on brain structure and function. The researchers evaluated the effects of estrogen and tamoxifen on positron emission tomography (PET) measures of brain glucose metabolism and magnetic resonance imaging (MRI) measures of hippocampal atrophy. Three groups of postmenopausal women were studied, women taking estrogen (ERT+), women with breast cancer taking tamoxifen, and women not taking estrogen or tamoxifen (ERT–). All subjects received a PET scan, an MRI scan, and cognitive testing. The tamoxifen group showed widespread areas of hypometabolism in the inferior and dorsal lateral frontal lobes relative to the other two groups. The ERT– group showed lower metabolism in the inferior frontal cortex and temporal cortex with respect to the ERT+ group. The tamoxifen group also showed significantly lower semantic memory scores than the other two groups. Finally, the tamoxifen group had smaller right hippocampal volumes than the ERT+ group, an effect that was of borderline significance. Both right and left hippocampal volumes were significantly smaller than the ERT+ group when a single outlier was removed. The ERT– group had hippocampal volumes that were intermediate to the other two groups (Fig. 13.2). These findings provide physiological and anatomical evidence for the neuroprotective effects of estrogen and support the notion of an antagonistic role of tamoxifen in both the frontal lobes and hippocampus.

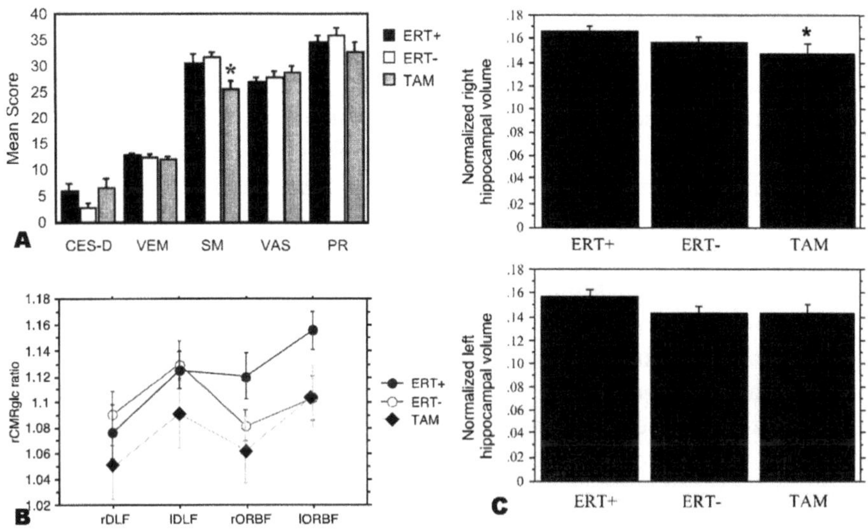

Fig. 13.2. A Neuropsychological test results. Mean scores for each group on the Center for Epidemiological Studies-Depression Scale (*CES-D*), verbal episodic memory (*VEM*), semantic memory (*SM*), verbal attention span (*VAS*), and pattern recognition (*PR*). **B** PET scan, region of interest (ROI) analysis. Regional cerebral glucose metabolism ratios for women taking estrogen, women not taking estrogen, and women taking tamoxifen. Regions are right and left dorsal lateral frontal cortex (*DLF*) and right and left orbital frontal cortex (*ORBF*). $P < 0.05$ between ERT+ and ERT- plus TAM in rORBF and lORBF. **C** Normalized hippocampal volumes (NHV). Mean NHV for women taking estrogen for each group. *Error bars* indicate standard deviations. *ERT+*, women taking estrogen; *ERT–*, women not taking estrogen; *TAM*, women taking tamoxifen. * TAM < ERT–, $p = 0.05$ (from Eberling et al. 2004)

Nevertheless, the authors point out that additional, well-controlled studies are warranted to further explore the association between tamoxifen and these measures.

13.2.4 Libido, Sexual Function

As previously mentioned, Morales et al. (2004) recently studied the effects of tamoxifen and third-generation aromatase inhibitors on menopausal symptoms of breast cancer patients. Patients taking tamoxifen had a significant decrease in sexual interest, and at a younger, premenopausal age tamoxifen was associated with hot flashes and vaginal dryness. Likewise, Modugno et al. (2003) studied the effects of raloxifene compared with placebo on sexual function in older postmenopausal women undergoing therapy for the treatment of osteoporosis in a subset of 943 women of the MORE trial (624 women with raloxifene and 319 with placebo). Subjects were administered the sexual function questionnaire (a modification of McCoy's Sex Scale Questionnaire) at baseline and again after 36 months of treatment, and they were informed that for this study, sexual activity was defined as "any activity that is sexually arousing to you – masturbation, oral sex, intercourse, etc." All women were asked to report their frequency of sexual activity and desire during the last 6 months. For sexually inactive women, the reason for inactivity was reported. For sexually active women, additional questions evaluated feelings during sexual activity, intensity of orgasms, and sexual problems. Overall, sexual function and changes in sexual function from baseline to study and between the raloxifene and placebo groups did not differ. In particular, there were no differences in sexual desire or frequency of sexual activity between the groups. Among sexually active women, there were no differences in enjoyment, satisfaction, orgasm, or reported sexual problems. Therefore, sexuality does not seem to be affected by treatment with raloxifene.

The results of the pilot study by Natale et al. (2004) in which mood, sleep, libido, and cognitive function were studied in 49 postmenopausal healthy women were similar. No significant differences were found in mood, well-being, libido, and indices of sexual activity.

13.3 Gallbladder and Hepatobiliar System

Several studies have shown that estrogens and their receptors play a role in the modulation of cholangiocyte proliferation. Alvaro et al. (2000) observed that cholangiocytes expressed both ER-alpha and ER-beta subtypes, whereas hepatocytes expressed only ER-alpha, and that the treatment with tamoxifen or ICI 182.780 of 3-week BDL rats inhibited cholangiocyte proliferation and induced overexpression of Fas antigen and apoptosis in cholangiocytes. Vickers et al. (2002) also evaluated the response of human cholangiocarcinoma cells to tamoxifen treatment through the Fas pathway by pretreatment with interferon-gamma. Tamoxifen exposure to human cholangiocarcinoma after pretreatment with INF-gamma allows for induction of apoptosis in vitro and significant inhibition tumor xenograft growth. The combination of these two compounds may provide a novel treatment regimen for cholangiocarcinoma. Likewise, Reddy et al. (2004) suggest tamoxifen as a novel treatment for primary biliary cirrhosis.

It is not, however, efficient in the treatment of hepatocarcinoma. Nowak et al. (2004), in a review by Cochrane, pointed out that the available data do not support the use of tamoxifen for patients with hepatocellular carcinoma. This same conclusion was reached by Gerard and Bleiberg (2004), who stated that hormonal therapy with tamoxifen or antiandrogens had shown no efficacy and might even be detrimental in patients with hepatocarcinoma.

Finally, and with respect to raloxifene, Grady et al. (2004), when analyzing the safety and adverse effects associated with raloxifene in the MORE study, noticed that this did not increase the risk for gallbladder disease.

13.4 Desmoids and Mesenteric Fibromatosis

Tonelli et al. (2003) studied the effects of 120 mg/d raloxifene on progressive desmoid tumors and mesenteric fibromatosis in 13 patients with familiar adenomatous polyposis, selected on the basis of intra-abdominal localization of the lesion, refractoriness to other medical treatments, and ER-alpha expression. The patients had a significant response to raloxifene therapy, with complete remission in 8 cases and partial response in 5 cases, evaluated by regression of symptoms and tumor size. Serum biochemical parameters did not show any significant changes, and side effects were never observed. These results support the efficacy of raloxifene on desmoid tumors and mesenteric fibromatosis contributing to a novel option in the pharmacological treatment of these neoplastic lesions.

13.5 Endocrine Functions

Most endocrine functions have already been commented on in previous chapters, so only the following will be mentioned here:

13.5.1 Insulin Sensitivity and Diabetes

Andersson et al. (2002) have shown in a randomized clinical trial that raloxifene does not affect insulin sensitivity or glycemic control in postmenopausal women with type-2 diabetes mellitus. It has favorable or neutral effects on selected surrogate markers of cardiovascular risk while decreasing hyperandrogenicity in these patients.

13.5.2 Thyroid Function

Estrogen may increase hepatic production of thyroxine-binding globulin (TBG) and decrease TBG clearance, thus increasing serum total thyroxine (tT_4) and, to a lesser extent, total triiodothyronine (tT_3). As a result, increased tT_4 and tT_3 are seen in states of excessive estrogen and/or progestin, such as pregnancy, HRT, and oral contraceptive usage. This phenomenon may cause problems in clinical diagnoses when tT_4 or tT_3 is used for these patients. Nevertheless, estrogen has been shown to increase thyroid-stimulating hormone (TSH) and to decrease free thyroxine (fT_4) through a mild inhibitory effect on the thyroid gland (Hsu et al. 2001). Compounds such as tamoxifen increase TSH without decreasing fT_4 (Zidan et al. 1999), but the effect of long-term raloxifene usage on TBG, T_3 uptake, tT_3, tT_4, fT_4, and TSH had not been well documented.

Therefore, Hsu et al. (2001) investigated whether raloxifene caused changes in serum concentrations of these markers comparing the effects of 1 year of treatment with either raloxifene or combined continuous estrogen and progesterone (CCEP) on the thyroid function test profiles, E2, and FSH. They studied 60 euthyroid postmenopausal women (age range 40–75 years) with relatively low bone mineral density. Fifty women received raloxifene (60 mg/d) before breakfast, and 10 women received combined conjugated equine estrogen (Premarin; 0.625 mg) and medroxyprogesterone acetate (Provera; 5 mg) daily. Fasting serum samples were collected for all participants at baseline and after 1 year of treatment. This study showed that the usual dosage of raloxifene administered for 1 year increased serum TBG. This increase in TBG is similar to the effects of CCEP and may then be associated with an increase in tT_4 and tT_3, whereas TSH and fT_4 were not significantly changed. The slight but insignificant decreases in fT_4 in both groups after 1 year of treatment were compatible with the findings that showed a mild suppression of thyroid function by tamoxifen and estrogen. The authors conclude that in patients treated with raloxifene, the results of tT_3 and tT_4 tests should be interpreted with caution because they could be falsely increased. Duntas et al. (2001), in another study on raloxifene and thyroid function, observed, however, that TBG levels and, consequently, thyroid function are not substantially affected by treatment with raloxifene.

13.6
Eye, Cataracts

Visual impairment and cataracts have been reported in patients undergoing long-term tamoxifen treatment (Gerner 1989). Similarly, it has been observed that tamoxifen and its derivatives are high-affinity blockers of specific chloride channels; this blockade appears to be independent of the interaction of tamoxifen with ERs and therefore reflects an alternative cellular target. But, since chloride channels in the lens of the eye were shown to be essential for maintaining normal lens hydration and transmittance, Zhang et al. (1994) studied organ culture and observed that these channels were blocked by tamoxifen, leading to lens opacity associated with cataracts at clinically relevant concentrations. The study suggested a molecular mechanism by which tamoxifen could cause cataract formation and, consequently, have implications for its clinical use. In a later paper, Zhang et al. (1995) suggested that ocular toxic side effects of antiestrogens would be minimized by use of the steroidal (ICI 182780) rather than nonsteroidal antiestrogens (tamoxifen).

Later, Gorin et al. (1998) estimated the prevalence of abnormalities in visual function and ocular structures associated with the long-term use of tamoxifen citrate in a sample of 303 women with breast cancer currently taking part in a randomized clinical trial to determine the efficacy of tamoxifen (20 mg/day) in preventing recurrences. There were no cases of vision-threatening ocular toxicity among the tamoxifen-treated participants, and, compared with non-treated participants, the tamoxifen-treated women had no differences in the activities of daily vision, visual acuity measurements, or other tests of visual function except for color screening. Nevertheless, intraretinal crystals and posterior subcapsular opacities were more frequent in the tamoxifen-treated group, leading the authors to conclude that women should have a thorough baseline ophthalmic evaluation within the first year of initiating tamoxifen therapy and receive appropriate followup evaluations.

Likewise, Paganini-Hill and Clark (2000) also studied 2653 women (but only information from 1297 women aged 57–75 years of age was analyzed) with primary breast cancer to evaluate the association of tamoxifen with cataracts and other eye problems. Women reporting treatment with tamoxifen were categorized as standard-term users (4–5 years), short-term users (< 4 years), or long-term users (6+ years) and compared to nonusers. The authors observed that standard-term and long-term users of tamoxifen reported developing cataracts more frequently than nonusers (18.2%, 21.4% vs. 14.8%). The relative risk was 1.40 (95% CI 0.94–2.10) for standard-term users and 1.70 (1.11–2.59) for long-term users. Yet tamoxifen was unrelated to frequency of glaucoma or macular degeneration or to Amsler grid test results. Thus this study suggested that five or more years of tamoxifen use increases risk of cataracts and that women choosing such therapy should be diligent about receiving regular ocular exams.

Bradbury et al. (2004), however, recently reanalyzed the relation between tamoxifen and cataracts and described it as "a null association," They used a nested, matched, case-control study design and data collected in the General Practice Research Database. They identified all women 30–79 years old who were diagnosed with breast cancer and treated with tamoxifen within 6 months, or with bladder cancer, colorectal cancer, or nonmelanoma skin cancer between January 1991 and December 1999. From this population they identified all newly diagnosed cases of cataract and matched four female controls to each case on age, index date, and study entry data. They assessed the risk of cataracts for current, past, and sometime users of tamoxifen and according to cumulative use of tamoxifen. The findings showed no increased risk for cataracts among breast cancer patients treated with tamoxifen (OR = 1, 0.7–1.4) compared to women with other cancers who were not prescribed tamoxifen, and there was no evidence of an increased risk with increasing cumulative dose. Consequently, the tamoxifen-cataract relationship is controversial, and the latest findings show an absence of evident relation.

In respect to other SERMs, Bishai et al. (1999) have communicated a case of intrauterine exposure to clomiphene (100 mg/d for approximately 4 weeks) and neonatal persistent hyperplastic primary vitreous. These same authors mention another described case in humans with congenital retinal aplasia.

Regarding raloxifene, no relation to ocular problems has been reported.

13.7 Other Effects

13.7.1 Arthritis

Creamer et al. (1994) reported cases of breast cancer where the use of tamoxifen was temporally related to the development of an inflammatory polyarthritis resembling rheumatoid arthritis. Cases of cyclical psoriatic arthritis, however, have positively responded to antiestrogen therapy (Stevens et al. 1993). Tsai and Liu (1992) have shown that tamoxifen concurrently injected with estradiol benzoate antagonizes the condrodestructive effects of estradiol at the early stage of knee osteoarthritis in rabbits.

13.7.2 Hemorheological Effects

Shand et al. (2002) have shown that, compared with placebo-treated subjects, long-term raloxifene treatment in postmenopausal women, at a dose of either 60 or 120 mg/d, was not associated with adverse changes in hemorheological factors (determinants of blood viscosity) that may contribute to venous thromboembolism.

13.7.3 Quality of Life (QoL)

The effect of raloxifene on QoL was investigated by Utian et al. (2004) in a prospective study using the Utian Quality of Life (UQoL) Scale in 74 women.

Although there were no treatment group differences, raloxifene was associated with an improvement from baseline in the occupational and health domains and in the overall score of the UQoL. The authors recommended more studies.

Palomba et al. (2004) have also studied the effects on cognigtion, mood, and QoL in 100 premenopausal women with symptomatic uterine leiomyomas treated with gonadotropin-releasing hormone agonist with or without raloxifene. The findings demonstrate that raloxifene is not able to prevent decreases in cognitive function and does not reduce the depresion and anxiety symptoms in women treated with GnRHa.

Finally, Fallowfield et al. (2004) analyzed the QoL of postmenopausal women in the Arimidex, Tamoxifen, Alone or in Combination (ATAC) Adjuvant Breast Cancer Trial. There were no differences among groups. Two years of treatment with these products had a similar overall QoL impact, showing gradual improvement over time.

References

1. Affinito P, Palomba S, Sorrentino C, Di Carlo C, Bifulco G, Arienzo MP, et al. (1999) Effects of postmenopausal hypoestrogenism on skin collagen. Maturitas 33:239–247
2. Agnusdei D (1999) Clinical efficacy of raloxifene in postmenopausal women. Eur J Obstet Gynecol Reprod Biol 85:43–46
3. Aldrighi JM, Quail DC, Levy-Frebault J, Aguas F, Kosian K, Carrido L, et al. (2004) Predictors of hot flushes in postmenopausal women who receive raloxifene therapy. Am J Obstet Gynecol 191:1979–1988
4. Alvaro D, Alpini G, Onori P, Perego L, Svegliata Baroni G, Franchitto A, et al. (2000) Estrogens stimulate proliferation of intrahepatic biliary epithelium in rats. Gastroenterology 119:1681–1691
5. Andersson B, Johannsson G, Holm G, Bengtsson BA, Sashegyi A, Pavo I, Mason T, Anderson PW (2002) Raloxifene does not affect insulin sensitivity or glycemic control in postmenopausal women with type 2 diabetes mellitus: a randomized clinical trial. J Clin Endocrinol Metab 87:122–128
6. Bergman A, Karram M, Bahatia N (1990) Changes in urethral cytology following estrogen administration. Gynecol Obstet Invest 29:211–213
7. Bernardi F, Pluchino N, Stomati M, Pieri M, Genazzani AR (2003) CNS: sex steroids and SERMSs. Ann NY Acad Sci 997:378–88
8. Bishai R, Arbour L, Lyons C, Koren G (1999) Intrauterine exposure to clomiphene and neonatal persistent hyperplastic primary vitreous. Teratology 60:143–145
9. Bradbury BD, Lash TL, Kaye JA, Jick SS (2004) Tamoxifen and cataracts: a null association. Breast Cancer Res Treat 87:189–196
10. Casper RF, McPherson R, Ste-Marie LG (1998) The Canadian Consensus Conference on menopause and osteoporosis. J Soc Obstet Gynaecol Can 20:1243–1272
11. Cohen FJ, Watts S, Shah A, Akers R, Plouffe L (2000) Uterine effects of three-year raloxifene therapy in postmenopausal women under age 60. Obstet Gynecol 95:104–110
12. Creamer P, Lim K, George E, Dieppe P (1994) Acute inflammatory polyarthritis in association with tamoxifen. Br J Rheumatol 33:998

13. Davies GC, Huster WJ, Lu Y, Plouffe L, Lakshmanan M (1999) Adverse events reported by postmenopausal women in controlled trials withs raloxifene. Obstet Gynecol 93:558–565
14. Duntas LH, Mantzou E, Koutras DA (2001) Lack of substantial effects of raloxifene on thyroxine-binding globulin in postmenopausal women: dependency on thyroid status. Thyroid 11:779–782
15. Eberling JL, Wu C, Tong-Turnbeaugh R, Jagust WJ (2004) Estrogen- and tamoxifen-associated effects on brain structure and function. NeuroImage 21:364–371
16. Fallowfield L, Cella D, Cuzick J, Francis S, Locker G, Howell A (2004) Quality of life of postmenopausal women in the Arimidex, Tamoxifen, Alone or in Combination (ATAC) Adjuvant Breast Cancer Trial. J Clin Oncol 22:4261–4271
17. Gerard B, Bleiberg H (2004) Treatment of hepatocarcinoma. Curr Oncol Rep 6:184–191
18. Gerner EW (1989) Ocular toxicity of tamoxifen. Ann Ophthalmol 21:420–423
19. Goldstein SR (2002) An update on non-uterine gynaecological effects on raloxifene. Eur J Cancer 38(Suppl 6):S65–S66
20. Goldstein SR, Nanavati N (2002) Adverse events that are associated with the selective estrogen receptor modulator levormeloxifene in an aborted phase III osteoporosis treatment study. Am J Obstet Gynecol 187:521–527
21. Goldstein SR, Scheele WH, Rajagopalan SK, Wilkie JL, Walsh BW, Parsons AK (2000) A 12-month comparative study of raloxifene, estrogen, and placebo on the post-menopausal endometrium. Obstet Gynecol 95:95–103
22. Goldstein SR, Neven P, Zhour L, Taylor YL, Ciaccia AV, Plouffe L Jr (2001) Raloxifene effects on frequency of surgery for pelvic floor relaxation. Obstet Gynecol 98:91–96
23. Gorin MB, Day R, Costantino JP, Fisher B, Redmond CK, Wickerham L, et al. (1998) Long-term tamoxifen citrate use and potential ocular toxicity. Am J Ophthalmol 126:338
24. Grady D, Brown JS, Vittinghoff E, Applegate W, Varner E, Snyder T (2001) Post-menopausal hormones and incontinence: the heart and estrogen/progestin replacement study. Obstet Gynecol 97:116–120
25. Grady D, Ettinger B, Moscarelli E, Plouffe L Jr, Sarkar S, Ciaccia A, Cummings S, Multiple Outcomes of Raloxifene Evaluation Investigators (2004) Safety and adverse effects associated with raloxifene: multiple outcome of raloxifene evaluation. Obstet Gynecol 104:837–844
26. Haskell SG, Richardson E (2004) The effect of raloxifene on cognitive function in postmenopausal women: a randomized clinical trial. Conn Med 68:355–358
27. Hendrix LS, McNeeley SG (2001) Effect of selective estrogen receptor modulators on reproductive tissues other than endometrium. Ann NY Acad Sci 949:243–250
28. Hsu S, Cheng WCh, Jang MW, Tsai KS (2001) Effects of long-term use of raloxifene, a selective estrogen receptor modulator, on thyroid function test profiles. Clin Chem 47:1865–1867
29. Jenkins V, Shilling V, Fallowfield L, Howell A, Hutton S (2004) Does hormone therapy for the treatment of breast cancer have a detrimental effect on memory and cognition? A pil study. Psychooncology 13:61–66
30. Lacreuse A, Wilson ME, Herndon JG (2002) Estradiol, but not raloxifene, improves aspects of spatial working memory in aged ovariectomized rhesus monkeys. Neurobiol Ag 23:589–600
31. Martino S, Cauley JA, Barrtt-Connor E, Powles TJ, Mershon J, Disch D, et al. (2004) Continuing outcomes relevant to Evista: Breast cancer incidence in postemenopausal osteoporotic women in a randomized trial of raloxifene. J Natl Cancer Inst 96:1751–1761
32. Miller CP (2002) SERMSs: evolutionary chemistry, revolutionary biology. Curr Pharm Des 8:2089–2111

33. Modugno F, Ness RB, Exing S, Cauley JA (2003) Effect of raloxifene on sexual function in older postmenopausal women with osteoporosis. Obstet Gynecol 101:353–361
34. Morales L, Neven P, Timmerman D, Christiaens MR, Vergote I, Van Limbergen E, et al. (2004) Acute effects of tamoxifen and third-generation aromatase inhibitors on menopausal symptoms of breast cancer patients. Anticancer Drugs 15:753–760
35. Mourits MJ, Bockermann I, de Vries EG, van der Zee AG, ten Hoor KA, van der Graaf WT, Sluiter WJ, Willemse PH (2002) Tamoxifen effects on subjective and psychosexual well-being, in a randomised breast cancer study comparing high-dose and standard-dose chemotherapy. Br J Cancer 86:1546–1550
36. Muchmore DB (2000) Raloxifene: a selective estrogen receptor modulator (SERM) with multiple target system effects. Oncologist 5:388–392
37. Natale V, Albertazzi P, Missiroli N, Pedrini D, Salgarello M (2004) Effects of raloxifene on mood, sleep, libido and cognitive function in postmenopausal healthy women: a pilot study. Maturitas 48:59–63
38. Neele SJM, Evertz R, Genazzani AR, Luisi M, Netelenbos C (2002) Raloxifene treatment increases plasma levels of β-endorphin in postmenopausal women: a randomized, placebo-controlled study. Fertil Steril 77:1110–1117
39. Nickelsen T, Lufkin EG, Riggs BL, Cox DA, Crook TH (1999) Raloxifene hydrochloride, a selective estrogen receptor modulator: safety assessment of effects on cognitive function and mood in postmenopausal women. Psychoneuroendocrinology 24:115–128
40. Nowak A, Findlay M, Culjak G, Stockler M (2004) Tamoxifen for hepatocellular carcinoma. Cochrane Database Syst Rev 3:CD001024
41. Paganini-Hill A, Clark LJ (2000) Eye problems in breast cáncer patients treated with tamoxifen. Breast Cancer Res Treat 60:167–172
42. Palomba S, Orio F Jr, Russo T, Falbo A, Amati A, Zullo F (2004) Gonadotropin-releasing hormone agonist with or without raloxifene effects on cognition, mood, and quality of life. Fertil Steril 82:480–482
43. Reddy A, Prince M, James OF, Jain S, Bassendine MF (2004) Tamoxifen: a novel treatment for primary biliary cirrhosis? Liver Int 24:194–197
44. Rekers H, Drogendijk AC, Valkenburg HA, Riphagen F (1992) The menopause, urinary incontinence and other symptoms of the genito-urinary tract. Maturitas 15:101–111
45. Robinson D, Cardozo LD (2003) The role of estrogens in female lower urinary tract dysfunction. Urology 62:45–51
46. Rutanen EM, Heikkinen J, Halonen K, Komi J, Lammintausta R, Ylikorkala O (2003) Effects of ospemifene, a novel SERM, on hormones, genital tract, climacteric symptoms, and quality of life in postmenopausal women: a double-blind, randomized trial. Menopause 10:433–439
47. Shand B, Gilchrist N, Blackwell T, March R (2002) The hemorheological effects of raloxifene in postmenopausal women with osteoporosis. Results of a 3-year placebo-controlled clinical trial. Clin Hemorheol Microcir 26:249–255
48. Sherwin BB (2002) Estrogen and cognitive aging in women. Trends Pharmacol Sci 23:527–534
49. Shilling V, Jenkins V, Fallowfield L, Howell A (2001) The effects of oestrogens and anti-oestrogens on cognition. Breast 10:484–491
50. Shively CA, Bethea CL (2004) Cognition, mood disorders, and sex hormones. ILAR J 45:189–199
51. Shumaker SA, Legault C, Rapp SR, Thal L, Wallace RB, Ockene JK, et al. and WHIMS Investigators (2003) Estrogen plus progestin and the incidence of dementia and mild cognitive impairment in postmenopausal women: the Women's Health Initiative Memory Study: a randomized controlled trial. J Am Med Assoc 289:2651–2662

52. Stevens HP, Ostlere LS, Black CM, Jacobs HS, Rustin MH (1993) Cyclical psoriatic arthritis responding to anti-oestrogen therapy. Br J Dermatol 129:458–460
53. Tonelli F, Ficari F, Valanzano R, Brandi ML (2003) Treatment of desmoids and mesenteric fibromatosis in familial adenomatous polyposis with raloxifene. Tumore 89:391–396
54. Tsai CL, Liu TK (1992) Inhibition of estradiol-induced early osteoarthritic changes by tamoxifen. Life Sci 50:1943–1951
55. Utian WH, Janata JW, Barbier S, Rosen AS, Mayer MH, Taylor MB (2004) Effect of raloxifene on quality of life: a prospective study using the Utian Quality of Life (UQOL) scale. Menopause 11:275–280
56. Vickers SM, Jhala NC, Ahn EY, McDonald JM, Pan G, Bland KI (2002) Tamoxifen (TMX)/Fas induced growth inhibition of human cholangiocarcinoma (HCC) by gamma interferon (IFN-gamma). Ann Surg 235:872–878
57. Yaffe K, Krueger K, Sarkar S, Grady D, Barrett-Connor E, Cox DA, Nickelsen T, Multiple Outcomes of Raloxifene Evaluation Investigators (2001) Cognitive function in postmenopausal women treated with raloxifene. N Engl J Med 344:1207–1213
58. Zec RF, Trivedi MA (2002) The effects of estrogen replacement therapy on neuropsychological functioning in postmenopausal women with and without dementia: a critical and theoretical review. Neuropsychol Rev 12:65–109
59. Zhang JJ, Jacob TJ, Valverde MA, Hardy SP, Mintening GM, Supúlveda FV, et al. (1994) Tamoxifen blocks chloride channels: a possible mechanism for cataract formation. J Clin Invest 94:1690–1697
60. Zhang JJ, Jacob TJ, Hardy SP, Higgins CF, Valverde MA (1995) Lens opacification by antioestrogens: tamoxifen vs ICI 182,780. Br J Pharmacol 115:1347–1348
61. Zidan J, Rubenstein W (1999) Effect of adjuvant tamoxifen therapy on thyroid function in postmenopausal women with breast cancer. Oncology 56:43–45

CHAPTER 14

The Role of SERMs in the Management of Postmenopausal Women

JOAQUIM CALAF I ALSINA

14.1 Introduction

Menopause is biological evidence of aging in women. The absence of menstruation is clinical evidence of the inability of individual females to reproduce. However, what seems to be bad news is in fact proof that individual women can protect themselves. The reproductive process in the female is a very demanding one, and, consequently, nature has provided a mechanism to interrupt reproductive activity when biologic structures giving support to pregnancy enter the aging process. Conversely, in the male, whose participation in reproduction is limited both in time and resources, such a limitative mechanism does not exist.

The interruption of menstrual activity is the consequence of the exhaustion of the follicular pool in the ovary. Thus follicular development and ovulation no longer occur, and, as a consequence, the theca-granulosa system as a functional unit secreting estrogens disappears. This leads to a progressive decrease in the circulating concentration of estrogens. Detectable levels after menopausal ovarian failure are the consequence of peripheral aromatization of androgenic precursors. Consequently, the degree of estrogen priming differs among individuals according to the importance of their androgenic metabolite secretion by the hiliar ovarian cells and/or the adrenal gland cells as well as the amount of aromatizing tissue, especially skin and fat, they have.

Estrogens are the most significant messengers in the coordination of the body's adaptive changes necessary to establish and maintain pregnancy. Thus, in women the majority of tissue systems are endowed with either or both of the presently identified estrogen receptors, alfa and beta. As a consequence, the resetting of the estrogenic control established after menopause leads to changes in tissue status, resulting in some cases in a higher risk for disease, either local or systemic.

All these estrogen-dependent changes coincide in time with the biological process of aging taking place irrespective of gender. A common tendency among gynecologists has been to attribute the majority of problems occurring after menopause to the absence of estrogens. This is as fallacious as ignoring the importance of estrogen deprivation in the onset and development of several female health problems. Thus any postmenopausal woman's healthcare provider must be mindful of the consequences of both aging and hypoestrogenemia.

The evident biological changes related to menopause elicit a feeling of vulnerability in women that makes them more receptive to measures aimed at detecting or preventing risk situations and, consequently, improving health status and life expectancy. This opens an "opportunity window" that must be used to enhance the introduction of a new lifestyle and reinforce the acceptance of pharmacological preventive measures when needed.

Counseling postmenopausal women entails the identification of individual threats and risks and the implementation of behavioral or pharmacological measures. In this paper we try to describe an analytical system for handling this process efficiently.

14.2 Identifying Troubles and Threats

For the clinician, the individual patient remains more important than the general framework. In the process of counseling postmenopausal women, an individual evaluation is mandatory. It is not unusual for some of the risk factors relevant for one disease to also have an impact on the incidence of other pathological processes. Frequently these changes are mediated by modifications in the synthesis, metabolization, or substitution of estrogen precursors or metabolites. This is clearly the case for obesity, diet, or smoking, where the production of precusor metabolites, their peripheral aromatization, and bioavailability through their binding to sex hormone binding globulin determines the final estrogenic priming. This situation leads to an increased risk of events as a result of the toxic and metabolic effects of some behavioral circumstances like smoking or sedentarism.

A thorough clinical evaluation with a systematic anamnesis and physical examination including body weight, height, waist/hip ratio, and blood pressure should precede any lab tests or instrumental examinations. In the process of detecting the "weak points" of a given woman, the application of specific risk scores can be of interest.

14.2.1 Cardiovascular Risk

Frequency and impact on mortality should be the major determinants when establishing priorities. Thus cardiovascular disease (CVD) must come first. Even if very irregular in its impact from country to country, CVD remains the leading killer of women in Europe, as is the case in most developed countries.

Different classification systems are available to estimate the individual risk of presenting a cardiovascular event in the next 10 years. One of the most frequently used is the Framingham score risk, for which there is also software available online (Third Report of the National Cholesterol Education Program 2002), but recently several organizations involved in cardiovascular care have produced guidelines to identify and manage these risk situations (Mosca 2004).

14.2.2 Menopausal Syndrome

Immediately after menopause vasomotor symptoms are the most relevant issues directely related to estrogen decrease. Frequently they appear in the year preceding the last menstrual period and as a consequence of the hormonal changes characterizing perimenopause. Hot flushes do not affect all postmenopausal women, and among those presenting the symptom the severity varies from severe to very light (Oldenhave et al. 1993; Dennerstein et al. 2002) (Fig. 14.1). The menopausal syndrome is closely related to estrogen deficiency and together with hot flushes includes changes in sleep quality, concentration and mood, and genitourinary complaints. There is no individual correlation between the presence and severity of some of the most representative symptoms (i.e., hot flushes) and circulating estradiol levels. Thus, being asymptomatic does not necessarily imply having a better estrogen priming; on the contrary, some women apparently able to produce a considerable amount of endogenous estrogens, as deduced from cervical mucus characteristics or endometrial thickness, complain of intense hot flushes.

If we consider the periods characterized by the higher prevalence of particular symptoms or threats as "opportunity windows" for specific treatments,

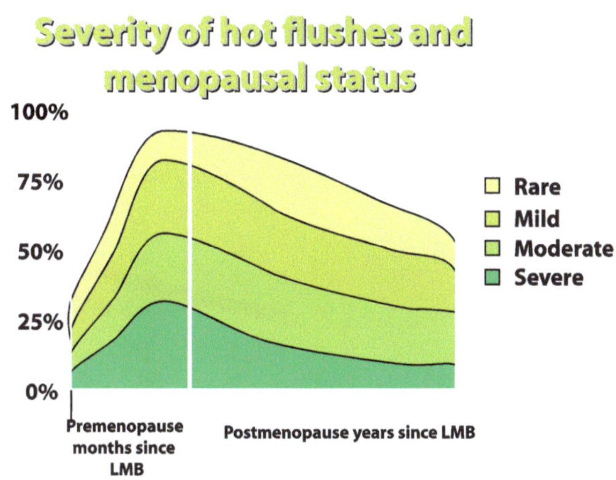

Fig. 14.1. Incidence of hot flushes immediately before, during, and after menopause stratified according to severity (redrawn from Oldenhave et al. 1993)

the period preceding and immediately following the last menstrual period can be identified as "the symptomatic window". The duration of this symptomatic period also has a very high interindividual variation, and even if the median is around 30 months after menopause, some women experience hot flushes well beyond their sixties. Vaginal dryness, if not treated, increases in incidence and severity over time, and vaginal tissue changes have their clinical expression in discomfort and pain during intercourse but also in urinary frequency and nocturia.

14.2.3 Osteoporosis

The individual ability to produce estrogens becomes more relevant when analyzing estrogen-dependent diseases like osteoporosis and breast cancer. The incidence of breast cancer and fracture are inversely related. Cauley's data also illustrate this negative correlation (Cauley et al. 1996).

Osteoporosis, the second most important threat to postmenopausal women, cannot be restricted to a "have or have not" condition. Bone health must rather be perceived as a continuum from normal bone to clinical fracture through osteopenia, osteoporosis, and subclinical fracture. Bone loss is the consequence of an increase in bone turnover, which is regulated by estrogens. Hypoestro-

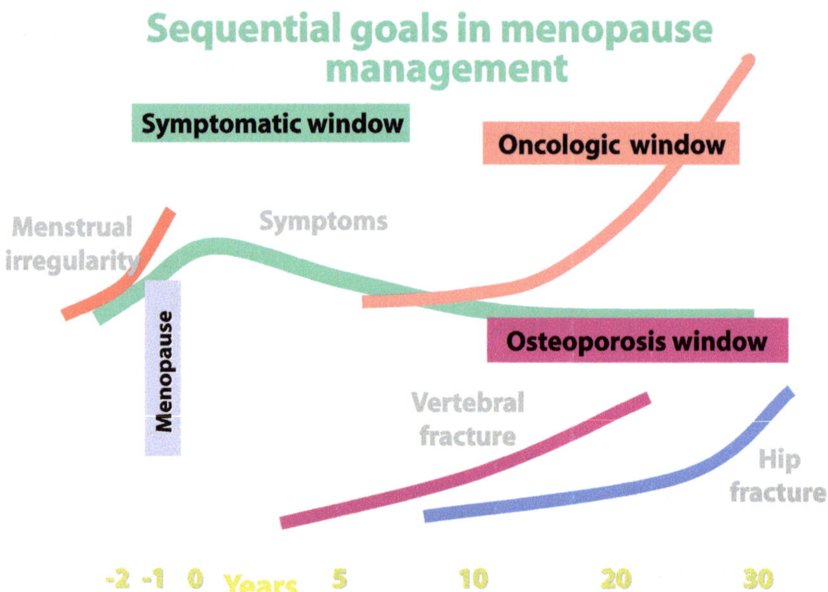

Fig. 14.2. Progressive appearance of clinical and subclinical consequences of hypoestrogenism and aging open different "opportunity windows" for intervention

genism favors uncoupled bone remodeling and, consequently, a decrease in bone density and quality. Clinical fractures are associated with a sevenfold increase in death risk (Cauley et al. 2000). Diagnosing fracture risk is difficult, and both risk scores and early densitometric screening by themselves have poor predictive values. Continuous evaluation, combining both tools, is probably the most efficient approach. The International Osteoporosis Foundation risk evaluation score can be used to determine early prescription of DEXA evaluation (International Osteoporosis Foundation online).

Vertebral and hip fractures have a different chronological incidence. Vertebral fractures begin to increase significantly after 65 years of age, whereas hip fracture incidence increases only 10 years later (U.S. Preventive Task Force 2002). This explains why the different studies with substances aimed at preventing fractures have been focused on populations of different age segments depending on the main outcome being measured. Studies showing an ability to prevent vertebral fracture have included populations in or near their sixties, whereas those focused on hip fracture prevention included patients at least 80 years old. For this reason we can consider that, starting at around age 60, we can open the “osteoporotic window” and that this window will remain open in the future (Fig. 14.2).

14.2.4 Breast Cancer

Postmenopausal breast cancer is, in the majority of cases, estrogen receptor positive (ER+) and, consequently, an estrogen-dependent disease. Estrogen circulating concentrations and lifetime exposure to estrogens are the most predictive risk factors for ER+ breast cancer (Cauley et al 1999). Gail’s score is the criterion used in the United States to indicate the use of tamoxifen to reduce breast cancer incidence. However, its external validity, and thus applicability in European countries with different breast cancer incidences, remains to be elucidated. Gail’s model, based on age, duration of reproductive life, family history, and the number of previous breast biopsies, is the most commonly used tool to estimate 5-year predicted risk (Gail et al. 1989). Scores of 1.67% or higher are considered to reflect high risk. As stated earlier, women with osteoporosis are considered to be at lower risk for breast cancer; this was also observed in an analysis of breast cancer incidence in the placebo group of the MORE study (Cauley et al. 2001). However, this was not the case for the women enrolled in CORE, a study designed to evaluate the efficacy of an additional 4 years of therapy in preventing invasive breast cancer in women who participated in the MORE trial (Martino et al. 2004; Delmas et al. 2005). Baseline risk estimation based on Gail’s method was 1.94%, and consequently these osteoporotic women should have been considered to be at high risk. In fact, the breast cancer incidence in the placebo group was 5.4 cases per 1000 women years, slightly higher than the 4.4 reported for the age group by the American National Cancer Institute (Kikuchi et al. 1997). Since age is a relevant component of Gail's score and being osteoporotic does not imply a lower risk of presenting breast cancer, we can also open, shortly after menopause, an "oncologic window" where the risk of having a breast cancer detected will increase with each passing year.

14.3 Intervention Tools

14.3.1 Lifestyle Optimization

The first step in establishing preventive interventions should be the implementation of adequate measures to correct any significant detected changes in lifestyle. The lifestyle changes with the greatest impact on health are cessation/avoidance of cigarette smoking, regular physical activity, a healthy diet low in inappropiate fats and high in calcium, and weight reduction or maintenance. Women can expect to live a third of their life after menopause. As stated above, the perimenopausal period, as any critical period in life, increases one's willingness to initiate an improvement process to increase one's health status and avoid disease. The task of the health counsellor is to take advantage of this susceptible status to positively modify lifestyle. Personalized recommendations must be at the frontline of health and life expectancy improvement measures; without such recommendations any pharmacological intervention will be less effective.

14.3.2 Hormone Therapy

Hormone therapy has proven highly effective in controlling the menopausal syndrome, especially severe hot flushes (MacLennan et al. 2004), even at doses significantly lower than those used until now (Speroff et al. 2000; Utian et al. 2001). Women's Health Initiative studies found that hormone replacement therapy, when administered as a primary prevention intervention for CVD in older women, increases the risk of heart disease and breast cancer. Even if a protective effect on fracture and colon cancer was observed, the risk-benefit ratio led to a recommendation of this treatment only for the short-term relief of menopausal symptoms (Rossouw et al. 2002; Anderson et al. 2004). The role of early administration of ovarian hormones to young postmenopausal women in the prevention of cardiovascular disease or late dementia remains to be elucidated. However, a protective effect on bone and, eventually, on lipid profile cannot be ruled out when these treatments are administered to symptomatic women.

14.3.3
Cardioprotective Treatments

Pharmacological measures to reduce CV risk are based on the identification and treatment of vulnerable risk factors. Among them hypertension, abnormal lipid profile, and hypercoagulant situations are at the origin of the majority of coronary events and stroke. Statins, thiazides, angiotensin-converting enzyme inhibitors, beta blockers, aspirin, and warfarin have independently shown their ability to prevent CV events (Mosca et al. 2004). Whether the prescription and control of these treatments is the task of the general practitioner or the gynecologist will depend on the organization of the health system in each country.

14.3.4
Bone Resorption Inhibitors

Prevention of osteoporosis and fracture can be achieved through limiting the resorption-remodeling process. Four main families of products can be effective in controlling bone resorption: estrogens, SERMs, bisphosphonates, and calcitonin. Large, prospective randomized trials have proven the effectiveness

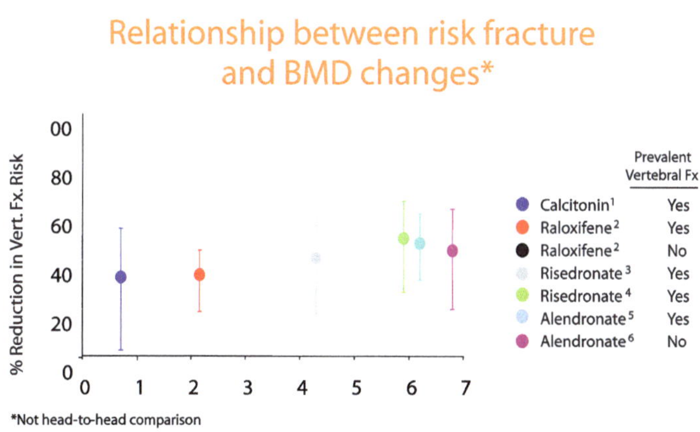

Fig. 14.3. The different anti resorptive substances have different effects on densitometric bone mineral density but similar impact on vertebral fracture incidence based on [1]Chesnut et al. 2000; [2]Ettinger et al. 1999; [3]Harris et al. 1999; [4]Reginster et al. 2000; [5]Black et al. 2000; [6]Cummings et al. 1998

of all four families in preventing vertebral fracture (Rossow et al. 2002; Anderson et al. 2004; Cummings et al. 1998; Ettinger et al. 1999; Harris et al. 1999). Only the studies on alendronate and risedronate showed their effectiveness in hip fracture prevention (Black et al. 2000; McClung et al. 2001). Although the effect of all these antiresorptives on bone mineral density (BMD) varies, their impact on vertebral fracture is similar. Given that reduced BMD increases the risk for fracture, the inference that an increase in BMD would be significantly associated with a vertebral fracture risk reduction has not been proven. Only a small proportion of risk reduction in fractures is explained by the increase in BMD (Delmas and Seeman 2004). As a consequence, the choice between the different antiresorptive alternatives must be established on the basis of their side effects and extrasqueletal benefits (Fig. 14.3).

14.3.5 Breast Cancer Risk

Any intervention diminishing the access of estrogens, either in time or in concentration, to the estrogen receptor in breast tissue can be expected to lower the future risk of presenting a breast cancer. Lifestyle interventions should include smoking cessation, weight reduction, and alcohol restriction (Manier et al. 2004). Hormonal treatment should be restricted to symptomatic women and at the lowest effective dose for the minimal necessary time. A large-scale prospective trial showed that in the United States breast cancer prevention could be achieved, in high-risk women, with the administration of tamoxifen for not more than 5 years (Fisher et al. 1998). Prospective studies conducted in Europe did not yield the same results, probably as a consequence of differences in population selection or study design (Cuzick et al. 2003). The efficiency of raloxifene as a breast cancer preventive tool is under evaluation in a "face-to-face" study with tamoxifen (Wickerman 2003). Ongoing studies will provide information on the value of aromatase inhibitors in the prevention of breast cancer in high-risk postmenopausal women (Cuzick 2003).

14.4 Adressing Health Expectancy Improvement

14.4.1 Poly Approach and Multitasking

Diseases are frequently multifactorial, especially those involved in the aging process. Also, the aging process itself is not the consequence of a single disease but rather of progressive impairment in multiple organs or systems. Thus a disease must frequently be approached with the simultaneous administration of several drugs and measures, and to maintain well-being we must address more than one threat. These are the basis of the "poly approach" concept and help elucidate the search for "multitasking" products.

Lifestyle interventions share the concepts of poly approach and multitasking, targeting a multifactorial disease through different pathways and with an intervention having an impact on the outcome of more than one disease. A clear example of this is physical activity. It has been shown effective in decreasing cardiovascular risk, improving bone health, and decreasing breast cancer risk (i.e., multitasking) but at the same time is only one of the lifestyle interventions necessary to improve cardiovascular prognosis together with smoking, diet, or weight control (i.e., poly approach). Also, it has been suggested that diet can dramatically change cardiovascular risk (Franco et al. 2004). This explains why counseling about the implementation of adequate lifestyle measures must be the first step in any planned intervention for life expectancy in health improvement.

14.4.2 Pharmacological Poly Approach

Cardiovascular adverse events are prominent examples of a disease that occurs as the consequence of simultaneous multiple dysfunctions (hypertension, dyslipemia, clotting disturbances, etc.). Patients at high cardiovascular risk frequently receive an ACE inhibitor, a statin, and aspirin to normalize the parameters epidemiologically related to cardiovascular events as a primary or secondary preventive measure. This has engendered the idea of improving compliance by pooling inside a single capsule up to six substances (statin, aspirin, folic acid, tiazide, ACE inhibitor, and beta blocker) in what has been known as the "poly pill". A mathematical calculation has allowed researchers to attribute to such intervention the ability to reduce cardiovascular disease by more than 80% (Wald and Law 2003) (Fig. 14.4).

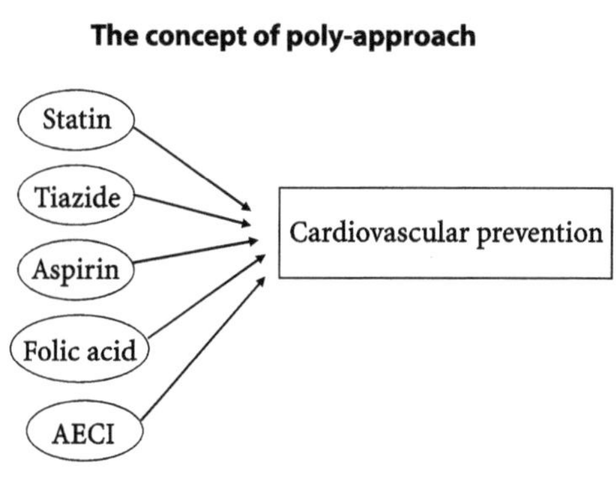

Fig. 14.4. Concept of poly approach: several products are administered simultaneously to cover different aspects of the etiology of a given disease

The probability that such an approach will reach clinical application is low. There are examples of previous attempts to similar nonselective interventions, long-term aspirin being perhaps the most significant, that have both advantages and inconveniences, the latter being especially relevant in the low-risk subgroups (Collaborative Group of Primary Prevention Project 2001). General opinion favors the idea of a wise selection of an individualized choice of drugs and measures to cover the needs of a given woman (Mulrow and Kussmaul 2005).

14.4.3 Multitasking Drugs

The idea of concentrating more than one outcome in a single therapeutic approach opens the door to the concept of multitasking substances. Several body organs and systems share regulating mechanisms. Thus, the ability to influence the very early steps of these biological processes can lead to multiple and different consequences, either positive or negative, for the administration of a drug. The identification of these "multitasking" substances will mean a clear improvement in the efficiency of preventive interventions.

Recent evidences show that substances conventionally used in cardiovascular prevention or treatment also influence all causes of mortality (Hippisley-Cox and Coupland 2005). Statins have shown a potential protective effect on both osteoporosis (Renjmark et al. 2004) and breast cancer (Cauley et al. 2003; Brower 2003; Mueck et al. 2003), even if the results are not always reproduced (LaCroix et al. 2003) (Fig. 14.5). Also, aspirin is expected to have a positive influence on breast cancer risk (Garcia-Rodriguez and Gonzalez-Perez 2004; Tait 2004) and is currently being included in prospective breast cancer prevention trials together with aromatase inhibitors (Cuzick 2005). Consequently we are facing a new scenario where, with the same efficacy for the main outcome, the effects of multitasking drugs will be preferred to those showing only monotasking effects (Calabro and Yeh 2004).

Estrogens are genuine, naturally engineered multitasking substances aimed at adapting the female body to the changes necessary to cover needs related to becoming pregnant and maintaining health during pregnancy. Administered after menopause they have a proven multitasking activity (bone, colon, breast, etc.), even if negative consequences outweigh the benefits in the populations studied. These evidences help to explain a very complex and comprehensive regulating system based on the practically universal distribution of estrogen receptors. The ability to selectively modify estrogen action at the level of different organs could change the global index by avoiding estrogen stimulation where undesirable and mimicking estrogen action where suitable.

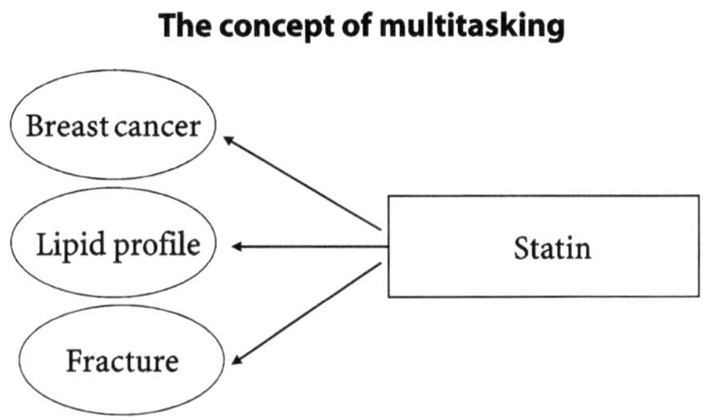

Fig. 14.5. Concept of multitasking: a single molecule influences evolution of different diseases through modulation of common pathway or information system

This profile fits perfectely the SERM concept. By designing molecules that exert specific effects on different organs and fine-tuning those molecules to a given woman's advantage, we would be able to influence health and survival expectancies.

Much progress has been made in this field over the last four decades (Chlebowski 2000). Tamoxifen is a substance able to block estrogen binding to estrogen receptors and, at the same time, itself induce protective effects on the breast and bone. It has, however, a negative estrogenic effect on thrombotic risk or endometrium cancer or by inducing hot flushes. It is now a first choice in preventive or adjuvant treatments in both pre- and postmenopausal women pending a final evaluation of the promising role of aromatase inhibitors.

Raloxifene represents a further step in the development of multitasking agents. The results obtained in large prospective studies have demonstrated a clear positive effect on bone density and prevention of vertebral fracture without any evidence of endometrial stimulation or cancer. A long-term study evaluating the effects of this substance on breast cancer risk among osteoporotic women has shown a sustained protective effect over 8 years of exposure (Martino et al. 2004), and a subanalysis of the MORE study has shown a significantly protective effect in a subgroup of high-cardiovascular-risk osteoporotic women (Barret-Connor et al. 2002). However, the ability to induce the appearance of hot flushes in recent postmenopausal women and the increase in the relative risk of venous thrombotic events remain negative aspects of this SERM.

New substances of this family are in development, and we cannot exclude the possibility that oriented modifications of the molecules of SERMs, statins, or prostaglandin inhibitors will be able to enhance their effect on the breast or bone, maintaining equivalent power in their genuine indication. Knowing that a perfect "multitasking" molecule is unlikely, we can expect to obtain the maximal benefit from a single pharmacological intervention with substances with relevant added positive effects.

14.5
Dynamic Decision-Making Diagram

Counseling a postmenopausal woman about improving her health and survival expectancies is a challenging task. Figure 14.6 represents a proposal for a decision-helping diagram. The main square framed by the two axes represents a given postmenopausal population from 50 to 80 years old. Fifty years is considered the average menopausal age, and the line before zero represents premenopause (note that on the abscissas the intervals are not in the same scale). On the ordinates the percentage of estimated women who might benefit from a given intervention is represented.

Healthy lifestyle is mandatory for all postmenopausal women together with adequate correction of detected risk factors. That is why this intervention is in the center of the diagram and concerns 100% of the women in this period. Then a decision must be made as to whether the woman's risk profile calls for any intervention beyond lifestyle improvement. The use of surrogate markers or risk scores can be useful in evaluating individual patients.

Local treatment should be offered to all women, especially those not receiving hormone treatment. Urogenital atrophy and vaginal dryness is frequent, but women have difficulties in expressing these symptoms, which is why the clinician should address this issue systematically.

For cardiovascular risk detecting and correcting factors like hypertension, obesity, insulin resistance, and type 2 diabetes or abnormal lipid profile, according to preestablished guidelines, can dramatically diminish the number of events.

During the symptomatic window, beginning even before menopause, hormonal treatment remains the best alternative, administered at the adequate

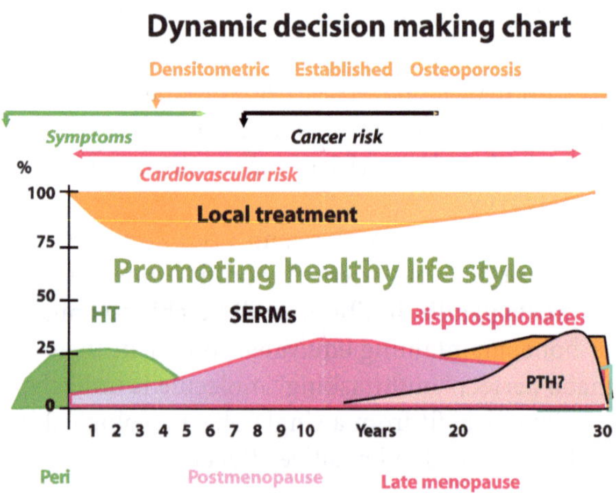

Fig. 14.6. Dynamic decision-making diagram to position different alternatives in management of postmenopausal women (see text)

dose and for the necessary period of time. We must remember that WHI showed a significant increase in breast cancer risk only after 5 years of exposure in older women and at higher doses than those usually necessary to control symptoms. Also, hormonal treatment is not contraindicated in severely symptomatic women with cardiovascular risk as long as an adequate cotreatment for this condition is administered. The hormonal treatment should be progressively withdrawn when approaching 5 years of exposure.

Regarding osteoporosis, the risk can change according to age, health status, and basal bone density or previous fracture detected. The alternatives for osteoporosis prevention and treatment can be divided according to their mechanism of action: those acting exclusively at the bone level, like bisphosphonates, strontium ranelate, or parathormone, or those modulating the normal bone remodeling regulatory system, closely related to estrogen priming, i.e., estrogens, SERMs, or calcitonin.

Women with osteoporosis, either densitometric or established, and some cases of osteopenia with increased fracture risk require pharmacological intervention. Any intervention for osteoporosis is expected to be long lasting. Thus it is difficult to expect that interventions in young postmenopausal women could be maintained for the remainder of one's life. The susceptibility to side effects changes either with the process of aging or the repeated use of a given product. Sequential treatment schedules, adapted to the risk profile of each period, would probably be more suitable.

In the early to mid postmenopausal period, either after estrogen treatment or in asymptomatic women, SERMs, and specifically raloxifene, appear to be the best alternative. They are well tolerated, have shown efficacy on the kinds of vertebral fractures, that appear more frequently in this period, and act through the natural mechanism of the bone remodeling process, i.e., the estrogen receptor. The probability of inducing hot flushes decreases with time following menopause and makes the onset of this undesired side effect a rare event (Fig. 14.7). As an added value they have proven to decrease the risk of ER+ breast cancer. If ongoing studies prove a positive effect on cardiovascular risk, they will have the attributes of a true multitasking agent for this period (Wickerham 2003). Putting benefits and risks together results in a very positive risk-benefit ratio (Mullins 2003).

As aging progresses the risk of thromboembolism increases, as does the incidence of hip fracture. The severity of osteoporosis in this period requires a very active antiresorptive agent, even if it limits very actively the bone renewal process. At the same time, we do not expect a very long-term exposure that might hamper the gastrointestinal functioning. It is appropriate at this point to initiate or shift to a bisphosphonate that could be maintained as long as necessary. This substance will also be adequate whenever there is a contraindication for early use of SERMS such as venous thrombosis, administration of

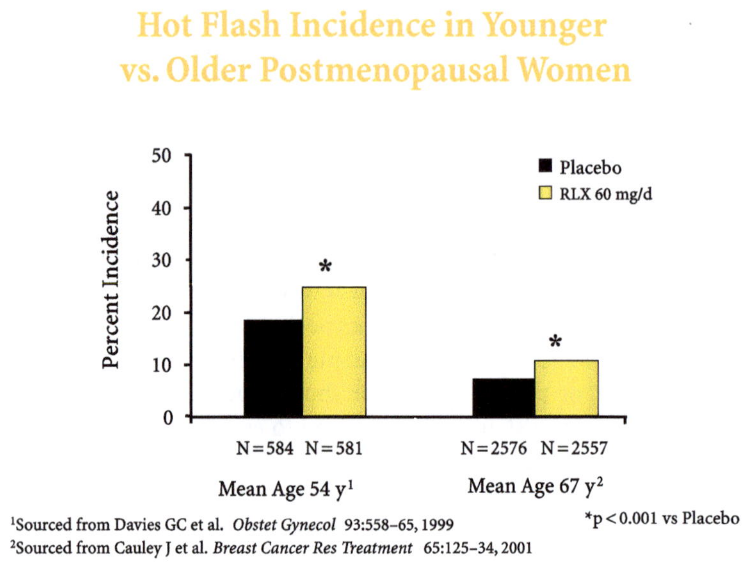

Fig. 14.7. Influence of raloxifen administration depends on age and time elapsed since menopause (redrawn from Davies et al. 1999 and Ettinger et al. 1999)

tamoxifen, or aromatase inhibitors in women with previous ER+ breast cancer or early symptomatic women not desiring hormonal treatment.

Finally, in very severe cases, the alternative to a bone remodeling agent such as teriparatide should be taken into consideration. The place for strontium ranelate, a substance without age-related contraindications, remains to be established as clinical experience in its use grows.

This is a proposal to help the clinician to counsel individual women. This process of individualization is crucial and is the best guarantee of a wise use of the different alternatives presently available for an efficient management of the postmenopausal period. Guidelines are only indications of the best choice for a majority of women, but, as health agents of our patients, we have the responsibility of determining how suitable they are for a given woman and introduce the appropriate corrections. In this context SERMs are an early alternative for osteoporosis prevention and treatment that provide an additive protective effect on the breast and are neutral on cardiovascular risk.

References

1. Anderson GL, Limacher M, Assaf AR et al. (2004) Effects of conjugated equine estrogens in postmenopausal women with hysterectomy. J Am Med Assoc 291:1701–1712
2. Barret-Connor E, Grady D, Sashegyi A et al. (2002) Raloxifene and cardiovascular events in osteoporotic postmenopausal women: four-year results from the MORE (Multiple Outcomes of Raloxifene Evaluation) randomized trial. J Am Med Assoc 287:847–857

3. Black DM, Thompson DE, Bauer DC, Ensrud K, Musliner T, Hochberg MC et al. (2000) Fracture risk reduction with alendronate in women with osteoporosis: the Fracture Intervention Trial. FIT Research Group. J Clin Endocrinol Metab 85:4118–4124
4. Brower V (2003) Of cancer and cholesterol: studies elucidate anticancer mechanism of statins. J Natl Cancer Inst 95(12):844–846
5. Calabro P, Yeh ET (2004) Multitasking of the 3-hydroxy-3methylglutaryl coenzime, a reductase inhibitor beyond cardiovascular diseases. Curr Atheroscleros Rep 6:36–41
6. Cauley J, Lucas FL, Kuller LH et al. (1996) Bone mineral density and risk of breast cancer in older women: the study of osteoporotic fractures. J Am Med Assoc 276:1404–1408
7. Cauley J, Lucas FL, Kuller LH et al. (1999) Elevated serum estradiol and testosterone concentrations are associated with a high risk of breast cancer. Ann Intern Med 130(4 Pt 1):270–277
8. Cauley J, Thompson DE, Ensrud KC et al. (2000) Risk of mortality following clinical fractures. Osteoporos Int 11:556–561
9. Cauley JA, Norton L, Lippman ME et al. (2001) Continued breast cancer risk reduction in postmenopausal women treated with raloxifene: 4-year results from the MORE trial. Breast Cancer Res Treat 65(2):125–134
10. Cauley JA, Zmuda JM, Lui LY et al. (2003) Lipid lowering drug use and breast cancer innolder women: a prospective study. J Womens Health 12(8):749–756
11. Chesnut CH III, Silverman S, Andriano K et al. (2000) A randomized trial of nasal spray salmon calcitonin in postmenopausal women with established osteoporosis: the prevent recurrence of osteoporotic fractures study. PROOF Study Group. Am J Med 109:267–276
12. Chlebowski RT (2000) Reducing the risk of breast cancer. N Engl J Med 343:191–198
13. Collaborative Group of the Primary Prevention Project (2001) Low-dose aspirin and vitamin E in people at cardiovascular risk: a randomised trial in general practice. Lancet 357:89–95
14. Cummings SR, Black DM, Thompson DE et al. (1998) Effect of alendronate on risk of fracture in women with low bone density but without vertebral fractures: results from the Fracture Intervention Trial. J Am Med Assoc 280:2077–2082
15. Cuzick J (2003) Aromatase inhibitors in prevention. Data from the ATAC trial and the design of IBIS II. Recent Results Cancer Res 163:96–103
16. Cuzick J (2005) Aromatase inhibitors for breast cancer prevention. J Clin Oncol 23:1636–1643
17. Cuzick J, Powles T, Veronesi U et al. (2003) Overview of the main outcomes in breast cancer prevention trials. Lancet 361:296–300
18. Davies CG, Huster WJ, Lu Y et al. (1999) Adverse events reported by menopausal women in controlled trials with raloxifene. Obstetr Gynecol 93:558–565
19. Delmas PD, Seeman E (2004) Changes in bone mineral density explain little of the reduction in vertebral or non vertebral fracture risk with anti-resorptive therapy. Bone 34:599–604
20. Delmas P, Cauley JA, Burshell AL et al. (2005) Breast cancer risk reduction over 8 years in postmenopausal women with osteopenia or osteoporosis receiving raloxifene. Bone 36:S436–S437
21. Dennerstein L, Guthrie J, Birkhäuser M et al. (2002) Symptoms and the menopause. International Position Paper on Women's Health and Menopause: a comprehensive approach. National Institutes of Health, pp 43–63
22. Ettinger B, Black DM, Mitlak BH et al. (1999) Reduction of vertebral fracture risk in postmenopausal women with osteoporosis treated with raloxifene: results from

a 3-year randomized clinical trial. Multiple Outcomes of Raloxifene Evaluation (MORE) Investigators. J Am Med Assoc 282:637–645
23. Fisher B, Constantino JP, Wickerham DL et al. (1998) Tamoxifen for prevention of breast cancer: report of the National Surgical Adjuvant Breast and Bowel Project P-1 study. J Natl Cancer Inst 90:1371–1388
24. Franco OH, Bonneux L, de Laet C et al. (2004) The Polymeal: a more natural, safer and probably tastier (than the polypill) strategy to reduce cardiovascular risk by more than 75%. Br Med J 329(7480):1447–1550
25. Gail MH, Brinton LA, Byar DP et al. (1989) Projecting individualized probabilities of developing breast cancer for white females who are being examined annually. J Natl Cancer Inst 81:1879–1986
26. Garcia Rodriguez LA, Gonzalez-Perez A (2004) Risk of breast cancer among users of aspirin and other anti-inflammatory drugs. Br Cancer J 91:525–529
27. Harris ST, Watts NB, Genant HK et al. (1999) Effects of risedronate treatment on vertebral and non-vertebral fractures in women with postmenopausal osteoporosis:a randomized controlled trial. Vertebral Efficacy With Risedronate Therapy (VERT) Study Group. J Am Med Assoc 282:1344–1352
28. Hippisley-Cox J, Coupland C (2005) Effect of combinations of drugs on all cause mortality in patients with ischaemic heart disease: nested case control analysis. Br Med J 330:1059–1063
29. International Osteoporosis Foundation (IOF) http://www.osteofund.org/index.php
30. Kikuchi Y, Hirata J, Kita T, Imaizumi E et al. (1997) SEER cancer statistics review. National Cancer Institute Bethesda MD
31. LaCroix AZ, Cauley JA, Pettinger M et al. (2003) Statin use, clinical fracture and bone density in postmenopausal women. Ann Int Med 139:97–104
32. MacLennan A, Lester S, Moore V (2004) Oral oestrogen replacement therapy versus placebo for hot flushes (Cochrane Review). In: The Cochrane Library, Issue 1. Wiley, Chichester
33. Manier J, Johansson R, Lenner P (2004) Smoking is associated with menopausal breast cancer in women with high levels of estrogens. Int J Cancer 112:324–328
34. Martino S, Cauley JA, Barrett-Connor E et al. (2004) Continuing outcomes relevant to Evista: breast cancer incidence in postmenopausal osteoporotic women in a randomized trial of raloxifene. J Natl Cancer Inst 96(23):1751–1761
35. McClung MR, Geusens P, Miller PD et al. (2001) Effect of risedronate on the risk of hip fracture in elderly women. N Engl J Med 344:333–340
36. Mosca L, Appel LJ, Benjamin EJ et al. (2004) Evidence-based guidelines for cardiovascular disease prevention in women. Circulation 109:672–693
37. Mueck AO, Seeeger H, Wallwiener D (2003) Effect of statins combined with estradiol on proliferation of human receptor-positive and receptor-negative breast cancer cells. Menopause 10(4):332–336
38. Mullins CD, Ohsfeldt RL (2003) Modeling the annual costs of postmenopausal prevention therapy: raloxifene, alendronate, or estrogen-progestin therapy. J Managed Care Pharm 9(2):150–158
39. Mulrow C, Kussmaul W (2005) The middle-aged and older American: wrong prototype for a preventive polypill. Ann Intern Med 142(6):467
40. Oldenhave A, Jaszmenni JB, Haspels AA et al. (1993) Impact of climacteric on well-being. A survey based on 5213 women 39 to 60 years old. Am J Obstetr Gynecol 168(3 Pt 1):772–780
41. Reginster J, Minne HW, Sorensen OH, Hooper M, Roux C, Brandi ML, Lund B, Ethgen D, Pack S, Roumagnac I, Eastell R (2000) Randomized trial of the effects of risedronate on

vertebral fractures in women with established postmenopausal osteoporosis. Vertebral Effica cy with Risedronate Therapy (VERT) Study Group. Osteoporos Int 11(1):83–91
42. Rejnmark L, Olsen ML, Johnsen SP et al. (2004) Hip fracture risk in statin users. A population based Danish case control study. Osteoporos Int 15(6):452–454
43. Rossouw JE, Anderson GL, Prentice RL et al. (2002) Risks and benefits of estrogen plus progestin in healthy postmenopausal women: principal results from the Women's Health Initiative
44. Speroff L, Symons J, Kempfert N et al. (2000) Femhrt study investigators. The effect of varying low-dose combinations of norethindrone acetate and ethinyl estradiol (femhrt) on the frequency and intensity of vasomotor symptoms. Menopause7:383–390
45. Tait CR (2004) Aspirin and breast cancer prevention: a link to ER status. Breast Cancer Res 6:211–212
46. Third Report of National Cholesterol Education Program (2002) Circulation 106:3143–3421. http://www.nhlbi.nih.gov/guidelines/cholesterol/index.htm
47. US Preventive Services Task Force (2002) Screening for osteoporosis in postmenopausal women. Originally in Ann Intern Med 137:526–528
48. Utian WH, Shoupe D, Bachmann G, Pinkerton JV, Pickar JH (2001) Relief of vasomotor symptoms and vaginal atrophy with lower doses of conjugated equine estrogens and medroxyprogesterone acetate. Fertil Steril 75:1065–1075
49. Wald NJ, Law MR (2003) A strategy to reduce cardiovascular disease by more than 80%. Br Med J 326(7404):1419
50. Wickerham DL (2003) Tamoxifen's impact as a preventive agent in clinical practice and an update on the STAR trial. Recent Results Cancer Res 163:87–95

Subject Index

MIX
Papier aus verantwortungsvollen Quellen
Paper from responsible sources
FSC® C105338

If you have any concerns about our products,
you can contact us on
ProductSafety@springernature.com

In case Publisher is established outside the EU,
the EU authorized representative is:
Springer Nature Customer Service Center GmbH
Europaplatz 3, 69115 Heidelberg, Germany

Printed by Libri Plureos GmbH
in Hamburg, Germany